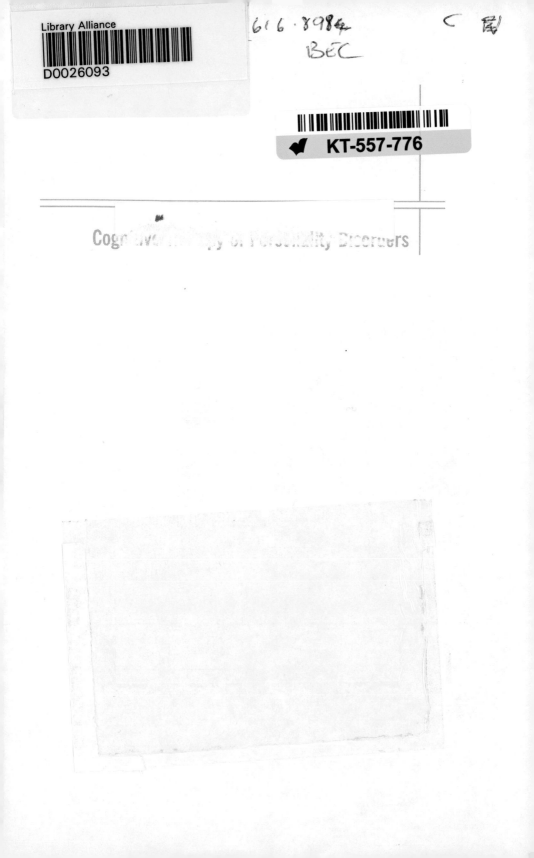
616.8984
BEC

C

Cognitive Therapy of Personality Disorders

Cognitive Therapy of Personality Disorders

SECOND EDITION

Aaron T. Beck

Arthur Freeman

Denise D. Davis

and Associates

THE GUILFORD PRESS
New York   London

© 2004 The Guilford Press
A Division of Guilford Publications, Inc.
72 Spring Street, New York, NY 10012
www.guilford.com

Paperback edition 2007

Printed in the United States of America

This book is printed on acid-free paper.

Last digit is print number: 9 8 7 6 5 4

Library of Congress Cataloging-in-Publication Data

Beck, Aaron T.
  Cognitive therapy of personality disorders / Aaron T. Beck, Arthur
Freeman, Denise D. Davis & associates.—2nd ed.
      p. cm.
  Includes bibliographical references and index.
  ISBN-10: 1-57230-856-7   ISBN-13: 978-1-57230-856-5 (hbk. : alk. paper)
  ISBN-10: 1-59385-476-5   ISBN-13: 978-1-59385-476-8 (pbk. : alk. paper)
  1. Personality disorders—Treatment. 2. Cognitive therapy. I. Freeman,
Arthur M.   II. Davis, Denise D.   III. Title.
  RC554.B43 2004
  616.85′8—dc22
                                                             2003017118

About the Authors

Aaron T. Beck, MD, is University Professor of Psychiatry at the University of Pennsylvania and President of the Beck Institute for Cognitive Therapy. He has authored more than 500 publications and has received numerous honors from professional and scientific organizations, including "America's Nobel," the Lasker Clinical Medical Research Award. Dr. Beck has worked extensively with personality disorders and has been an investigator on two studies using cognitive therapy with borderline personality disorder.

Arthur Freeman, EdD, ABPP, ACT, is Visiting Professor at Governors State University, University Park, Illinois, and Clinical Professor at the Philadelphia College of Osteopathic Medicine. He has been the president of the Association for Advancement of Behavior Therapy and of the International Association for Cognitive Psychotherapy. He is a Distinguished Founding Fellow of the Academy of Cognitive Therapy and has earned diplomates in Clinical Psychology, Behavioral Psychology, and Family Psychology from the American Board of Professional Psychology. Dr. Freeman's research and clinical interests include marital and family therapy, and cognitive-behavioral treatment of depression, anxiety, and personality disorders.

Denise D. Davis, PhD, is a Founding Fellow of the Academy of Cognitive Therapy and has collaborated with Drs. Beck and Freeman and other associates of the Beck Center since completing an extramural postdoctoral fellowship there in 1984. A contributor to the first edition of this volume as well as to numerous other chapters, articles, and workshops on cognitive therapy, Dr. Davis was a founding editor of the journal *Cognitive and Behavioral Practice*. She currently serves as Assistant Director of Clinical Training in Psychology at Vanderbilt University and has also maintained an independent practice of cognitive therapy for 20 years.

Contributing Authors

James Pretzer, PhD, Cleveland Center for Cognitive Therapy, Cleveland, Ohio; Department of Psychiatry, Case Western Reserve University School of Medicine, Cleveland, Ohio

Barbara Fleming, PhD, Cleveland Center for Cognitive Therapy, Cleveland, Ohio; Department of Psychiatry, Case Western Reserve University School of Medicine, Cleveland, Ohio

Arnoud Arntz, PhD, Department of Medical, Clinical and Experimental Psychology, Maastricht University, Maastricht, the Netherlands

Andrew Butler, PhD, Beck Institute for Cognitive Therapy and Research, Bala Cynwyd, Pennsylvania; Department of Psychiatry, University of Pennsylvania School of Medicine, Philadelphia, Pennsylvania

Gina Fusco, PsyD, Philadelphia College of Osteopathic Medicine, Philadelphia, Pennsylvania; Alternative Behavioral Services, Yardley, Pennsylvania

Karen M. Simon, PhD, Cognitive Behavioral Therapy of Newport Beach, Newport Beach, California

Judith S. Beck, PhD, Beck Institute for Cognitive Therapy and Research, Bala Cynwyd, Pennsylvania; Department of Psychiatry, University of Pennsylvania School of Medicine, Philadelphia, Pennsylvania

Anthony Morrison, ClinPsyD, Department of Psychology, University of Manchester, Manchester, United Kingdom

Christine A. Padesky, PhD, Center for Cognitive Therapy, Huntington Beach, California, *www.padesky.com*

Julia Renton, ClinPsyD, Bolton, Salford and Trafford Mental Health Trust, Manchester, United Kingdom

Authors are listed by the extent of their contributions, and alphabetically within equivalent groups.

Preface

In the more than two decades since Aaron T. Beck and his colleagues published *Cognitive Therapy of Depression,* cognitive therapy has developed in an almost exponential fashion. From the early work of treating depression, the model has been advanced and applied to the treatment of all the commonly seen clinical syndromes, including anxiety, panic disorder, eating disorders, and substance abuse, as well as disturbances of thinking associated with psychoses. Outcome studies have demonstrated its efficacy in a wide range of clinical disorders. In addition to its application to practically all the clinical populations, with modifications, cognitive therapy has been applied to all ages (children, adolescents, geriatric patients) and has been used in a variety of settings (outpatient, inpatient, couples, groups, and families).

The interest in and development of the clinical work in treating those patients with personality disorders have grown with the clinical sophistication and skill of the cognitive therapists. The first edition of this volume was the first cognitive approach to focus specifically on this diverse and difficult group. Our second edition reflects both our growing clinical sophistication and the expanding potential of cognitive therapy to effectively treat these disorders that often have been regarded as untreatable.

The work in cognitive therapy has drawn interest from around the world, and centers for cognitive therapy (or cognitive therapy study groups) have been established on every continent except Antarctica.

Prochaska and Norcross (2003) stated the following in the fifth edition of their *Systems of Psychotherapy*:

> Probably the safest prediction about cognitive therapy's direction is that it is moving up. Cognitive-behavioral therapies in general, and Beckian cognitive therapy in particular, are the fastest growing and most heavily researched orientations on the contemporary scene. The reasons for its current popularity are manifest: cognitive therapy is manualized, relatively brief, extensively evaluated, medication compatible, and problem focused. Let us put it this way: if we were forced to purchase stock in any of the psychotherapy systems, Beck's cognitive therapy would be the blue-chip growth selection for the next five years. (p. 369)

The interest in cognitive approaches among therapists has increased 600% since 1973 (Norcross, Prochaska, & Gallagher, 1989).

The original impetus for this volume came from therapists trained at the Center for Cognitive Therapy at the University of Pennsylvania or those who received training from these individuals. The content of the present work has grown organically from early case discussions and seminars led by Beck over many years. When we decided to write a book that would allow a sharing of the understandings gained from our work, we realized that it would be impossible for one or two people to be expert in treating all the various personality disorders. We therefore enlisted a distinguished and talented group of therapists trained at the Center for Cognitive Therapy to coauthor the text, all writing in their specific areas of expertise. We rejected the notion of an edited text that offered a series of disparate (or redundant) presentations. In the interest of uniformity and consistency in presentation, we decided in favor of a volume that would represent a total collaborative production of all the contributors.

Different authors took responsibility for different specific topics or clinical applications. The draft material on each topic was then circulated to stimulate cross-fertilization and facilitate consistency and was then returned to the original author(s) for revisions and further development. Finally, the entire manuscript was reviewed and edited by one of the authors to ensure continuity in style, language, and content. Although the book is the product of a team of authors, each author takes responsibility for the content. The major authors of each of the chapters are, however, identified below. The integration, final editing, continuity of the volume, and management of the second edition revision project is the work of Denise D. Davis.

As we considered the reasons to pursue a revised edition of this volume, a number of issues influenced our decision. First, cognitive therapy of the personality disorders has continued to expand in the 14 years since the first edition. Our experience as cognitive therapists has grown, as we see even more clearly both the value and the challenge of this potentially powerful therapeutic approach. Much has been gained in the way of new empirical evidence. Several of the authors who contributed to the first edition were ready to add the richness and depth of an additional decade of experience to their original clinical applications. We were also able to enlist the help of several new authors who have made major contributions in their areas of expertise in recent years, adding a fresh and up-to-date perspective to enhance the core of our original work. Finally, we wanted to expand the original offering in the areas of clinical assessment, and through more discussion of the role of emotions and the therapy relationship in cognitive therapy with personality disorders.

We have organized the volume into two sections. The first offers a broad overview of historical, theoretical, and therapeutic aspects. This section is followed by the clinical application chapters that detail the individualized treatment of specific personality disorders. The clinical chapters are arranged according to the three clusters described in the revised fourth edition of the *Diagnostic and Statistical Manual of Mental Disorders* (DSM-IV-TR; American Psychiatric Association, 2000). Cluster A, those disorders that are described as "odd or eccentric," includes the paranoid, schizoid, and schizotypal personality disorders. Cluster B includes the antisocial, borderline, histrionic, and narcissistic personality disorders, which are described as "dramatic, emotional, or erratic." Cluster C includes the "anxious or fearful persons" that fall into the categories of dependent, avoidant, and obsessive–compulsive personality disorders. After much consideration, the passive–aggressive personality disorder was included in our second edition, despite being removed from the DSM-IV-TR list of personality disorders and placed with proposed new categories awaiting further study. We agreed on the special clinical relevance of passive–aggressive or negativistic personality adjustment. Furthermore, our research demonstrated the unique set of dysfunctional beliefs associated with the clinical diagnosis of this disorder.

The material in Part I was developed by Aaron T. Beck, Arthur Freeman, Andrew Butler, Denise D. Davis, and James Pretzer. In Chapter 1, Freeman and Pretzer begin by outlining the cognitive-behavioral approach to the general problems of referral, diagnosis, and treatment of personality-disordered patients. A discussion of the concept of schema formation and its effect on behavior offers the reader an introduction to this vital issue, which is expanded in later chapters. The chapter then discusses the clinical studies and research done to date that is relevant to cognitive-behavioral treatment of personality.

In Chapter 2, Beck offers an explication of how personality processes are formed and serve adaptive functions in the individual's life. Starting with an evolutionary focus, Beck elaborates on how the schemas (and the idiosyncratic combinations of schemas) contribute to the formation of various disorders. The basic strategies for adaptation are then outlined, along with the basic beliefs/attitudes for each of the personality disorders. The processing of information and specific types of distortion of the available information are then tied to the schematic characteristics, including the density, activity, and valence of the schemas. Within each personality disorder, certain beliefs and strategies predominate and form a characteristic profile. Beck identifies the typical overdeveloped and underdeveloped strategies for each disorder. The strategies may, he posits, be derivative from or compensate for particular developmental experiences. By offering cognitive profiles, including the view of self, view of others, core and conditional beliefs, and main compensatory strategies, he places the disorders in a perspective that allows the application of the broad range of cognitive and behavioral interventions.

In Chapter 3, Andrew Butler discusses assessment concerns relevant to personality disorders, including the conceptual, methodological, and strategic issues inherent in understanding these complex domains of psychopathology. Cognitive measures of personality pathology are discussed, with illustrations of the specific measure developed within recent years, the Personality Belief Questionnaire. In Chapter 4, Beck and Freeman review the general principles for the cognitive therapy of personality disorders. The core schemas can be inferred by first looking at the patient's automatic thoughts. By using imagery and reawakening of past traumatic experiences, therapists can also activate the core schemas. The beliefs embedded in these schemas can then be examined within the therapeutic context. The chapter outlines basic cognitive therapy strategies with particular emphasis on the development of case conceptualization. Therapeutic collaboration, guided discovery, and the importance of transference and countertransference are discussed. The chapter concludes with an overview of specific cognitive and behavioral techniques for modifying schemas.

The last chapter in this section, Chapter 5, is newly formulated to highlight the cognitive approach to the therapeutic relationship in treating personality disorders. Building on the previous work by Beck and Freeman concerning the various reasons for therapeutic noncollaboration, Denise Davis adds further considerations of culture and managed care. In addition, she discusses an expansion of the interpersonal domain in the context of treating personality disorders and offers a conceptualization of transference and countertransference that is grounded in the cognitive therapy model. This chapter illustrates specific strategies for a cognitive therapy approach to both patient and therapist emotions. This overview of the emotional and interpersonal features of cognitive intervention is complemented by a specific discussion of therapeutic relationship issues and collaboration strategy within each of the subsequent chapters on specific personality disorders in Part II.

Each of the disorder-specific chapters in Part II follows a format of first describing the key features and ways the disorder is likely to present in a clinical context, followed by a summary of historical perspectives on the disorder. Key research and empirical data are noted, followed by a brief discussion of differential diagnostic issues. From there, each author offers a specific conceptualization to explain the disorder within the cognitive model, followed by an overview of how treatment can be approached with patients who present with these features. The specific beliefs and strategies that affect collaboration, and the possible ways to address these challenges, are elaborated within a section on collaboration strategy, followed by abundant and detailed illustration of specific interventions. Finally, suggestions for maintaining progress are offered. Although each of these authors followed a similar outline, a wealth of different ideas for applying the cognitive model are contained in these respective chapters.

Chapter 6, revised by the original author, James Pretzer, begins the clinical applications section with an introduction to the problem of the paranoid personality disorder. This infrequently studied group presents several idiosyncratic problems, not the least being a high degree of interpersonal suspicion. The schizoid and schizotypal personality disorders are detailed in a new Chapter 7 by Anthony Morrison and Julia Renton. These authors offer well-grounded and practical recommendations for differentiating these disorders, for clinically treating the thoughts and beliefs that contribute to the characteristic odd and eccentric social adjustment of these patients, and for engaging this typically disengaged person in a treatment collaboration. The Cluster B disorders of the dramatic, emotional, and erratic personality are introduced with Arthur Freeman and Denise Davis's reformulation of Davis's original consideration of the antisocial personality in Chapter 8. Specific issues of confronting these patients' particular tendencies toward avoidance and manipulation, setting limits, involving patients in homework, and teaching functional skills are elaborated.

A new Chapter 9 on the borderline personality is presented by Arnoud Arntz, who summarizes the sizable empirical and theoretical contributions in this area over the past decade. The pertinent issues of treatment of borderline psychopathology are aptly illustrated using the cognitive approach to schema modification. Barbara Fleming updates her original discussion of the histrionic personality disorder in Chapter 10, including a fascinating summary of the sexist influences historically associated with this disorder. She reconceptualizes the disorder in cognitive terms and illustrates a treatment protocol that clearly addresses the psychopathology of dramatic and excessive emotions. Denise Davis recasts her original discussion of the narcissistic personality in Chapter 11 with cognitive understanding of this self-inflating disorder. Key beliefs and assumptions are delineated, along with a model for engaging this challenging problem and pinpointing the primary operative beliefs that may be amenable to modification.

In Chapter 12, Barbara Fleming returns to revamp her original work on the dependent personality disorder, introducing the Cluster C—anxious and fearful patients. The dependent patient's beliefs relative to competence, abandonment, and independence are addressed in a variety of ways to encourage the development of more adaptive and independent functioning. Therapist frustration is a key issue that Fleming addresses, as dependent patients are particularly prone to superficial compliance and therapist flattery in the interest of maintaining their dependent relationship with the therapist. Strategies to titrate and manage patient dependency are detailed. Christine A. Padesky and Judith S. Beck return to collaborate on Chapter 13, treatment of the avoidant personality disorder. Themes of self-deprecation, expectation of rejection, and a belief that unpleasant emotions or encounters are intolerable guide these authors in applying their renowned clinical expertise. As in the first edition, treatment of the anxiety component and need for specific skill training are emphasized. Their original case example is expanded, with more detailed illustrations of techniques and an expanded range of ideas for possible interventions.

In Chapter 14, Karen M. Simon returns to update and expand the original chapter on obsessive–compulsive personality disorder. Although this disorder comprises traits that are highly valued by society, including performance, emotional control, self-discipline, perseverance, reliability, and politeness, Simon illustrates how these constructive strategies become dysfunctional rigidity, perfectionism, rumination, dogmatism, and indecision. Associated problems of depression, sexual problems, and psychosomatic difficulties are addressed. New contributor Gina Fusco considers the passive–aggressive or negativistic personality in Chapter 15. This chapter reviews the history of the conceptual issues surrounding the somewhat controversial disorder, and Fusco focuses on the primary issues of ambivalence, dependency, and poor assertion that typically impair the adaptive functioning of passive–aggressive individuals. Through the use of clinical examples, Fusco amply describes the cognitive approach to resolving therapy impasses and moving toward more constructive changes.

Finally, in Chapter 16, James Pretzer presents a summary of key issues and looks ahead to the future frontiers of the cognitive approach to treating personality disorders.

Acknowledgments

There are five significant events in the publication of a book. The first is the thrill and excitement of the initial conceptualization and development of the concept for the book. During this early stage ideas are offered, developed, modified, discarded, re-evaluated, and reformulated. Both editions of this volume began, as so much of our work has begun, from clinical necessity coupled with scientific curiosity. The personality-disordered patient was part of virtually every therapist's work at our Center. The idea for this book grew out of the weekly clinical seminars led by Aaron T. Beck. As the idea developed, the input and clinical insights of our colleagues at the University of Pennsylvania and the various Centers for Cognitive Therapy around the United States were sought and must be acknowledged here. Many of them became coauthors and had a significant impact on the direction and content of both the first and the current edition of this volume. Their brilliance and clinical acumen have given this work a particular sparkle.

The second major point for some books is the decision whether or not to undertake any substantial revision of the original work, producing a subsequent edition. Significant discussion and consideration took place between the publisher and the authors before determining the course of this particular project. In executing the decision to proceed with a second edition, a decision was made to create the role of an authorship project manager, to ensure the timeliness and consistency of the final product.

The third major event in the birth of a book is the collection and collation of the manuscript. Ideas have now been concretized and set to paper. It is at this point that the shaping process is begun. For the second edition of this volume, Denise D. Davis served as authorship project manager and reviewer of all of the manuscripts, shaping, editing, and polishing the revised volume from consideration to completion.

The fourth major point occurs when the draft manuscript is mailed to the publisher. Seymour Weingarten, Editor-in-Chief of The Guilford Press, has been a friend of cognitive therapy for many years. (It was Seymour's wisdom and foresight that led him to publish *Cognitive Therapy of Depression* over two decades ago.) His support, encouragement, and prompting have helped both the first and second editions of this volume move toward the finished state. Carolyn Graham, Craig Thomas, and the rest of the staff at Guilford have provided constant support and guidance in bringing this second edition to completion.

Although modern technology has reduced much of our need for additional technical assistance in producing the final manuscript draft, we wish to offer our personal thanks to those who contributed the support that allowed us to complete this major endeavor.

Cognitive therapy has grown from its humble beginnings to become the fastest growing psychotherapy in the world. I am particularly proud of this revised edition of *Cognitive Therapy of Personality Disorders* because it represents the collaborative effort of many of the most productive members of my professional family (including, of course, my daughter Judith). I want to express my appreciation to the various contributors to the book and particularly to Denise Davis and Art Freeman, who brought the revised edition to fruition.   —AARON T. BECK

In 1977, I began working at the Center for Cognitive Therapy at the University of Pennsylvania, thereby beginning a quarter century of collaboration with Tim Beck. This was a turning point in my life, both personally and professionally. Tim has been colleague, counselor, collaborator, supporter, critic, and friend. Denise Davis has been a valued colleague for two decades. She has likewise been a friend and collaborator. My wife, Sharon, is a life partner in every way. Her love, creativity, and caring are energizing and supportive.   —ARTHUR FREEMAN

Tim Beck and Art Freeman have provided many years of encouragement and inspired leadership in the development of cognitive therapy. I want to express my personal thanks to Tim and Art for their friendship and always generous collaboration. Their confidence is indeed a treasured gift. The contributors to this volume have all been wonderful, enlightening, and responsive to what may have seemed like endless requests. I am grateful for the opportunity to learn from their work. I also wish to thank my outstanding collaborator in life, Charles Sharbel, for the joy, space, and support that made my work on this project possible.

—DENISE D. DAVIS

Finally, we all wish to thank the patients with whom we have worked over the years for allowing us to share the burden they carried. It was their pain and anguish that motivated us to develop the theory and techniques that are called cognitive therapy. They taught us much, and we hope that we have helped them to lead fuller, more complete lives.

The fifth and final stage of the book comes with publication. Given all that has come before, this final stage is almost anticlimactic. Our work is now in the hands of you, our colleagues, who we hope will profit from this volume, along with the patients with whom you work.

AARON T. BECK
ARTHUR FREEMAN
DENISE D. DAVIS

Contents

PART I

HISTORY, THEORY, AND RESEARCH

CHAPTER 1

Overview of Cognitive Therapy of Personality Disorders

The therapy of patients with various disorders of personality has been discussed in the clinical literature since the beginning of the recorded history of psychotherapy. Freud's classic cases of Anna O (Breuer & Freud, 1893–1895/1955) and the Rat Man (Freud, 1909/1955) can be rediagnosed within current criteria as personality disorders. With the development of the first *Diagnostic and Statistical Manual of Mental Disorders* (DSM-I) of the American Psychiatric Association (1952) through to the present version of the manual (DSM-IV-TR; American Psychiatric Association, 2000), the definitions and parameters for understanding these serious and chronic states have been gradually expanded and refined. The general literature on the psychotherapeutic treatment of personality disorders has emerged more recently and is growing quickly. The main theoretical orientation in the treatment literature for personality disorders has been, until recently, psychoanalytic (Chatham, 1985; Goldstein, 1985; Horowitz, 1977; Kernberg, 1975, 1984; Lion, 1981; Masterson, 1985; Reid, 1981; Saul & Warner, 1982; Waldinger & Gunderson, 1987).

THE COGNITIVE-BEHAVIORAL APPROACH TO PERSONALITY DISORDERS

More recently, behavioral (Linehan, 1987a, 1993; Linehan, Armstrong, Suarez, Allmon, & Heard, 1991) and cognitive-behavioral therapists (Fleming & Pretzer, 1990; Freeman, Pretzer, Fleming, & Simon, 1990;

McGinn & Young, 1996; Pretzer & Beck, 1996) have conceptualized and developed a cognitive-behavioral treatment approach to personality disorders. When first introduced for the treatment of affective disorders, cognitive approaches drew on the ideas of the "ego analysts," derived from the works of Adler, Horney, Sullivan, and Frankl. Though their therapeutic innovations were seen as radical by psychoanalysts, the earliest cognitive therapies were in many ways "insight therapies," in that the therapy used largely introspective techniques designed to change a patient's overt "personality" (Beck, 1967; Ellis, 1962). Beck, Ellis, and their colleagues were among the first to use a wide range of behavioral treatment techniques, including structured *in vivo* homework. They have consistently emphasized the impact of cognitive and behavioral techniques not only on symptoms but also on the cognitive "schemas" or controlling beliefs. Schemas provide the instructions to guide the focus, direction, and qualities of daily life and special contingencies.

Cognitive therapy theorists and psychoanalysts conceptually agree on the notion that it is usually more productive to identify and modify "core" problems in treating personality disorders. The two perspectives differ in their views of the nature of this core structure, the difference being that the psychoanalytic perspective sees these structures as unconscious and not easily available to the patient. The cognitive perspective holds that the products of this process are largely in the realm of awareness (Ingram & Hollon, 1986) and with special strategies may be even more accessible to consciousness. Dysfunctional feelings and conduct (according to the cognitive therapy theory) are largely due to the function of certain schemas that produce consistently biased judgments and a concomitant tendency to make cognitive errors in certain types of situations. The basic premise of the cognitive therapy model is that attributional bias, rather than motivational or response bias, is the main source of dysfunctional affect and conduct in adults (Hollon, Kendall, & Lumry, 1986; Zwemer & Deffenbacher, 1984). Other work has shown that clinically relevant cognitive patterns are related to psychopathology in children in a way that parallels the cognitive and affective relationship patterns typically found among adults (Quay, Routh, & Shapiro, 1987; Ward, Friedlander, & Silverman, 1987) and that effective cognitive therapy can follow similar lines in children and adults (DiGiuseppe, 1989).

It is rare that personality problems are the chief complaint of a patient presenting for treatment. Instead, difficulties with depression, anxiety, or external situations compel the patient into treatment. Personality-disordered patients will often see the difficulties they encounter in dealing with other people as generally independent of their own behavior or input. They will frequently describe being victimized by others or, more globally, by "the system." Such patients are apt to have little idea about how they got to be the way they are, how they contribute to their own problems, or how to change. Other patients are very much aware of the self-defeating elements of their problems (e.g., overdependence, inhibition, and excessive avoidance) but remain unaware of the personality aspects or the role of personal volition in change.

Heuristic signs that may point to the possibility of Axis II problems include the following scenarios:

1. A patient or significant other reports, "Oh, he (she) has always done that since he (she) was a little boy (girl)," or the patient may report, "I've always been this way."
2. The patient is not compliant with the therapeutic regimen. Although noncompliance is common in many problems, for many reasons, persistent noncompliance should be used as a signal for further exploration of Axis II features.
3. Therapy seems to have come to a sudden stop for no apparent reason. The clinician working with this patient can often help the patient to reduce problems of anxiety or depression, only to be blocked in further therapeutic work by the personality disorder.
4. The patient seems entirely unaware of the effect of his or her behavior on others. Such patients report the responses of others but fail to address any provocation or dysfunctional behavior that they might contribute.
5. The patient gives "lip service" to the tasks of therapy by expressing interest and intention to change but fails to follow through on agreed actions. The importance of change is acknowledged, but the patient manages to avoid making any actual changes.
6. The patient's personality problems appear to be acceptable and natural for him or her. The patient sees the problems as a fundamental aspect of his or her "self" and makes statements such as, "This is who I am; this is how I have always been. I can't imagine being any other way."

Actions that the therapist views as evidence of an Axis II disorder may have been functional behavior for the patient across many life situations. However, this function in one setting may have caused great personal cost in other areas—for example, a perfectionistic computer programmer worked diligently at her job, but with little satisfaction from the work. She was under pressure at work due to late completion of tasks, and generally isolated from others because of working late into the evening and on weekends, trying to get work done according to her "standards." Her compulsive personality traits had previously been rewarded in school, as teachers gave her the best grades, the most attention, and the highest awards for outstanding performance based on her neat, perfect work. Another patient, a 66-year-old military veteran with both obsessive–compulsive and dependent personality disorders, stated, "The best time of my life was in the army. I didn't have to worry about what to wear, what to do, where to go, or what to eat." His rule orientation and compliance with orders facilitated a successful career in military service but made civilian adjustment more challenging.

Given the chronic nature of the problems of the personality-disordered patient and the price paid in terms of isolation, dependence on others, or external approbation, one must question why these dysfunctional behaviors are maintained. They may cause difficulty at work, at school, or within personal or family life. In some instances, they are reinforced by society (e.g., the adage to "always do your best"). Often, compelling schemas that a patient "knows" are erroneous are the most refractory to change. Two factors seem most important in explaining the tenacious hold of dysfunctional schemas. First, as DiGiuseppe (1986) has pointed out, the problem may be partly due to the difficulty people (including scientifically oriented therapists) have in making a "paradigm shift" from a sometimes accurate hypothesis to a less familiar one. Second, as Freeman (1987; Freeman & Leaf, 1989) has noted, people often find ways to adjust to and extract short-term benefits from fundamentally biased schemas that also restrict or burden their long-term capacity to deal with the challenges of life. With respect to the paradigm shift, DiGiuseppe (1989) recommends therapeutic use of various examples of the error that a particular schema produces, so that its biasing effect can be seen in terms of impact on important areas of the patient's life. Further, the consequences of an unbiased alternative should be repeatedly explicated.

The second problem is not so tractable. When patients adjust their lives to compensate for their anxieties, for example, change necessarily involves facing that anxiety and altering their previous adjustment. This stance is typically very difficult to embrace. Consider, for example, the compulsive computer programmer previously mentioned. Given this patient's history and general life adjustment, we would not expect her to seek or embrace homework assignments involving the risks of making mistakes or performing at a merely adequate level on some tasks. Before she could enter into these therapeutic tasks, the therapist might expect to have to reshape her initial expectations about treatment goals, time course, and procedures of therapy; help her to achieve some relatively immediate and practical gains; and develop a collaborative relationship with mutual trust and respect.

An unfortunate life history may contribute to the compelling quality of biased schemas and the development of personality disorders. An example appears in the data reported by Zimmerman, Pfohl, Stangl, and

Coryell (1985). They studied a sample of women who had been hospitalized for acute depressive episodes, coded as DSM-III Axis I disorders. When they divided their sample into three groups, distinguished by differential severity of negative life events or psychosocial stress (Axis IV), all three groups were similar on symptomatic measures of depression. Despite their similarity in presenting symptoms, these three groups did differ significantly in terms of other indications of severity and difficulty of treatment. Among the 30% of all patients who attempted suicide during the course of the study, the attempt rate was four times as high in the high-stress as in the low-stress group. Personality disorders were evident in 84.2% of the high-stress group, 48.1% of the moderate-stress group, and only 28.6% of the low-stress group. The investigators interpreted their finding that frequent negative life events were associated with personality disorder and case severity as at least partly due to the chronicity of the events and the patients' response to this chronicity. If unusually frequent negative events have occurred in someone's life, a pessimistic bias about one's self, world, and future is quite likely. In contrast, individuals who successfully escape or avoid life stressors may live in a relatively secure personal world and may have very low rates of *clinically evident* personality disorders.

The effectiveness of cognitive therapy at any given point in time depends on the degree to which patients' expectations about therapeutic goals are congruent with those of their therapists (Martin, Martin, & Slemon, 1987). Mutual trust and acknowledgment of the patient's requests by the therapist are important (Wright & Davis, 1994), as they are in any medical setting (Like & Zyzanski, 1987). The collaborative nature of goal setting is one of the most important features of cognitive therapy in general (Beck, Rush, Shaw, & Emery, 1979; Freeman et al., 1990). One of the most important considerations in working with personality-disordered patients is to anticipate the anxiety that will be provoked by a therapeutic process that challenges their identity and sense of self. Although their schematic structure may be unrewarding and lonely, change means that such patients are in new territory, where the land is alien. They are being asked not just to change a single chain of behaviors, or reframe a simple perception, but rather to give up who they are and how they have defined themselves for many years, and across many contexts. It is crucial to recognize that this will likely provoke anxiety, and both patient and therapist must be apprised of this potential. A variety of anxiety management tools can be tapped to address this occurrence (e.g., Beck & Emery, with Greenberg, 1985), including a calm, confident, and reassuring approach by the therapist (see Chapter 5).

The strategies needed to work effectively with personality-disordered patients can be conceptualized as a tripartite approach. To take a strictly cognitive approach and try to logically separate patients from their distortions will not work. Having the patient abreact within the session to fantasies and recollections will not be successful by itself. Developing a warm, supportive, and available relationship with the patient is not sufficient to alter the behavioral, cognitive, and affective elements of dysfunctional schemas. We believe it is essential to address all three areas (cognitive, behavioral, and affective) and to use three components in treatment (cognitive, expressive, and relational).

CLINICAL STUDIES AND EMPIRICAL RESEARCH

When the first edition of this text was published, research into the role of cognition in personality disorders and into the effectiveness of cognitive therapy as a treatment for personality disorders was in its infancy. There were many clinical reports regarding cognitive therapy with personality disorders and only a limited number of empirical studies. In the intervening years, the situation has improved considerably. There still is a need for much more empirical research, but we now have a respectable amount of empirical research into both cognitive conceptualizations of personality disorders and the effectiveness of cognitive therapy as a treatment for individuals with personality disorders.

The Validity of Cognitive Conceptualizations of Personality Disorder

Cognitive conceptualizations of personality disorders are of recent vintage, and consequently only limited research into the validity of these conceptualizations has been reported thus far. Two early studies examined the overall relationship between dysfunctional cognitions and personality disorders. O'Leary et al. (1991) examined dysfunctional beliefs and assumptions in borderline personality disorder. Subjects with borderline personality disorder scored significantly higher on a measure of the overall level of dysfunctional beliefs than did normal controls, and their scores were among the highest of any diagnostic group reported up to that time. Furthermore, their scores were not related to the presence or absence of a concurrent major depression, to history of a previous major depression, or to clinical status. In another study, Gasperini et al. (1989) investigated the relationship between mood disorders, personality disorders, the Automatic Thoughts Questionnaire (ATQ), and the Self Control Schedule (SCS) through factor analyses. They found that the first factor that emerged from the factor analysis of ATQ and SCS items reflected the presence of a "Cluster B" personality disorder (narcissistic, histrionic, borderline, and antisocial), whereas the second factor reflected the presence of a "Cluster C" personality disorder (compulsive, dependent, avoidant, and passive–aggressive). Although "Cluster

A" personality disorders (paranoid, schizoid, and schizotypal) were unrelated to any of the factors that emerged from the factor analysis, few of the subjects in this study received Cluster A diagnoses, and the lack of relationship could easily be due to this alone. Both of these early studies provide support for the general proposition that dysfunctional cognitions play a role in personality disorders, but they have only a limited bearing on the conceptualizations presented in this volume because they did not examine the specific relationships between dysfunctional cognitions and personality disorders that contemporary authors have hypothesized.

More recent studies have examined the relationships between the sets of beliefs that have been hypothesized to play a role in each of the personality disorders (Beck, Freeman, & Associates, 1990; Freeman et al., 1990) and diagnostic status. Arntz, Dietzel, and Dreessen (1999) found that the subscale of the Personality Disorder Beliefs Questionnaire which was hypothesized to contain beliefs characteristic of borderline personality disorder did indeed discriminate subjects with borderline personality disorder from subjects with Cluster C personality disorders. Beck et al. (2001) used a similar measure, the Personality Belief Questionnaire, which contained nine subscales designed to assess the beliefs hypothesized to play a role in each of the nine DSM-III personality disorders. They found that for avoidant, dependent, obsessive–compulsive, narcissistic, and paranoid personality disorders, subjects with that personality disorder preferentially endorsed the beliefs hypothesized to play a role in that disorder and scored significantly higher on the relevant subscale than did psychiatric patients without a personality disorder. The other personality disorders were not examined in this study due to a lack of subjects. These findings support the hypothesis that dysfunctional beliefs are related to personality disorders in ways that are consistent with cognitive theory, but do not provide grounds for conclusions about causality or about the effectiveness of cognitive therapy as a treatment for individuals with personality disorders.

The Effectiveness of Cognitive Therapy with Personality Disorders

Cognitive therapy has been found to provide effective treatment for a wide range of Axis I disorders. However, research into the effectiveness of cognitive-behavioral approaches to treating individuals with personality disorders is more limited. Table 1.1 provides an overview of the available evidence regarding the effectiveness of cognitive-behavioral interventions with individuals diagnosed as having personality disorders. It is immediately apparent from this table that there have been many uncontrolled clinical reports which assert that cognitive-behavioral therapy can provide effective treatment for personality disorders. However, there

TABLE 1.1. The Effectiveness of Cognitive-Behavioral Treatment with Personality Disorders

Personality disorder	Uncontrolled clinical reports	Single-case design studies	Studies of effects of personality disorders on treatment outcome	Controlled outcome studies
Antisocial	+	−	+	*a*
Avoidant	+	+	±	±
Borderline	±	−	+	±
Dependent	+	+	+	
Histrionic	+		−	
Narcissistic	+	+		
Obsessive–compulsive	+	−		
Paranoid	+	+		
Passive–aggressive	+		+	
Schizoid	+			
Schizotypal				

Note. +, Cognitive-behavioral interventions found to be effective; −, cognitive-behavioral interventions found not effective; ±, mixed findings. *a*Cognitive-behavioral interventions were effective with antisocial personality disorder subjects only when the individuals were depressed at pretest.

are fewer controlled outcome studies to provide support for these assertions, which has led some to be concerned about the risks associated with a rapid expansion of theory and practice that has outstripped the empirical research (Dobson & Pusch, 1993). Fortunately we do have some empirical support for current clinical practice.

Effects of Comorbid Personality Disorders on the Treatment of Axis I Disorders

Many individuals with personality disorders enter treatment seeking help with an Axis I disorder and are not particularly interested in treatment for their Axis II disorder. Is it feasible to treat the Axis I problem without addressing the Axis II disorder? Quite a few studies have examined the effectiveness of cognitive-behavioral treatment for Axis I disorders in subjects who are also diagnosed as having personality disorders. A number of studies have found that the presence of an Axis II diagnosis greatly decreases the likelihood of treatment being effective. For example, Turner (1987) found that socially phobic patients without personality disorders improved markedly after a 15-week group treatment for social phobia and maintained their gains at a 1-year follow-up. However, patients with personality disorder diagnoses in addition to social phobia showed little or no improvement both posttreatment and at the 1-year follow-up. Similarly, Mavissakalian and Hamman (1987) found that

75% of agoraphobic subjects rated as being low in personality disorder characteristics responded well to a time-limited behavioral and pharmacological treatment for agoraphobia, while only 25% of the subjects rated as being high in personality disorder characteristics responded to this treatment. Other studies have found that subjects with personality disorders in addition to their Axis I problems respond to cognitive-behavioral treatment but respond more slowly (Marchand, Goyer, Dupuis, & Mainguy, 1998).

However, other research demonstrates that the impact of comorbid personality disorders on the treatment of Axis I disorders is more complex than this. Some studies have found that the presence of personality disorder diagnoses did not influence outcome (Dreesen, Arntz, Luttels, & Sallaerts, 1994) or that subjects with personality disorder diagnoses present with more severe symptomatology but respond equally well to treatment (Mersch, Jansen, & Arntz, 1995). Other studies have found that personality disorder diagnoses influenced outcome only under certain conditions (Fahy, Eisler, & Russell, 1993; Felske, Perry, Chambless, Renneberg, & Goldstein, 1996; Hardy et al., 1995), that clients with personality disorders are likely to terminate treatment prematurely but that those who persist in treatment can be treated effectively (Persons, Burns, & Perloff, 1988; Sanderson, Beck, & McGinn, 1994), and that some personality disorders predicted poor outcome while others did not (Neziroglu, McKay, Todaro, & Yaryura-Tobias, 1996). Kuyken, Kurzer, De Rubeis, Beck, and Brown (2001) found that it was not the presence of a personality disorder diagnosis per se that influenced outcome but that the presence of maladaptive avoidant and paranoid beliefs predicted poor treatment outcome.

Interestingly, some studies provide evidence that focused treatment for Axis I disorders can have beneficial effects on comorbid Axis II disorders. For example, in their study of the treatment of agoraphobia, Mavissakalian and Hamman (1987) found that four of seven subjects who initially met diagnostic criteria for a single personality disorder diagnosis before treatment no longer met criteria for a personality disorder diagnosis following treatment. In contrast, subjects diagnosed as having more than one personality disorder did not show similar improvement.

Taken together, the results of these studies suggest that cognitive-behavioral treatment for an Axis I disorder when an Axis II disorder is also present sometimes is ineffective, sometimes is effective, and sometimes results in improvement in the Axis II disorder as well. Little is known regarding the factors that determine whether treatment for the Axis I disorder will be effective or not. One major limitation of the studies that have examined the effectiveness of cognitive-behavioral treatment for Axis I disorders with individuals who also have personality disorders is that the treatment approaches used in these studies typically did not take the presence of personality disorders into account. This leaves unanswered the question whether treatment protocols designed to account for the presence of personality disorders would prove to be more effective.

Uncontrolled Studies of Cognitive-Behavioral Treatment of Axis II Disorders

A number of studies have focused specifically on cognitive-behavioral treatment of individuals with personality disorders. Turkat and Maisto (1985) used a series of single-case design studies to investigate the effectiveness of individualized cognitive-behavioral treatment for personality disorders. Their study provides evidence that some clients with personality disorders could be treated effectively, but the investigators were unsuccessful in treating many of the subjects in their study.

A recent study has attempted to test the efficacy of the intervention approach advocated by Beck et al. (1990) using a series of single case studies with repeated measures (Nelson-Gray, Johnson, Foyle, Daniel, & Harmon, 1996). The nine subjects for this study were diagnosed with major depressive disorder and one or more co-occurring personality disorders. Each subject was assessed pretherapy, posttherapy, and at a 3-month follow-up for level of depression and for the number of diagnostic criteria present for his or her primary personality disorder. After receiving 12 weeks of treatment, six of the eight subjects who completed the 3-month follow-up manifested a significant decrease in level of depression, two subjects manifested a significant decrease on both measures of personality disorder symptomatology, two failed to show improvement on either measure, and four showed mixed results. As the authors note, 12 weeks is a much shorter course of treatment than Beck et al. (1990) would expect to be required for most clients with personality disorders.

Finally, Springer, Lohr, Buchtel, and Silk (1995) report that a short-term cognitive-behavioral therapy group produced significant improvement in a sample of hospitalized subjects with various personality disorders and that a secondary analysis of a subset of subjects with borderline personality disorder revealed similar findings. They also report that clients evaluated the group as being useful in their life outside the hospital.

Formal Outcome Studies of Cognitive-Behavioral Treatment of Axis II Disorders

At least three personality disorders have been the subject of controlled outcome studies. In a study of the treatment of opiate addicts in a methadone maintenance program, Woody, McLellan, Luborsky, and O'Brien (1985) found that subjects who met DSM-III diagnostic criteria for both major depression and antisocial personality disorder responded well to both cognitive therapy and a supportive–expressive psychotherapy systematized by Luborsky (Luborsky, McLellan, Woody, O'Brien, & Auerbach, 1985). The subjects showed statistically significant improvement on 11 of 22 outcome variables used, including psychiatric symptoms, drug use, employment, and illegal activity. Subjects who met criteria for antisocial personality disorder but not major depression showed little response to treatment, improving on only 3 of 22 variables. This pattern of results was maintained at a 7-month follow-up. Although subjects not diagnosed as antisocial personality disorder responded to treatment better than the sociopaths did, depressed sociopaths did only slightly worse than the nonsociopaths, but the nondepressed sociopaths did much worse.

Early studies of the treatment of avoidant personality disorder found that both short-term social skills training and social skills training combined with cognitive interventions were equally effective in increasing the frequency of social interaction and decreasing social anxiety (Greenberg & Stravynski, 1985; Stravynski, Marks, & Yule, 1982). Initially, the equivalence of the two treatments in this study was interpreted as demonstrating the "lack of value" of cognitive interventions (Stravynski et al., 1982). However, it should be noted that the two treatments were equally effective, that all treatments were provided by a single therapist (who was also principal investigator), and that only one of many possible cognitive interventions (disputation of irrational beliefs) was used. In a subsequent study, Greenberg and Stravynski (1985) reported that the avoidant client's fear of ridicule appears to contribute to premature termination in many cases, and they suggested that interventions that modify relevant aspects of the clients' cognitions might add substantially to the effectiveness of intervention. A more recent outcome study (Felske et al., 1996) found that patients with avoidant personality disorder improved significantly with an exposure-based cognitive-behavioral treatment approach. However, these patients were more severely impaired than patients with social phobia who did not meet criteria for avoidant personality disorder. Despite their improvement over the course of treatment, avoidant personality patients continued to be more impaired than those with social phobia who received the same treatment. The authors suggest that comorbid depression may partially explain this limited response to treatment.

Dialectical behavior therapy is a cognitive behavioral treatment approach which Linehan and her colleagues developed specifically as a treatment for borderline personality disorder (Linehan, 1987a, 1987b, 1993). This approach combines a cognitive-behavioral perspective with concepts derived from dialectical materialism and from Buddhism. The result is a somewhat complex theoretical framework and a contemporary cognitive-behavioral, problem-solving approach to treatment. It includes an emphasis on collaboration, skill training, and contingency clarification and management with a number of features designed to address issues believed to be important in treating individuals with borderline personality disorder (for a detailed presentation of this treatment approach, see Linehan, 1993).

In a series of papers (Linehan et al., 1991; Linehan, Heard, & Armstrong, 1993; Linehan, Tutek, & Heard, 1992), Linehan and her colleagues have reported a controlled comparison of the effects of dialectical behavior therapy with the effects of "treatment as usual" in the community mental health system in a sample of chronically parasuicidal borderline patients. Following 1 year of treatment, the patients in the dialectical behavior therapy condition were found to have a significantly lower dropout rate and significantly less self-injurious behavior than subjects receiving "treatment as usual" (Linehan et al., 1991). The dialectical behavior therapy subjects also were found to have significantly better scores on measures of interpersonal and social adjustment, anger, work performance, and anxious rumination (Linehan et al., 1992). However, the two groups showed only modest overall improvement in depression or other symptomatology and did not differ significantly in these areas (Linehan et al., 1991). Throughout a 1-year follow-up, the dialectical behavior therapy subjects were found to have significantly higher global functioning. During the initial 6 months of the follow-up study they showed less parasuicidal behavior, less anger, and higher self-rated social adjustment. During the second 6 months, they had fewer days of hospitalization, and better interviewer-rated social adjustment.

These findings are quite encouraging given that the patients not only met diagnostic criteria for borderline personality disorder but also were chronically parasuicidal, had histories of multiple psychiatric hospitalizations, and were unable to maintain employment due to their psychiatric symptoms. These subjects clearly were more disturbed than many individuals who meet diagnostic criteria for a personality disorder but are not parasuicidal, are rarely hospitalized, and are able to maintain productive employment.

Comparisons with Other Treatment Approaches

Only limited research compares cognitive therapy with other approaches in the treatment of individuals with personality disorders. In a study of the treatment of heroin addicts with and without antisocial personality disorder, Woody et al. (1985) found that both cognitive therapy and supportive–expressive psychotherapy were effective for antisocial subjects who were depressed at the beginning of treatment, and that neither approach was effective with antisocial subjects who were not depressed. In a large, multisite outcome study, the National Institute of Mental Health Treatment of Depression Collaborative Program found a nonsignificant trend for cognitive therapy to have advantages over other treatment approaches with patients with personality disorders. Patients with personality disorders did slightly better than other patients in cognitive therapy, but they did worse than other patients in interpersonal psychotherapy and pharmacotherapy (Shea et al., 1990). However, this trend was not statistically significant. A small study comparing treatments for panic disorder (Black, Monahan, Wesner, Gabel, & Bowers, 1996) found that cognitive therapy produced a greater decline in scores on a self-report measure of personality disorder characteristics than did either psychotrophic medication (fluvoxamine) or a pill placebo. Finally, Hardy et al. (1995) found that individuals with Cluster B personality disorders had significantly poorer outcomes in interpersonal psychotherapy than in cognitive therapy (they did not assess Cluster A or Cluster C personality disorders). These four studies are encouraging, but they clearly do not provide adequate grounds for drawing conclusions about how cognitive therapy compares with other treatments for individuals with personality disorders.

The Effect of Personality Disorders on "Real Life" Clinical Practice

In clinical practice, most therapists do not apply a standardized treatment protocol with a homogeneous sample of individuals who share a common diagnosis. Instead, clinicians face a variety of clients and take an individualized approach to treatment. A study of the effectiveness of cognitive therapy under such "real-world" conditions provides important support for the clinical use of cognitive therapy with clients who are diagnosed as having personality disorders. Persons et al. (1988) conducted an interesting empirical study of clients receiving cognitive therapy for depression in private practice settings. The subjects were 70 consecutive individuals seeking treatment from Dr. Burns or Dr. Persons in their own private practices. Both are established cognitive therapists who have taught and published extensively, and in this study both therapists conducted cognitive therapy as they normally do. This meant that treatment was open-ended, it was individualized rather than standardized, and medication and inpatient treatment were used as needed.

The primary focus of the study was on identifying predictors of dropout and treatment outcome in cognitive therapy for depression. However, it is interesting for our purposes to note that 54.3% of the subjects met DSM-III criteria for a personality disorder diagnosis and that the investigators considered the presence of a personality disorder diagnosis as a potential predictor of both premature termination and therapy outcome. The investigators found that patients with personality disorders were significantly more likely to drop out of therapy prematurely than patients without personality disorders, but those patients with personality disorder diagnoses who persisted in therapy through the completion of treatment showed substantial improvement. In fact, clients with personality disorders who persisted in treatment did not differ significantly in degree of improvement from patients without personality disorders. Similar findings have been reported by Sanderson et al. (1994) in a study of cognitive therapy for generalized anxiety disorder. Subjects diagnosed with a comorbid personality disorder were more likely to drop out, but treatment was effective in reducing both anxiety and depression for those who completed a minimum course.

IMPLICATIONS FOR CLINICAL PRACTICE

The past two decades have seen advances in theory and practice regarding cognitive therapy with personality disorders that outstrip the empirical research (Dobson & Pusch, 1993). Although this discrepancy provides grounds for legitimate concern, it is hardly feasible to suspend theoretical and clinical work until more empirical research is completed. The practicing clinician faces a difficult situation in that one can hardly refuse to provide treatment for a class of disorders which may be present in as many as 50% of clients seen in many outpatient settings. Fortunately, there is a growing body of evidence that cognitive-behavioral treatment can be effective for clients with personality disorders. As will be illustrated in the chapters to follow, the development and validation of these treatment strategies for personality disorders is at the vanguard of cognitive therapy.

CHAPTER 2

Theory of Personality Disorders

Cognitive therapy for any disorder depends on the conceptualization of the disorder and its adaptation to the unique features of a specific case. This chapter presents an overall theory of personality disorders within the broad context of their origin, development, and function of personality. This exposition focuses initially on how personality processes are formed and operate in the service of adaptation. Before presenting a synopsis of our theory of personality disorder, we review our concepts of personality and then relate them to the disorders.

We start the discourse with a speculative explanation of how the prototypes of our personality patterns could be derived from our phylogenetic heritage. Those genetically determined "strategies" that facilitated survival and reproduction would presumably be favored by natural selection. Derivatives of these primitive strategies can be observed in an exaggerated form in the symptom syndromes, such as anxiety disorders and depression, and in personality disorders, such as the dependent personality disorder.

Our discussion then progresses along the continuum from evolutionary-based strategies to a consideration of how information processing, including affective processes, is antecedent to the operation of these strategies. In other words, evaluation of the particular demands of a situation precedes and triggers an adaptive (or maladaptive) strategy. How a situation is evaluated depends in part, at least, on the relevant underlying beliefs. Those beliefs are embedded in more or less stable structures, labeled "schemas," that select and synthesize incoming data. The psychological sequence progresses then from evaluation to affective and motivational arousal, and finally to selection and implementation of a relevant strategy. We regard the basic structures (schemas) on which these cognitive, affective, and motivational processes depend as the fundamental units of personality.

Personality "traits" identified by adjectives such as "dependent," "withdrawn," "arrogant," or "extraverted" may be conceptualized as the overt expression of these underlying structures. By assigning meanings to events, the cognitive structures start a chain reaction culminating in the kinds of overt behavior (strategies) that are attributed to personality traits. Behavioral patterns that we commonly ascribe to personality traits or dispositions ("honest," "shy," "outgoing") consequently represent interpersonal strategies developed from the interaction between innate dispositions and environmental influences.

Attributes such as dependency and autonomy, which are conceptualized in motivational theories of personality as basic drives, may be viewed as a function of a conglomerate of basic schemas. In behavioral or functional terms, the attributes may be labeled "basic strategies." These specific functions may be observed in an exaggerated way in some of the overt behavioral patterns attributed, for example, to the dependent or schizoid personality disorders.

Our presentation then moves on to the topic of activation of the schemas (and modes) and their expression in behavior. Having laid the groundwork for our theory of personality, we go on to review the relation of these structures to psychopathology. The pronounced activation of dysfunctional schemas lies at the core of the so-called Axis I disorders, such as depression. The more idiosyncratic, dysfunctional schemas displace the more reality-oriented, adaptive schemas in functions such as information processing, recall, and prediction. In depression, for example, the mode that is organized around the theme of self-negation becomes dominant; in anxiety disorders, the personal danger mode is hyperactive; in panic disorders, the mode relevant to imminent catastrophe is mobilized.

The typical dysfunctional beliefs and maladaptive strategies expressed in personality disorders make individuals susceptible to life experiences that impinge upon their cognitive vulnerability. Thus, the dependent personality disorder is characterized by a sensitivity to loss of love and help; the narcissistic by trauma to self-esteem; the histrionic by failure to manipulate others to provide attention and support. The cognitive vulnerability is based on beliefs that are extreme, rigid, and imperative. We speculate that these dysfunctional beliefs have originated as the result of the interaction between the individual's genetic predisposition and exposure to undesirable influences from other people and specific traumatic events.

THE EVOLUTION OF INTERPERSONAL STRATEGIES

Our view of personality takes into account the role of our evolutionary history in shaping our patterns of thinking, feeling, and acting. We can better understand personality structures, functions, and processes if we examine attitudes, feelings, and behavior in the light of their possible relation to ethological strategies.

Much of the behavior we observe in nonhuman animals is generally regarded as "programmed." The underlying processes are programmed and are expressed in overt behavior. The development of these programs frequently depends on the interaction between genetically determined structures and experience. Similar developmental processes may be assumed to occur in humans (Gilbert, 1989). It is reasonable to consider the notion that long-standing cognitive–affective–motivational programs influence our automatic processes: the way we construe events, what we feel, and how we are disposed to act. The programs involved in cognitive processing, affect, arousal, and motivation may have evolved as a result of their ability to sustain life and promote reproduction.

Natural selection presumably brought about some kind of fit between programmed behavior and the demands of the environment. However, our environment has changed more rapidly than have our automatic adaptive strategies—largely as a result of our own modifications of our social milieu. Thus, strategies of predation, competition, and sociability that were useful in the more primitive surroundings do not always fit into the present niche of a highly individualized and technological society, with its own specialized cultural and social organization. A bad fit may be a factor in the development of behavior that we diagnose as a "personality disorder."

Regardless of their survival value in more primitive settings, certain of these evolutionary-derived patterns become problematic in our present culture because they interfere with the individual's personal goals or conflict with group norms. Thus, highly developed predatory or competitive strategies that might promote survival in primitive conditions may be ill suited to a social milieu and may eventuate in an "antisocial personality disorder." Similarly, a kind of exhibitionistic display that would have attracted helpers and mates in the wild may be excessive or inappropriate in contemporary society. In actuality, however, these patterns are most likely to cause problems if they are inflexible and relatively uncontrolled.

The symptom syndromes—Axis I disorders—can also be conceptualized in terms of evolutionary principles. For example, the fight–flight pattern, although presumably adaptive in archaic emergency situations of physical danger, may form the substrate of either an anxiety disorder or a chronic hostile state. The same response pattern that was activated by the sight of a predator, for example, is also mobilized by threats of psychological traumas such as rejection or devaluation (Beck & Emery, with Greenberg, 1985). When this psychophysiological response—perception of danger and arousal of the autonomic nervous system—is triggered by exposure to a broad spectrum of potentially aversive interpersonal situations, the vulnerable individual may manifest a diagnosable anxiety disorder.

Similarly, the variability of the gene pool could account for individual differences in personality. Thus, one individual may be predisposed to freeze in the face of danger, another to attack, a third to avoid any potential sources of danger. These differences in overt behavior, or strategies—any of which may have survival value in certain situations—reflect relatively enduring characteristics that are typical of certain "personality types" (Beck et al., 1985). An exaggeration of these patterns may lead to a personality disorder; for example, the avoidant personality disorder may reflect a strategy of withdrawing from or avoiding any situation involving the possibility of social disapproval.

Why do we apply the term "strategy" to characteristics that have been traditionally labeled "personality traits" or "patterns of behavior"? Strategies in this sense may be regarded as forms of programmed behavior that are designed to serve biological goals. Although the term implies a conscious, rational plan, it is not used in that sense here but, rather, as it is employed by ethologists—to denote highly patterned stereotyped behaviors that promote individual survival and reproduction (Gilbert, 1989). These patterns of behavior may be viewed as having an ultimate goal of survival and reproduction: "reproductive efficacy" or "inclusive fitness." These evolutionary strategies were described 200 years ago by Erasmus Darwin (1791, cited in Eisely, 1961), grandfather of Charles Darwin, as expressions of hunger, lust, and security.

Although animals are not aware of the ultimate goal of these biological strategies, they are conscious of subjective states that reflect their mode of operation: hunger, fear, or sexual arousal, and the rewards and punishments for their fulfillment or nonfulfillment (namely, pleasure or pain). We are prompted to eat to relieve the pangs of hunger but also to obtain satisfaction. We seek sexual relations in order to reduce sexual tension as well as to gain gratification. We "bond" with other people to relieve loneliness but also to achieve the pleasure of camaraderie and intimacy. In sum, when we experience internal pressure to satisfy certain short-range wishes, such as obtaining pleasure and relieving tension, we may, to some degree at least, be fulfilling long-range evolutionary goals.

In humans, the term "strategy" can be analogously applied to forms of behavior that may be either adaptive or maladaptive, depending on the circumstances. Egocentricity, competitiveness, exhibitionism, and avoidance of unpleasantness may all be adaptive in certain situations but grossly maladaptive in others. Because we can observe only the overt behavior of other people, the question arises as to how our conscious internal states (thoughts, feelings, and wishes) are related to the strategies. If we examine the cognitive and affective patterns, we see a specific relationship between certain beliefs and attitudes on the one hand and behavior on the other.

One way to illustrate this relationship is to examine the exaggerated processes observed in individuals with various personality disorders and to compare specific typical attitudes associated with these disorders with the corresponding strategies. As indicated in Table 2.1, it is possible to demonstrate a typical attitude associated with each of the traditional personality disorders. It can be seen that the specific strategy representative of a particular disorder would flow logically from this characteristic attitude.

Table 2.1 does not include the borderline and schizotypal personality disorders. These two disorders do not show a typical idiosyncratic set of beliefs and strategies, as do the rest. The borderline disorder, for example, consists of a wide variety of typical beliefs and patterns of behavior that are characteristic of the broad range of personality disorders. Schizotypal disorder is characterized more precisely by peculiarities in thinking rather than an idiosyncratic content.

The first column in Table 2.1 lists the personality disorder; the second presents the corresponding attitude underlying the overt behavior; the third column translates the idiosyncratic behavioral pattern of the personality disorder into a strategy. It follows logically that a dependent personality disorder characterized by clinging behavior would stem from a cognitive substrate based in part on the fear of abandonment; avoidant behavior from a fear of being hurt; and passive–aggressive patterns from

TABLE 2.1. Basic Beliefs and Strategies Associated with Traditional Personality Disorders

Personality disorder	Basic belief/attitudes	Strategy (overt behavior)
Dependent	"I am helpless."	Attachment
Avoidant	"I may get hurt."	Avoidance
Passive–aggressive	"I could be controlled."	Resistance
Paranoid	"People are dangerous."	Wariness
Narcissistic	"I am special."	Self-aggrandizement
Histrionic	"I need to impress."	Dramatics
Obsessive–compulsive	"I must not err."	Perfectionism
Antisocial	"Others are to be taken."	Attack
Schizoid	"I need plenty of space."	Isolation

a concern about being dominated. The clinical observations from which these formulations are derived are discussed in subsequent chapters.

We suggest that such strategies may be analyzed in terms of their possible antecedents in our evolutionary past. The dramatic behavior of the histrionic personality, for example, may have its roots in the display rituals of nonhuman animals; the antisocial in predatory behavior; and the dependent in the attachment behavior observed throughout the animal kingdom (cf. Bowlby, 1969). By viewing people's maladaptive behavior in such terms, we can review it more objectively and reduce the tendency to stamp it with pejorative labels such as "neurotic" or "immature."

The concept that human behavior can be viewed productively from an evolutionary perspective was developed fully by McDougall (1921). He elaborated at length on the transformation of "biological instincts" into "sentiments." His writing paved the way for some of the current biosocial theorists such as Buss (1987), Scarr (1987), and Hogan (1987). Buss has discussed the different types of behaviors displayed by humans, such as competitiveness, dominance, and aggression, and traced their similarity to the behaviors of other primates. Particularly, Buss focuses on the role of sociability in humans and other primates.

Hogan postulates a phylogenetic heritage, according to which biologically programmed mechanisms emerge in developmental sequence. He views culture as providing the opportunity through which genetic patterns may be expressed. He regards the driving force of adult human activity, such as the investment in acceptance, status, power, and influence, as analogous to that observed in primates and other social mammals, as well as in humans. He emphasizes the importance of "fitness" in his evolutionary theory of human development.

Scarr specifically emphasizes the role of genetic endowment in determining personality. She states:

> Over development, different genes are turned on and off, creating maturational change in the organization of behavior as well as maturation changes in patterns of physical growth. Genetic differences among individuals are similarly responsible for determining what experiences people do and do not have in their environments. (Scarr, 1987, p. 62)

INTERACTION BETWEEN THE GENETIC AND INTERPERSONAL

The processes highlighted in the personality disorders can also be clarified by studies in the field of developmental psychology. Thus, the kind of clinging behavior, shyness, or rebelliousness observed in the growing child may persist through the developmental period (J. Kagan, 1989).

We predict that these patterns persist into late adolescence and adulthood and may find continued expression in certain of the personality disorders, such as the dependent, avoidant, or passive–aggressive types.

Regardless of the ultimate origin of the genetically determined prototypes of human behavior, there is strong evidence that certain types of relatively stable temperaments and behavioral patterns are present at birth (J. Kagan, 1989). These innate characteristics are best viewed as "tendencies" that can become accentuated or diminished by experience. Furthermore, a continuous, mutually reinforcing cycle can be set up between an individual's innate patterns and the patterns of other significant people.

For example, an individual with a large potential for care-eliciting behavior may evoke the care-producing behavior of other people, so that his or her innate patterns are maintained long beyond the period that such behavior is adaptive (Gilbert, 1989). For example, Sue, a patient whom we discuss in detail later, was described by her mother as having been more clinging and demanding of attention than her siblings practically from the time of birth. Her mother responded by being especially nurturant and protective. Throughout her developmental period and into adulthood, Sue succeeded in attaching herself to stronger people who would respond to her expressed desires for continuous affection and support. Another aspect was her belief that she was unlovable. She was picked on by older brothers, which laid the foundation for a later belief: "I cannot maintain the affection of a man." Because of these beliefs, she tended to avoid situations in which she could be rejected.

Until now we have been speaking of "innate tendencies" and "behavior" as though those characteristics can account for individual differences. Actually, our theory stipulates that integrated cognitive–affective–motivational programs decide an individual's behavior and differentiate that individual from other people. In older children and in adults, shyness, for example, is a derivative of an infrastructure of attitudes such as "It's risky to stick your neck out," a low threshold for anxiety in interpersonal situations, and a motivation to hang back with new acquaintances or strangers. These beliefs may become fixed as a result of the repetition of traumatic experiences that seem to confirm them.

Despite the powerful combination of innate predispositions and environmental influences, some individuals manage to change their behavior and modify the underlying attitudes. Not all shy children grow into shy adults. The influences of key people and purposeful experiences in cultivating more assertive behaviors, for example, may shift a shy person toward greater assertiveness and gregariousness. As we see in subsequent chapters in this book, even strongly maladaptive patterns may be modified by focusing therapy on testing these attitudes and forming or strengthening more adaptive attitudes.

Our formulation until now has addressed, briefly, how innate endowment can interact with environmental influences to produce quantitative distinctions in characteristic cognitive, affective, and behavioral patterns to account for individual differences in personality. Each individual has a unique personality profile, consisting of varying degrees of probability of responding in a particular way to a particular degree to a particular situation.

A person entering a group including unfamiliar people may think, "I'll look stupid," and will hang back. Another person may respond with the thought, "I can entertain them." A third may think, "They're unfriendly and may try to manipulate me," and will be on guard. When differing responses are characteristic of individuals, they reflect important structural differences represented in their basic beliefs (or schemas). The basic beliefs, respectively, would be: "I am vulnerable because I am inept in new situations," "I am entertaining to all people," and "I am vulnerable because people are unfriendly." Such variations are found in normal, well-adjusted people, and provide a distinctive coloring to their personalities. However, these kinds of beliefs are far more pronounced in the personality disorders; in the example just mentioned, they characterize the avoidant, histrionic, and paranoid disorders, respectively. Individuals with personality disorders show the same repetitive behaviors in many more situations than do other people. The typical maladaptive schemas in personality disorders are evoked across many or even most situations, have a compulsive quality, and are less easy to control or modify than their counterparts in other people. Any situation that has a bearing on the content of their maladaptive schemas will activate those schemas in preference to more adaptive ones. For the most part, these patterns are self-defeating in terms of many of these individuals' important goals. In sum, relative to other people, their dysfunctional attitudes and behaviors are overgeneralized, inflexible, imperative, and resistant to change.

ORIGIN OF DYSFUNCTIONAL BELIEFS

Given that the personality patterns (cognition, affect, and motivation) of people with personality disorders deviate from those of other people, the question arises: How do these patterns develop? To address this question—albeit briefly—we need to return to the nature–nurture interaction. Individuals with a particularly strong sensitivity to rejection, abandonment, or thwarting may develop intense fears and beliefs about the catastrophic meaning of such events. A patient, predisposed by nature to overreact to the more commonplace kinds of rejection in childhood, may develop a negative self-image ("I am unlovable"). This image may be reinforced if the rejection is particularly powerful, occurs at a particularly vulnerable time, or is repeated. With repetition, the belief becomes structuralized.

The patient mentioned earlier, Sue, developed an image of herself as inept and inadequate because she was always criticized by her siblings whenever she made a mistake. To protect herself as much as possible from pain and suffering, she tended to avoid situations in which this could occur. Her overgeneralized attitude was, "If I allow myself to be vulnerable in any situation, I will get hurt."

INFORMATION PROCESSING AND PERSONALITY

The way people process data about themselves and others is influenced by their beliefs and the other components of their cognitive organization. When there is a disorder of some type—a symptom syndrome (Axis I)[1] or a personality disorder (Axis II)—the orderly utilization of these data becomes systematically biased in a dysfunctional way. This bias in interpretation and the consequent behavior is shaped by dysfunctional beliefs.

Let us return to the example of Sue, who had both dependent and avoidant personality disorders and felt great concern about being rejected. In a typical scenario, she heard noises coming from the next room, where her boyfriend, Tom, was attending to some chores. Her perception of the noise provided the raw data for her interpretation. This perception was embedded in a specific context—her knowledge that Tom was in the next room putting up some pictures. The fusion of the stimulus and the context constituted the basis for information.

Because raw sensory data, such as noises, have limited informational value in themselves, they need to be transformed into some kind of meaningful configuration. This integration into a coherent pattern is the product of structures (schemas) operating on the raw sensory data within the specific context. Sue's instant thought was, "Tom is making a lot of noise." In most instances, people might conclude their information processing at this point, with the storing of this inference in short-term memory. But because Sue was rejection-prone, she was disposed to infer important meanings from such situations. Consequently, her information processing continued and she attached a personalized meaning: "Tom is making a lot of noise *because he's angry at me.*"

---

[1]Throughout this volume, we follow the revised fourth edition of the *Diagnostic and Statistical Manual of Mental Disorders* (American Psychiatric Association, 2000). The conventional syndromes, such as major depressive disorder or generalized anxiety disorder, manifested by strong subjective symptom complexes, are classified as Axis I, and personality disorders as Axis II.

Such an attribution of causality is produced by a higher order of structuring that attaches significance to events. A component (schema) of this higher-level system would be her belief: "If an intimate of mine is noisy, it means he's angry at me." This type of belief represents a conditional schema ("If . . . then") in contrast to a basic schema ("I am unlovable").

In this case, it was possible that Tom was angry at Sue. However, because Sue's basic belief was very strong, she was apt to make this interpretation whenever an intimate such as Tom was noisy, whether or not he actually was angry. Furthermore, prominent in the hierarchy of her beliefs was the formula, "If an intimate is angry, he will reject me," and, at a more generalized level, "If people reject me, I will be all alone," and "Being alone will be devastating." Beliefs are organized according to a hierarchy that assigns progressively broader and more complex meanings at successive levels.

This example illustrates a relatively new concept in cognitive psychology—namely, that information processing is influenced by a "feedforward" mechanism (Mahoney, 1984). At the most basic level, Sue had a belief that she was unlovable. This belief was manifested by a disposition to assign a consistent meaning when a relevant event occurred (Beck, 1964, 1967). The belief took a conditional form: "If men reject me, it means I'm unlovable." For the most part, this belief was held in abeyance if she was not exposed to a situation in which personal rejection by a man could occur. This belief (or schema) would supersede other more reasonable beliefs (or schemas) that might be more appropriate, however, when a situation relevant to this belief occurred (Beck, 1967). If there were data that could conceivably indicate that Tom was rejecting her, then her attention became fixed on the notion of her unlovability. She molded information about Tom's behavior in a way to fit this schema, even though other formulas might fit the data better—for example, "Loud hammering is a sound of exuberance." Because Sue's rejection schema was hypervalent, it was triggered in preference to other schemas, which seemed to be inhibited by the hypervalent schema.

Of course, Sue's psychological processes continued beyond her conclusion about being rejected. Whenever a schema of personal loss or threat is activated, there is a consequent activation of an "affective schema"; such a schema led in Sue's case to intense sadness. A negative interpretation of an event is linked to an affect that is congruent with it.

Although phenomena such as thoughts, feelings, and wishes may flash only briefly into our consciousness, the underlying structures responsible for these subjective experiences are relatively stable and durable. Furthermore, these structures are not in themselves conscious, although we can, through introspection, identify their content. Nonetheless, through conscious processes such as recognition, evaluation, and testing of their interpretations (basic techniques of cognitive therapy), people can modify the activity of the underlying structures and, in some instances, substantially change them.

CHARACTERISTICS OF SCHEMAS

It seems desirable at this point to review the place of schemas in personality and to describe their characteristics.

The concept of "schema" has a relatively long history in 20th-century psychology. The term, which can be traced to Bartlett (1932, 1958) and Piaget (1926, 1936/1952), has been used to describe those structures that integrate and attach meaning to events. The content of the schemas may deal with personal relationships, such as attitudes toward the self or others, or impersonal categories (e.g., inanimate objects). These objects may be concrete (a chair) or abstract (my country).

Schemas have additional structural qualities, such as breadth (whether they are narrow, discrete, or broad), flexibility or rigidity (their capacity for modification), and density (their relative prominence in the cognitive organization). They also may be described in terms of their valence—the degree to which they are energized at a particular point in time. The level of activation (or valence) may vary from latent to hypervalent. When schemas are latent, they are not participating in information processing; when activated, they channel cognitive processing from the earliest to the final stages. The concept of schemas is similar to the formulation by George Kelly (1955) of "personal constructs."

In the field of psychopathology, the term "schema" has been applied to structures with a highly personalized idiosyncratic content that are activated during disorders such as depression, anxiety, panic attacks, and obsessions and become prepotent. When hypervalent, these idiosyncratic schemas displace and probably inhibit other schemas that may be more adaptive or more appropriate for a given situation. They consequently introduce a systematic bias into information processing (Beck, 1964, 1967; Beck et al., 1985).

The typical schemas of the personality disorders resemble those that are activated in the symptom syndromes, but they are operative on a more continuous basis in information processing. In dependent personality disorder, the schema "I need help" will be activated whenever a problematic situation arises, whereas in depressed persons it will be prominent only during the depression. In personality disorders, the schemas are part of normal, everyday processing of information.

Personality may be conceptualized as a relatively stable organization composed of systems and modes. Systems of interlocking structures (schemas) are responsible for the sequence extending from the reception of a stimulus to the end point of a behavioral response. The integration of environmental stimuli and the formation of an adaptive response depend on these interlocking systems of specialized structures. Separate but related systems are involved in memory, cognition, affect, motivation, action, and control. The basic processing units, the schemas, are organized according to their functions (and also according to content). Different types of schemas have different functions. For example, the cognitive schemas are concerned with abstraction, interpretation, and recall; the affective schemas are responsible for the generation of feelings; the motivational schemas deal with wishes and desires; the instrumental schemas prepare for action; and the control schemas are involved with self-monitoring and inhibiting or directing actions.

Some subsystems composed of cognitive schemas are concerned with self-evaluation; others are concerned with evaluation of other people. Other such subsystems are designed to store memories, either episodic or semantic, and provide access to them. Still other subsystems function to prepare for forthcoming situations and provide the basis for expectancies, predictions, and long-range forecasts.

When particular schemas are hypervalent, the threshold for activation of the constituent schemas is low: They are readily triggered by a remote or trivial stimulus. They are also "prepotent"; that is, they readily supersede more appropriate schemas or configurations in processing information (Beck, 1967). In fact, clinical observation suggests that schemas that are more appropriate to the actual stimulus situation are actively inhibited. Thus, in clinical depression, for example, the negative schemas are in ascendancy, resulting in a systematic negative bias in the interpretation and recall of experiences as well as in short-term and long-term predictions, whereas the positive schemas become less accessible. It is easy for depressed patients to see the negative aspects of an event but difficult to see the positive. They can recall negative events much more readily than positive ones. They weigh the probabilities of undesirable outcomes more heavily than positive outcomes.

When a person goes into a clinical depression (or anxiety disorder), there is a pronounced "cognitive shift." In energy terms, the shift is away from normal cognitive processing to a predominance of processing by the negative schemas that constitute the depressive mode. The terms "cathexis" and "countercathexis" have been used by psychoanalytic writers to describe the deployment of energy to activate unconscious patterns (cathexis) or to inhibit them (countercathexis). Thus, in depression, the depressive mode is cathected; in generalized anxiety disorder, the danger mode is cathected; in panic disorder, the panic mode is cathected (Beck et al., 1985).

THE ROLE OF AFFECT IN PERSONALITIES

Discussion of cognitive and behavioral patterns may seem to slight the subjective aspects of our emotional life—our feelings of sadness, joy, terror, and anger. We are aware that we are likely to feel sad when we are separated from a loved one or experience a loss of status, to be pleased when we receive expressions of affection or reach a goal, and to be angry when we are unfairly treated. How do these emotional—or affective—experiences fit into the scheme of personality organization? What is their relationship to basic cognitive structures and strategies? According to our formulation, the affects related to pleasure and pain play a key role in the mobilization and maintenance of the crucial strategies. The survival and reproductive strategies appear to operate in part through their attachment to the pleasure–pain centers. As pointed out previously, activities that are directed toward survival and reproduction lead to pleasure when successfully consummated and to "pain" when thwarted. The appetitive urges related to eating and sex create tension when stimulated and gratification when fulfilled. Other emotional structures producing anxiety and sadness, respectively, reinforce the cognitive signals that alert us to danger or accentuate the perception that we have lost something of value (Beck et al., 1985). Thus, the emotional mechanisms serve to reinforce behaviors directed toward survival and bonding through the expectation and experience of various types of pleasure. At the same time, complementary mechanisms serve to dampen potentially self-defeating or dangerous actions through the arousal of anxiety and dysphoria (Beck et al., 1985). Other automatic mechanisms, those associated with the control system and involved in modulating behavior, will be discussed presently.

FROM PERCEPTION TO BEHAVIOR

Among the basic components of the personality organization are sequences of different kinds of schemas that operate analogously to an assembly line. For purposes of simplification, these structures may be viewed as operating in a logical linear progression. For example, exposure to a dangerous stimulus activates the relevant "danger schema," which begins to process the information. In sequence, then, the affective, motivational, action, and control schemas are activated. The person interprets the situation as dangerous (cognitive schema), feels anxiety (affective schema), wants to get away (motivational schema), and becomes mobilized to run away (action or instrumental schema). If the person judges that running away is counterproductive, he or she may inhibit this impulse (control schema).

In Axis I disorders, a specific mode becomes hypervalent and leads, for example, to preoccupation with loss, danger, or combat. In the case of depression, a chain reaction is set up: cognitive →affective →motivational →motor. In personally meaningful situations, the interpretation and the affect feed into the "effector loop" or action system. For instance, after her interpreting a rejection, a sad expression would sweep across Sue's face. This process, which occurred automatically, might have served phylogenetically as a form of communication—as a distress signal, for example. Concomitantly, "action schemas" were triggered: Her own particular strategy for dealing with rejection was activated, and she experienced an impulse to go into the next room and ask Tom to reassure her. She was mobilized to act according to her stereotyped strategy. At this point, she might or might not yield to her impulse to run to Tom.

THE INTERNAL CONTROL SYSTEM

We know that people do not give in to every impulse, whether it is to laugh, cry, or hit somebody. Another system—the "control system"—is operative in conjunction with the action system to modulate, modify, or inhibit impulses. This system also is based on beliefs, many or most of which are realistic or adaptive. Although the impulses constitute the "wants," these beliefs constitute the "do's" or the "do nots" (Beck, 1976). Examples of such beliefs are "It is wrong to hit somebody weaker or bigger than you." "You should defer to authorities." "You should not cry in public." These beliefs are automatically translated into commands: "Don't hit." "Do what you're told." "Don't cry." The prohibitions thus exercise a counterforce to the expression of the wishes. Sue had specific personal beliefs—here, in particular, "If I ask Tom too much for reassurance, he will get mad at me" (a prediction). Hence, she inhibited her wish to run into the next room and ask him whether he still loved her.

In therapy, it is important to identify those beliefs (e.g., "I'm unlikable") that shape the personal interpretations; those in the instrumental system that initiate action (e.g., "Ask him if he loves me"); and those in the control system that govern anticipations and consequently facilitate or inhibit action (Beck, 1976). The control or regulatory system plays a crucial—and often unrecognized—role in personality disorder and consequently deserves further elaboration. The control functions can be divided into those concerned with self-regulation—that is, inner-directed—and those involved with relating to the external, primarily social, environment. The self-directed regulatory processes of particular relevance to the personality disorders are concerned with the way people communicate with themselves. The internal communications consist of self-monitoring, self-appraisal and self-evaluation, self-warnings, and self-instructions (Beck, 1976). When exaggerated or deficient, these processes become more conspicuous. People who monitor themselves too much tend to be inhibited—we see this in the avoidant personality, as well as in anxiety states—whereas too little inhibition facilitates impulsivity.

Self-appraisals and self-evaluations are important methods by which people can determine whether they are "on course." Whereas self-appraisal may simply represent observations of the self, self-evaluation implies making value judgments about the self: good–bad, worthwhile–worthless, lovable–unlovable. Negative self-evaluations are found overtly in depression but may operate in a more subtle fashion in most of the personality disorders.

In normal functioning, this system of self-evaluations and self-directions operates more or less automatically. People may not be aware of these self-signals unless they specifically focus their attention on them. These cognitions may then be represented in a particular form labeled "automatic thoughts" (Beck, 1967). As noted earlier, these automatic thoughts become hypervalent in depression, and they are expressed in notions such as "I am worthless" or "I am undesirable."

The self-evaluations and self-instructions appear to be derived from deeper structures: namely, the self-concepts or self-schemas. In fact, exaggerated negative (or positive) self-concepts may be the factors that move a person from being a "personality type" into having a "personality disorder." For example, the development of a rigid view of the self as helpless may move a person from experiencing normal dependency wishes in childhood to "pathological" dependency in adulthood. Similarly, an emphasis on systems, control, and order may predispose a person to a personality disorder in which the systems become the master instead of the tool—namely, obsessive–compulsive personality disorder.

In the course of maturation, we develop a medley of rules that provide the substrate for our self-evaluations and self-directions. These rules also form the basis for setting standards, expectations, and plans of action for ourselves. Thus, a woman who has a rule with a content such as "I must always do a perfect job" may be continuously evaluating her performance, praising herself for attaining a specific goal, and criticizing herself for falling short of the mark. Because the rule is rigid, she cannot operate according to a practical, more flexible rule, such as "The important thing is to get the job done, even if it isn't perfect." Similarly, people develop rules for interpersonal conduct: The do's and don't's may lead to marked social inhibition, such as we find in avoidant personalities. These people also will feel anxious at even entertaining thoughts of violating a rule such as "Don't stick your neck out."

TRANSITION TO AXIS II DISORDER

When people develop an Axis I disorder, they tend to process information selectively and in a dysfunctional way. Basic beliefs that the patient held prior to developing depression or anxiety become much more plausible and pervasive, solidifying the cognitive foundation of the Axis II disorder. Beliefs such as "If you aren't successful, you are worthless," or "A good parent should always satisfy her children's needs," become more absolute and extreme. Moreover, certain aspects of the negative self-image become accentuated and broadened, so that the patient begins to perseverate in the thought "I am worthless," or "I am a failure." Negative thoughts that were transient and less powerful prior to the depression become prepotent and dominate the patient's feelings and behavior (Beck, 1963).

Some of the more specific conditional beliefs become broadened to include a much broader spectrum of situations. The belief or attitude "If I don't have somebody to guide me in new situations, I won't be able to cope" becomes extended to "If somebody strong isn't accessible at all times, I will flounder." As the depression increases, these beliefs may be broadened to "Since I'm helpless, I need somebody to take charge and take care of me." The beliefs thus become more absolute and more extreme.

The ease with which these patients accept their dysfunctional beliefs during depression or anxiety disorders suggests that they have temporarily lost the ability to reality-test their dysfunctional interpretations. For example, a depressed patient who gets the idea "I am a despicable human being" seems to lack the capacity to look at this belief, to weigh contradictory evidence, and to reject the belief even though it is unsupported by evidence. The cognitive disability seems to rest on the temporary loss of access to and application of the rational modes of cognition by which we test our conclusions. Cognitive therapy aims explicitly to "reenergize" the reality-testing system. In the interim, the therapist serves as an "auxiliary reality tester" for the patient.

Depressed patients differ also in the way that they automatically process data. Experimental work (Gilson, 1983) indicates that they rapidly and efficiently incorporate negative information about themselves but are blocked in processing positive information. Dysfunctional thinking becomes more prominent, and it becomes more difficult to apply the corrective, more rational cognitive processes.

As pointed out earlier, the way people use data about themselves and others is influenced by their personality organization. When there is a disorder of some type—a clinical (symptom) syndrome (Axis I) or personality disorder (Axis II)—the orderly processing of these data becomes systematically biased in a dysfunctional way. The bias in interpretation and the consequent behavior is shaped by the patients' dysfunctional beliefs and attitudes.

THE COGNITIVE SHIFT

The shift in the cognitive functions in the transition from a personality disorder into an anxiety state and then to depression is illustrated by Sue's experience. As far back as Sue could remember, she had questions about her acceptability. When her relationship with Tom was threatened, these sporadic self-doubts became transformed into continuous worry. As she moved into depression, her belief that she might be undesirable shifted to the belief that she *was* undesirable.

Similarly, Sue's attitude about the future shifted from a chronic uncertainty to a continuous apprehension, and ultimately—as she became more depressed—to hopelessness about her future. Further, she tended to catastrophize about the future when anxious but accepted the catastrophe as though it had already occurred when she became depressed.

When she was not clinically depressed or anxious, Sue was capable of accessing some positive information about herself: She was a "good person," a considerate and loyal friend, and a conscientious worker. As she became anxious, she could credit herself with these positive qualities, but they seemed less relevant—perhaps because they apparently did not assure her of a stable relationship with a man. With the onset of her depression, however, she had difficulty in acknowledging or even thinking of her positive assets; even when she was able to acknowledge them, she tended to disqualify them, as they were discordant with her self-image.

We have already noted that patients' dysfunctional beliefs become more extreme and rigid as the affective disorders develop. Prior to this, Sue would only occasionally endorse the belief "I can never be happy without a man." As her anxiety and depression developed, this belief moved to "I will always be unhappy if I don't have a man."

The progression of cognitive dysfunction from the personality disorder to anxiety and then to depression is illustrated by the gradual impairment of reality testing. When in an anxious state, Sue was able to view some of her catastrophic concerns with some objectivity. She could see that the thought "I will always be alone and unhappy if this relationship breaks up" was only a thought. When she became depressed, the idea that she would indeed always be unhappy was no longer simply a possibility; it was, for her, reality—a fact.

In therapy, the long-standing beliefs that form the matrix of the personality disorder are the most difficult to change. The beliefs that are associated only with the affective and anxiety disorders are subject to more rapid amelioration because they are less stable. Thus, it is possible for a person to shift from a depressive mode to a more normal mode with psychotherapy, chemotherapy, or simply with the passage of time. There is a shift in energy—or cathexis—from one mode to the other. When this shift takes place, the features of the "thinking disorder" in depression (systematic negative bias, overgeneralization, personalization) greatly diminish. The "normal" mode of the personality disorder is more stable than the depressive or anxious mode. Because the schemas in the normal mode are denser and more heavily represented in the cognitive organization, they are less amenable to change. These schemas give the normal personality and the personality disorder their distinctive characteristics. Within each personality disorder, certain beliefs and strategies are predominant and form a characteristic profile.

COGNITIVE PROFILES

One simple way to approach the personality disorders is to think of them in terms of certain vectors. Following the formulation of Horney (1950), we can view these interpersonal strategies in terms of how personality types relate to and act toward other people, how they use interpersonal space. Individuals may move or place themselves against, toward, away from, above, or under others. The dependent moves *toward* and often *below* (submissive, subservient). Another "type" *stays still* and may obstruct others: the passive–aggressive. The narcissists position themselves *above* others. The compulsive may move *above* in the interest of control. The schizoid moves *away,* and the avoidant moves *closer* and then *backs off.* The histrionic personalities use the space to *draw others* toward them.[2] As we shall see, these vectors may be regarded as the visible manifestations of specific interpersonal strategies associated with specific personality disorders. This simplified sketch presents one way of looking at personality types and personality disorders—in terms of the way individuals position themselves in relation to other people. Insofar as this patterning is regarded as dysfunctional, the diagnosis of personality disorder is deemed to be justified when it leads to (1) problems that produce suffering in the patient (e.g., avoidant personality) or (2) difficulties with other people or with society (e.g., antisocial personality). However, many people with a diagnosed personality disorder do not re-

---

[2]As noted previously, the borderline and schizotypal disorders are not included in our differentiation of strategies because these two disorders are not as well characterized by a specific thought content.

gard themselves as having such a disorder. Individuals generally regard their personality patterns as undesirable only when they lead to symptoms (e.g., depression or anxiety) or when they seem to interfere with important social or occupational aspirations (as in the case of the dependent, avoidant, or passive–aggressive personalities).

When confronted with situations that interfere with the operation of their idiosyncratic strategy—for example, when a dependent person is separated from or threatened with separation from a significant other, or the obsessive–compulsive is thrown into an unmanageable situation— then the person may develop symptoms of depression or anxiety. Other people with personality disorders may regard their own patterns as perfectly normal and satisfactory for them but acquire a diagnostic label because their behavior is viewed negatively by other people, as in the case of narcissistic, schizoid, or antisocial personalities.

The observable behaviors (or strategies), however, are only one aspect of the personality disorders. Each disorder is characterized not only by dysfunctional or asocial behavior but by a composite of beliefs and attitudes, affect, and strategies. It is possible to provide a distinctive profile of each of the disorders based on their typical cognitive, affective, and behavioral features. Although this typology is presented in pure form, it should be kept in mind that specific individuals may show features of more than one personality type.

OVERDEVELOPED AND UNDERDEVELOPED PATTERNS

Individuals with a personality disorder tend to show certain patterns of behavior that are hypertrophied, or overdeveloped, and other patterns that are underdeveloped. The obsessive–compulsive disorder, for example, may be characterized by an excessive emphasis on control, responsibility, and systematization and a relative deficiency in spontaneity and playfulness. As illustrated in Table 2.2, the other personality disorders similarly show a heavy weighting of some patterns and a light representation of others. The deficient features are frequently the counterparts of the strong features. It is as though when one interpersonal strategy is overdeveloped, the balancing strategy fails to develop properly. One can speculate that as a child becomes overinvested in a predominant type of behavior, it overshadows and perhaps weakens the development of other adaptive behaviors.

As will be shown in the subsequent chapters on each of the personality disorders, certain overdeveloped strategies may be a derivative from or compensation for a particular type of self-concept and a response to particular developmental experiences. Also, as indicated previously, genetic predisposition may favor the development of a particular type of pattern in preference to other possible patterns. Some children, for example, appear to be oriented toward entertaining, whereas others appear shy and inhibited from the early stages of development. Thus, the narcissistic personality may develop as an individual fights fiercely to overcome a deep sense of unworthiness. The obsessive–compulsive personality may develop in response to chaotic conditions in childhood—as a way of bringing order to a disordered environment. A paranoid personality may be formed in response to early experiences of betrayal or deception; a passive–aggressive personality may develop in response to manipulation by others. The dependent personality often represents a fixation on a close attachment that, for a variety of reasons, may have

TABLE 2.2. Typical Overdeveloped and Underdeveloped Strategies

Personality disorder	Overdeveloped	Underdeveloped
Obsessive–compulsive	Control Responsibility Systematization	Spontaneity Playfulness
Dependent	Help seeking Clinging	Self-sufficiency Mobility
Passive–aggressive	Autonomy Resistance Passivity Sabotage	Intimacy Assertiveness Activity Cooperativeness
Paranoid	Vigilance Mistrust Suspiciousness	Serenity Trust Acceptance
Narcissistic	Self-aggrandizement Competitiveness	Sharing Group identification
Antisocial	Combativeness Exploitativeness Predation	Empathy Reciprocity Social sensitivity
Schizoid	Autonomy Isolation	Intimacy Reciprocity
Avoidant	Social vulnerability Avoidance Inhibition	Self-assertion Gregariousness
Histrionic	Exhibitionism Expressiveness Impressionism	Reflectiveness Control Systematization

been reinforced by family members rather than normally attenuated over the developmental period. Similarly, a histrionic personality may be evoked from experiences of being rewarded for successful exhibitionism—for example, entertaining others to get approval and affection. It should be noted that different pathways may lead to personality disorders. Narcissistic, obsessive–compulsive, paranoid, and even antisocial personality disorder, for example, may develop either as a compensation or as a fear (i.e., as a result of a sense of chaos, manipulation, or victimization) as a result of reinforcement of the relevant strategies by significant others or through both methods.

One cannot overlook the importance of identification with other family members. Some individuals *seem* to adopt certain dysfunctional patterns of their parents or siblings and build on them as they grow older. In other individuals, personality disorders seem to evolve from the inheritance of a strong predisposition. Thus, research by J. Kagan (1989) indicates that a shyness exhibited early in life tends to persist. It is possible that an innate disposition to shyness could be so reinforced by subsequent experience that instead of simply being nonassertive, the individual develops into an avoidant personality. It is useful to analyze the psychological characteristics of individuals with personality disorders in terms of their views of themselves and others, their basic beliefs, their basic strategies, and their main affects. In this way, therapists can obtain specific cognitive–behavioral–emotive profiles that help them to understand each disorder and that facilitate treatment.

SPECIFIC COGNITIVE PROFILES

Avoidant Personality Disorder

People diagnosed as having avoidant personality disorder, using the DSM-IV-TR criteria, have the following key conflict: They would like to be close to others and to live up to their intellectual and vocational potential, but they are afraid of being hurt, rejected, and unsuccessful. Their strategy (in contrast to the dependent) is to back off—or avoid getting involved in the first place.

Self-view: They see themselves as socially inept and incompetent in academic or work situations.

View of others: They see others as potentially critical, uninterested, and demeaning.

Beliefs: Not infrequently, persons with this disorder have these *core* beliefs: "I am no good . . . worthless . . . unlovable. I cannot tolerate unpleasant feelings." These beliefs feed into the next (higher) level of *conditional* beliefs: "If people got close to me, they would discover the 'real me' and would reject me—that would be intolerable." Or, "If I undertake something new and don't succeed, it would be devastating."

The next level, which dictates their behavior, consists of *instrumental* or self-instructional beliefs such as "It is best to stay clear of risky involvement," "I should avoid unpleasant situations at all costs," "If I feel or think of something unpleasant, I should try to wipe it out by distracting myself or taking a fix (drink, drug, etc.)."

Threats: The main threats are of being discovered to be a "fraud," being put down, demeaned, or rejected.

Strategy: Their main strategy is to avoid situations in which they could be evaluated. Thus, they tend to hang back on the fringes of social groups and avoid attracting attention to themselves. In work situations, they tend to avoid taking on new responsibilities or seeking advancement because of their fear of failure and of subsequent reprisals from others.

Affect: The main affect is dysphoria, a combination of anxiety and sadness, related to their deficits in obtaining the pleasures they would like to receive from close relationships and the sense of mastery from accomplishment. They experience anxiety, related to their fear of sticking their necks out in social or work situations.

Their low tolerance for dysphoria prevents them from developing methods for overcoming their shyness and asserting themselves more effectively. Because they are introspective and monitor feelings continually, they are acutely sensitive to their feelings of sadness and anxiety. Ironically, despite their hyperawareness of painful feelings, they shy away from identifying unpleasant thoughts—a tendency that fits in with their major strategy and is labeled "cognitive avoidance." Their low tolerance for unpleasant feelings and their sensitivity to failure and rejection pervade all of their actions. Unlike the dependent person, who handles fear of failure by leaning on others, the avoidant person simply lowers expectations and stays clear of any involvement that incurs a risk of failure or rejection.

Dependent Personality Disorder

Individuals with dependent personality disorder have a picture of themselves as helpless and therefore try to attach themselves to some stronger figure who will provide the resources for their survival and happiness.

Self-view: They perceive themselves as needy, weak, helpless, and incompetent.

View of others: They see the strong "caretaker" in an idealized way: as nurturant, supportive, and competent. In contrast to the avoidant personality, who stays clear of "entangling relationships" and consequently does not gain social support, the dependent personality can function quite well as long as a strong figure is accessible.

Beliefs: These patients believe that "I need other people—specifically, a strong person—in order to survive." Further, they believe that their happiness depends on having such a figure available. They believe that they need a steady, uninterrupted flow of support and encouragement. As one dependent patient put it, "I cannot live without a man." Or, "I can never be happy unless I am loved."

In terms of the hierarchy of beliefs, their *core* belief is likely to be "I am completely helpless," or "I am all alone." Their *conditional* beliefs are "I can function only if I have access to somebody competent," "If I am abandoned, I will die," "If I am not loved, I will always be unhappy." The *instrumental* level consists of imperatives such as "Don't offend the caretaker," "Stay close," "Cultivate as intimate a relationship as possible," "Be subservient in order to bind him or her."

Threat: The main threat or trauma is concerned with rejection or abandonment.

Strategy: Their main strategy is to cultivate a dependent relationship. They will frequently do this by subordinating themselves to a "strong" figure and trying to placate or please this person.

Affect: Their main affect is anxiety—the concern over possible disruption of the dependent relationship. They periodically experience heightened anxiety when they perceive that the relationship actually is strained. If the figure they depend on is removed, they may sink into a depression. On the other hand, they experience gratification or euphoria when their dependent wishes are granted.

Passive–Aggressive Personality Disorder

Even though this disorder is not included in DSM-IV-TR, we have found that a significant number of patients have behaviors and beliefs indicative of this disorder. Individuals with passive–aggressive personality disorder have an oppositional style, which belies the fact that they do want to get recognition and support from authority figures. The chief problem is a conflict between their desire to get the benefits conferred by authorities on the one hand and their desire to maintain their autonomy on the other. Consequently, they try to maintain the relationship by being passive and submissive, but, as they sense a loss of autonomy, they are inclined to resist or even to subvert the authorities.

Self-view: They may perceive themselves as self-sufficient but vulnerable to encroachment by others. (They are, however, drawn to strong figures and organizations because they crave social approval and support. Hence, they are frequently in a conflict between their desire for attachment and their fear of encroachment.)

View of others: They see others—specifically, the authority figures—as intrusive, demanding, interfering, controlling, and dominating, but at the same time capable of being approving, accepting, and caring.

Beliefs: Their *core* beliefs have to do with notions such as "Being controlled by others is intolerable," "I have to do things my own way," or "I deserve approval because of all I have done."

Their conflicts are expressed in beliefs such as "I need authority to nurture and support me" versus "I need to protect my identity." (The same kind of conflicts are often expressed by borderline patients.) The *conditional* belief is expressed in terms such as "If I follow the rules, I lose my freedom of action." Their *instrumental* beliefs revolve around postponing action that is expected by an authority, or complying superficially but not substantively.

Threat: The main threat or fears revolve around loss of approval and abridgement of autonomy.

Strategy: Their main strategy is to fortify their autonomy through devious opposition to the authority figures while ostensibly courting the favor of the authorities. They try to evade or circumvent the rules in a spirit of covert defiance. They are often subversive in the sense of not getting work done on time, not attending classes, and so on—ultimately self-defeating behavior. Yet, on the surface, because of their need for approval, they may seem to be compliant and cultivate the goodwill of the authorities. They often have a strong passive streak. They tend to follow the line of least resistance; they often avoid competitive situations and are interested more in solitary pursuits.

Affect: Their main affect is unexpressed anger, which is associated with rebellion against an authority's rules. This affect, which is conscious, alternates with anxiety when they anticipate reprisals and are threatened with cutting off of "supplies."

Obsessive–Compulsive Personality Disorder

The key words for obsessive–compulsives are "control" and "should." These individuals make a virtue of justifying the means to achieve the end to such an extent that the means becomes an end in itself. To them, "orderliness is godliness."

Self-view: They see themselves as responsible for themselves and others. They believe they have to depend on themselves to see that things get done. They are accountable to their own perfectionistic conscience. They are driven by the "shoulds." Many of the people with this disorder have a core image of themselves as inept or helpless. The deep concern about being helpless is linked to a fear of being overwhelmed, unable to function. In these cases, their overemphasis on systems is a compensation for their perception of defectiveness and helplessness.

View of others: They perceive others as too casual, often irresponsible, self-indulgent, or incompetent. They liberally apply the "shoulds" to others in an attempt to shore up their own weaknesses.

Beliefs: In the serious obsessive–compulsive disorder, the *core* beliefs are "I could be overwhelmed," "I am basically disorganized or disoriented," "I need order, systems, and rules in order to survive." Their *conditional* beliefs are "If I don't have systems, everything will fall apart," "Any flaw or defect in performance will produce a landslide," "If I or others don't perform at the highest standards, we will fail," "If I fail in this, I am a failure as a person," "If I have a perfect system, I will be successful/happy." Their *instrumental* beliefs are imperative: "I must be in control," "I must do virtually anything just right," "I know what's best," "You have to do it my way," "Details are crucial," "People *should* do better and try harder," "I have to push myself (and others) all the time," "People should be criticized in order to prevent future mistakes." Frequent automatic thoughts tinged with criticalness are "Why can't they do it right?" or "Why do I always slip up?"

Threats: The main threats are flaws, mistakes, disorganization, or imperfections. They tend to "catastrophize" that "things will get out of control" or that they "won't be able to get things done."

Strategy: Their strategy revolves around a system of rules, standards, and "shoulds." In applying rules, they evaluate and rate other people's performance as well as their own. In order to reach their goals, they try to exert maximum control over their own behavior and that of others involved in carrying out their goals. They attempt to assert control over their own behavior by "shoulds" and self-reproaches, and over other people's behavior by overly directing, or disapproving and punishing them. This instrumental behavior amounts to coercing and slave driving themselves or others.

Affect: Because of their perfectionistic standards, these individuals are particularly prone to experience regrets, disappointment, and anger toward themselves and others. The affective response to their anticipation of substandard performance is anxiety or anger. When serious "failure" does occur, they may become depressed.

Paranoid Personality Disorder

The key word for paranoid personality disorder is "mistrust." It is conceivable that, under certain circumstances, wariness, looking for hidden motives, or not trusting others may be adaptive—even life-saving—but the paranoid personality adopts this stance in most situations, including the most benign.

Self-view: The paranoid personalities see themselves as righteous and vulnerable to mistreatment by others.

View of others: They see other people essentially as devious, deceptive, treacherous, and covertly manipulative. They believe that other people actively desire to interfere with them, put them down, discriminate against them—but in a hidden way in an innocent guise. Some patients may think that others form secret coalitions against them.

Beliefs: The *core* beliefs consist of notions such as "I am vulnerable to other people," "Other people cannot be trusted," "They have bad intentions (toward me)," "They are deceptive," "They're out to undermine me or depreciate me." The *conditional* beliefs are "If I am not careful, people will manipulate, abuse, or take advantage of me," "If people act friendly, they are trying to use me," "If people seem distant, it proves they are unfriendly." The *instrumental* (or self-instructional) beliefs are "Be on guard," "Don't trust anybody," "Look for hidden motives," "Don't get taken in."

Threats: The main fears are concerned with being diminished in some way: manipulated, controlled, demeaned, or discriminated against.

Strategy: With this notion that other people are against them, the paranoid personalities are driven to be hypervigilant and always on guard. They are wary, suspicious, and looking all the time for cues that will betray the "hidden motives" of their "adversaries." At times, they may confront these "adversaries" with allegations about being wronged and consequently provoke the kind of hostility that they believed had already existed.

Affects: The main affect is anger over the presumed abuse. Some paranoid personalities, however, may also experience constant anxiety over the perceived threats. This painful anxiety is often the prod for their seeking therapy.

Antisocial Personality Disorder

The antisocial personalities may assume a variety of forms: the expression of antisocial behavior may vary considerably (see DSM-IV-TR; American Psychiatric Association, 2000) from conniving, manipulating, and exploiting to direct attack.

Self-view: In general, these personalities view themselves as loners, autonomous, and strong. Some of them see themselves as having been abused and mistreated by society and therefore justify victimizing others because they believe that they have been victimized. Other patients may simply cast themselves in the predatory role in a "dog-eat-dog" world in which breaking the rules of society is normal and even desirable.

View of others: They see other people as either exploitative and thus deserving of being exploited in retaliation, or as weak and vulnerable and thus deserving of being preyed upon.

Beliefs: The *core* beliefs are "I need to look out for myself," "I need to be the aggressor or I will be the victim." The antisocial personality also believes that "Other people are patsies or wimps," or "Others are exploitative, and therefore I'm entitled to exploit them back." This person believes that he or she *is* entitled to break rules: Rules are arbitrary and designed to protect the "haves" against the "have nots." This view is in contrast to that of people with narcissistic personalities, who believe that they are such special, unique individuals and that they are above the rules—a prerogative that they believe everybody should easily recognize and respect.

The *conditional* belief is "If I don't push others around (or manipulate, exploit, or attack them), I will never get what I deserve." The *instrumental* or imperative beliefs are "Get the other guy before he gets you," "It's your turn now," "Take it, you deserve it."

Strategy: The main strategies fall into two classes. The overt antisocial personality will openly attack, rob, and defraud others. The more subtle type–the "con artist"—seeks to inveigle others and, through shrewd, subtle manipulations, to exploit or defraud them.

Affect: When a particular affect is present, it is essentially anger—over the injustice that other people have possessions that they (the antisocial personalities) deserve.

Narcissistic Personality Disorder

The key word for narcissistic personality disorder is "self-aggrandizement."

Self-view: The narcissistic personalities view themselves as special and unique—almost as princes or princesses. They believe that they have a special status that places them above ordinary people. They consider themselves superior and entitled to special favors and favorable treatment; they are above the rules that govern other people.

View of others: Although they may regard other people as inferior, they do not do this in the same sense as do the antisocial personalities. They simply see themselves as prestigious and as elevated above the average person; they see others as their vassals and potential admirers. They seek recognition from others primarily to document their own grandiosity and preserve their superior status.

Beliefs: The *core* narcissistic beliefs are as follows: "Since I am special, I deserve special dispensations, privileges, and prerogatives," "I'm superior to others and they should acknowledge this," "I'm above the rules." Many of these patients have covert beliefs of being unlovable or helpless. These beliefs emerge after a significant failure and form core elements in the patients' depression.

The *conditional* beliefs are, "If others don't recognize my special status, they should be punished," "If I am to maintain my superior status, I should expect others' subservience." On the other hand, they have negatively framed beliefs such as, "If I'm not on top, I'm a flop." Thus, when they experience a significant defeat, they are prone to a catastrophic drop in self-esteem. The *instrumental* belief is, "Strive at all times to demonstrate your superiority."

Strategy: Their main plans revolve around activities that can reinforce their superior status and expand their "personal domain." Thus, they may seek glory, wealth, position, power, and prestige as a way of continuously reinforcing their superior image. They tend to be highly competitive with others who claim an equally high status and will resort to manipulative strategies to gain their ends.

Unlike the antisocial personality, they do not have a cynical view of the rules that govern human conduct; they simply consider themselves exempt from them. Similarly, they do regard themselves as part of society, but at the very top stratum.

Affect: Their main affect is anger when other people do not accord them the admiration or respect to which they believe they are entitled, or otherwise thwart them in some way. They are prone to becoming depressed, however, if their strategies are foiled. For example, psychotherapists have treated several "inside traders" on Wall Street who became depressed after their manipulations were discovered and they were publicly disgraced. They believed that by tumbling from their high position, they had lost everything.

Histrionic Personality Disorder

The key word for histrionic personalities is "expressiveness," which embodies the tendency to dramatize or romanticize all situations and to try to impress and captivate others.

Self-view: They view themselves as glamorous, impressive, and deserving of attention.

View of others: They view others favorably as long as they can elicit their attention, amusement, and affection. They try to form strong alliances with others, but with the proviso that they be at the center of the group and that others play the role of attentive audience. In contrast to narcissistic personalities, they are very much involved in their minute-to-minute interactions with other people, and their self-esteem depends on their receiving continuous expressions of appreciation.

Beliefs: The person with a histrionic disorder often has *core* beliefs such as "I am basically unattractive," or "I need other people to admire me in order to be happy." Among the compensatory beliefs are "I am very lovable, entertaining, and interesting," "I am entitled to admiration," "People are there to admire me and do my bidding," "They have no right to, deny me my just deserts."

Conditional beliefs include the following: "If I entertain or impress people I am worthwhile," Unless I captivate people, I am nothing," "If I can't entertain people, they will abandon me," "If people don't respond, they are rotten," "If I can't captivate people, I am helpless."

Histrionic people tend to be global and impressionistic in their thinking, a factor that is reflected in their *instrumental* belief, "I can go by my feelings." If the obsessive–compulsives are guided by rationally or intellectually derived systems, the histrionics are guided primarily by feelings. Histrionics who feel angry may use this as sufficient justification for punishing another person. If they feel affection, they consider it a justification for pouring on affection (even though they may switch over to another type of expression a few minutes later). If they feel sad, this is sufficient rationale for them to cry. They tend to dramatize their ways of communicating their sense of frustration or despair, as in the "histrionic suicide attempt." These general patterns are reflected in imperatives such as "Express your feelings," "Be entertaining," "Show people that they have hurt you."

Strategy: They use dramatics and demonstrativeness to bind people to them. When they do not succeed, however, they believe they are being treated unfairly, and they try to coerce compliance through theatrical expressions of their pain and anger: crying, assaultive behavior, and impulsive suicidal acts.

Affect: The most prominent positive affect is gaiety, often mixed with mirth and other high spirits when they are successfully engaging other people. They generally experience an undercurrent of anxiety, however, that reflects their fear of rejection. When thwarted, their affect can change rapidly to anger or sadness.

Schizoid Personality Disorder

The key word for schizoid personality disorder is "isolation." These persons are the embodiment of the autonomous personality. They are willing to sacrifice intimacy in order to preserve their detachment and autonomy. On the other hand, they view themselves as vulnerable to being controlled if they allow others to get too close to them.

Self-view: They see themselves as self-sufficient and as loners. They prize mobility, independence, and solitary pursuits. They would rather make decisions by themselves and carry out solo activities than be involved in a group.

View of others: They see other people as intrusive and controlling.

Beliefs: Their *core* beliefs consist of notions such as "I am basically alone," "Close relationships with other people are unrewarding and messy," "I can do things better if I'm not encumbered by other people" "Close relationships are undesirable because they interfere with my freedom of action."

The *conditional* beliefs are "If I get too close to people, they will get their hooks into me," "I can't be happy unless I have complete mobility." The *instrumental* beliefs are "Don't get too close," "Keep your distance," "Don't get involved."

Strategy: Their main interpersonal strategy is to keep their distance from other people, insofar as this is feasible. They may get together with others for specific reasons, such as vocational activities or sex, but otherwise prefer to distance themselves. They are readily threatened by any actions that represent encroachment on their space.

Affect: As long as schizoids keep their distance, they may experience a low level of sadness. If they are forced into a close encounter, they may become very anxious. In contrast to histrionic personalities, they are not inclined to show their feelings either verbally or through facial expressions; consequently they convey the impression that they do not have strong feelings.

THINKING STYLES

The personality disorders may also be characterized by their cognitive styles, which may be a reflection of the patients' behavioral strategies. These cognitive styles deal with the *manner* in which people process information, as opposed to the specific *content* of the processing. Several of the personality types have such distinctive cognitive styles that it is worthwhile to describe them.

People with histrionic personality disorder use the strategy of "display" to attract people and satisfy their own desires for support and closeness. When the strategy of impressing or entertaining people is unsuccessful, they show an open display of "dramatics" (weeping, rage, etc.) to punish the offenders and coerce them to comply. The processing of information shows the same global, impressionist quality. These individuals "miss the trees for the forest." They make stereotyped, broad, global interpretations of a situation at the expense of crucial details. They are likely to respond to their gestalt of the situation, based on inadequate information. People with histrionic disorder are also prone to attach a pattern to a situation even though it does not fit. For example, if other people seem unresponsive to their entertaining, they judge the situation in its entirety—"They are rejecting me"—rather than seeing the specifics that might account for other people's behavior. Thus, they are oblivious to the fact that the other people may be fatigued, bored, or preoccupied with other things. This impressionistic quality is also evident in the way they put a gloss on every experience: Events are romanticized into high drama or grand tragedy. Finally, because they are more attuned to the subjective rather than the objective measuring of events, they tend to use their feelings as the ultimate guide as to their interpretation. Thus, if they feel bad in an encounter with another person, this means the other person is bad. If they feel euphoric, the other person is wonderful.

People with obsessive–compulsive personality, in marked contrast to histrionics, "miss the forest for the trees." These persons focus so much on details that they miss the overall pattern; for example, a person with this disorder may decide on the basis of a few flaws in another person's performance that the other person has failed, even though the flaws may have simply represented some variations in an overall successful performance. Further, in contrast to histrionics, people with obsessive–compulsive personality disorder tend to minimize subjective experiences. Thus, they deprive themselves of some of the richness of life and of access to feelings as a source of information that enhances the significance of important events.

The thinking style of people with avoidant personality disorder differs from that of the aforementioned individuals. Just as they tend to avoid situations that will make them feel bad, they also employ a mechanism of "internal avoidance." As soon as they start to have an unpleasant feeling, they try to damp it down by diverting their attention to something else or by taking a quick fix, such as having a drink. They also avoid thoughts that might produce unpleasant feelings.

The cognitive styles of the other personality disorders are not as sharply delineated as those of the disorders just described.

SUMMARY OF CHARACTERISTICS

Table 2.3 lists the characteristics of nine personality disorders. The first two columns list the view of the self and view of others, the next column gives the specific beliefs, and the last column lists the specific strategies. It can be seen from this table how the self-view, the view of others, and the beliefs lead into the specific strategy. Although the strategy, or behavior, provides the basis for making the diagnosis of personality disorder, it

TABLE 2.3. Cognitive Profiles of Personality Disorders

Personality disorder	View of self	View of others	Main beliefs	Main strategy
Avoidant	Vulnerable to depreciation, rejection Socially inept Incompetent	Critical Demeaning Superior	"It's terrible to be rejected, put down." "If people know the 'real' me, they will reject me." "I can't tolerate unpleasant feelings."	Avoid evaluative situations Avoid unpleasant feelings or thoughts
Dependent	Needy Weak Helpless Incompetent	(Idealized) Nurturant Supportive Competent	"I need people to survive, be happy." "I need to have a steady flow of support, encouragement."	Cultivate dependent relationships
Passive–aggressive	Self-sufficient Vulnerable to control, interference	Intrusive Demanding Interfering Controlling Dominating	"Others interfere with my freedom of action." "Control by others is intolerable." "I have to do things my own way."	Passive resistance Surface submissiveness Evade, circumvent rules
Obsessive–compulsive	Responsible Accountable Fastidious Competent	Irresponsible Casual Incompetent Self-indulgent	"I know what's best." "Details are crucial." "People *should* do better, try harder."	Apply rules Perfectionism Evaluate, control "Shoulds," criticize, punish
Paranoid	Righteous Innocent, noble Vulnerable	Interfering Malicious Discriminatory Abusive motives	"Others' motives are suspect." "I must always be on guard." "I cannot trust people."	Be wary Look for hidden motives Accuse Counterattack
Antisocial	A loner	Vulnerable	"I'm entitled to *break* rules."	Attack, rob

	View of Self	View of Others	Beliefs	Strategy
	Autonomous Strong	Exploitative	"Others are patsies, wimps." "I'm better than others."	Deceive, manipulate
Borderline	Vulnerable (to rejection, betrayal, domination) Deprived (of needed emotional support) Powerless Out of control Defective Unlovable Bad	(Idealized) Powerful, loving, perfect (Devalued) Rejecting, controlling, betraying, abandoning	"I can't cope on my own." "I need someone to rely on." "I cannot bear unpleasant feelings." "If I rely on someone I'll be mistreated, found wanting, and abandoned." "The worst possible thing would be to be abandoned." "It's impossible for me to control myself." "I deserve to be punished."	Subjugate own needs to maintain connection Protest dramatically, threaten, and/or become punitive toward those that signal possible rejection Relieve tension through self-mutilation and self-destructive behavior Attempt suicide as an escape
Narcissistic	Special, unique Deserve special rules; superior Above the rules	Inferior Admirers	"Since I'm special, I *deserve* special rules." "I'm above the rules." "I'm better than others."	Use others Transcend rules Manipulate Compete
Histrionic	Glamorous Impressive	Seducible Receptive Admirers	"People are there to serve or admire me." "People have no right to deny me my just deserts." "I can go by my feeling."	Use dramatics, charm; temper tantrums, crying; suicide gestures
Schizoid	Self-sufficient Loner	Intrusive	"Others are unrewarding." "Relationships are messy, undesirable."	Stay away
Schizotypal	Unreal, detached, loner Vulnerable, socially conspicuous Supernaturally sensitive and gifted	Untrustworthy Malevolent	(Idiographic, odd, superstitious, magical thinking; for instance, beliefs in clairvoyance, telepathy, or "sixth sense" are central in the belief structure.) "It's better to be isolated from others."	Watch for and neutralize mal-evolent attention from others Stay to self Be vigilant for supernatural forces or events

is important for a full understanding of the nature of the disorder to clarify the self-concept, concept of others, and beliefs. These cognitive components are involved in information processing and, when activated, trigger the relevant strategy.

An avoidant person, Jill, for example, *viewed herself* as socially inept and was vulnerable, therefore, to depreciation and rejection. Her view *of others* as critical and demeaning complemented this sense of vulnerability. Her *belief* that rejection was terrible added enormous valence to her sensitivity and tended to blow up the significance of any anticipated rejection or actual rejection. In fact, this particular belief tended to screen out positive feedback. Her anticipation of rejection made her feel chronically anxious around people, and her magnification of any signs of nonacceptance made her feel bad.

Two other beliefs contributed to her hanging back from involvements: namely, that (1) if she got close to people, they would recognize her as inferior and inadequate; and (2) she could not tolerate unpleasant feelings, which led her to try to avoid their arousal. Hence, as a result of the pressure of her various beliefs and attitudes, she was propelled toward the only strategy that would accommodate her serious concerns— namely, to avoid any situations in which she could be evaluated. In addition, because of her low tolerance for unpleasant feelings or thoughts, she chronically turned off any thoughts that could evoke unpleasant feelings. In therapy she had difficulty in making decisions, identifying negative automatic thoughts, or examining her basic beliefs, because these would lead to such feelings.

Figure 2.1 illustrates the basic flow. A similar flow chart can be constructed for each of the other personality disorders. The chart should incorporate the distinctive beliefs and the resultant behavior patterns. The person with dependent personality disorder, for example, differs from one with avoidant personality in that the former tends to idolize other potentially nurturant persons and believes that they will help and support him or her. Thus, he or she is drawn to people. Passive–aggressive individuals want approval but cannot tolerate any semblance of control, so they tend to thwart others' expectations of them, and thus defeat themselves. Obsessive–compulsive persons idealize order and systems and are driven to control others (as well as themselves). The paranoid individual is extremely vigilant of other people because of a basic mistrust and suspiciousness and is inclined to accuse them (either overtly or mentally) of discrimination. The antisocial personality asserts that he or she is entitled to manipulate or abuse others, because of a belief that he or she has been wronged, or that others are wimps, or that we live in a "dog-eat-dog" society. Narcissists see themselves as above ordinary mortals and seek glory through any

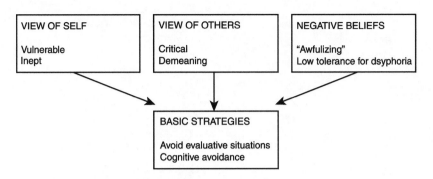

FIGURE 2.1. Relationship of views and beliefs to basic strategies.

methods that can safely be used. Histrionic individuals try to draw others to them by being entertaining but also through temper tantrums and dramatics to coerce closeness when their charm is ineffective. The schizoid person, with the belief that relationships are unrewarding, keeps his or her distance from other people.

The understanding of the typical beliefs and strategies of each personality disorder provides a road map for therapists. They should keep in mind, however, that most individuals with a specific personality disorder will manifest attitudes and behaviors that overlap other disorders. Consequently, it is important for therapists to expose these variations in order to make a complete evaluation.

CHAPTER 3

Assessment of Personality Disorders

Personality disorders represent a challenging but important target for clinical assessment and intervention. Along with the significant impairment and distress associated with these disorders, theoretical formulations and empirical findings suggest that personality disorders, maladaptive traits, or associated cognitive schemas increase the risk of Axis I disorders and influence the development, maintenance, and expression of Axis I symptoms (cf. Beck, Freeman, & Associates 1990; Gunderson, Triebwasser, Phillips, & Sullivan, 1999). Thus, assessing for presence and type of personality pathology may yield important information regarding the etiology of comorbid conditions and inform treatment decisions relevant to both Axis II and Axis I. Furthermore, when treatment progress is slow or stalled, it may indicate the presence of an undiagnosed personality disorder or inadequate assessment and conceptualization of personality pathology.

This chapter begins with a review of the conceptual and methodological issues associated with assessment of personality pathology, followed by a review of commonly used assessment procedures and instruments. Special attention is given to self-report questionnaires that have been developed since the first edition of this book for assessing the cognitive basis of personality disorders.

CONCEPTUAL AND METHODOLOGICAL ISSUES

Assessment of personality disorders requires a working knowledge of both the general definition of a personality disorder and disorder-specific criteria. Because the specific criteria for the various Axis II disorders are covered elsewhere in this book we do not address them here. The general criteria for a personality disorder diagnosis are worth emphasizing, however, particularly because they can get overlooked or be underappreciated if clinicians become mainly focused on the content of a patient's personality structure.

As defined by the fourth edition of the *Diagnostic and Statistical Manual of the Mental Disorders* (DSM-IV; American Psychiatric Association, 1994), a personality disorder is "an enduring pattern of inner experience and behavior that deviates markedly from the expectations of the individual's culture, is pervasive and inflexible, has an onset in adolescence or early adulthood, is stable over time, and leads to distress or impairment" (p. 633). The pattern is manifested in two (or more) of the following areas: (1) cognition (i.e., ways of perceiving and interpreting self, other people, and events), (2) affectivity (i.e., the range, intensity, lability, and appropriateness of emotional response), (3) interpersonal functioning, and (4) impulse control.

Given this definition, clinicians should keep two critical questions in mind when determining whether a personality disorder diagnosis is warranted:

1. Do the relevant inner experiences and behaviors represent inflexible, pervasive, and long-standing patterns and not just transient or episodic effects related to a patient's current psychiatric state?
2. Do these long-standing patterns create significant distress or significantly impair functioning across multiple domains (e.g., social and occupational)?

Such judgments are ultimately left to the clinician as no distinct cutting points have been proposed or identified empirically to establish the boundaries between pathological and normal personality, between personality disorders and Axis I disorders, or between the various personality disorders themselves (Zimmerman, 1994).

Categorical versus Dimensional Approaches

Although DSM-IV represents a categorical approach in which personality disorders represent qualitatively distinct clinical syndromes, it also acknowledges the potential value of dimensional approaches for conceptualizing and measuring personality disorders. One such approach is simply to quantify the degree to which the criteria for each personality disorder are present and then present this information in the form of a profile. An alternative dimensional approach is to quantify traits that are relevant to personality disorders and lie along a continuum from normal to pathological. This trait-dimensional approach is consistent with the increasingly advocated view that personality disorders have "fuzzy" and rather arbitrary boundaries between each other and with normal personality (Pfohl, 1999).

The strategies one uses for assessing personality pathology will depend in part on the choice of categorical versus dimensional approaches. For pragmatic reasons, such as entering an Axis II diagnosis in a clinical report, clinicians often find the categorical approach preferable. The categorical approach also has the advantages of clarity and ease in communication and familiarity among clinicians (Widiger, 1992). However, several drawbacks to the categorical approach have been noted, including (1) a high degree of comorbidity and mixed diagnoses observed among personality disorders, (2) the lack of clear thresholds for distinguishing between patients with and without specific personality disorders, (3) the temporal instability of personality disorder diagnoses, and (4) a notable lack of agreement on the appropriate conceptualization of the various personality disorders (L. Clark, 1999). Another commonly observed problem with the categorical approach used in DSM is the polythetic derivation of diagnoses. Diagnoses are made based on the presence of a minimum number of criteria drawn from a larger list of prototypical criteria. Thus, different individuals can be given the same Axis II diagnosis while having different profiles of criteria for that disorder. Categorical (present/absent) assessments also provide less clinical information than dimensional assessments, which can yield idiographic patient profiles.

Psychometrically, dimensional judgments of personality have consistently shown better reliability than categorical judgments (Heumann & Morey, 1990; Pilkonis, Heape, Ruddy, & Serrao, 1991; Trull, Widiger, & Guthrie, 1990). In practice, there is no reason why categorical and dimensional approaches cannot be integrated. For instance, dimensional assessment can provide detailed information as to a patient's profile of personality functioning, and this same information can be useful in making a categorical diagnosis on Axis II.

Distinguishing Axis I from Axis II Disorders

Coexistence of Axis I and Axis II disorders is commonplace. For instance, van Velzen and Emmelkamp (1996) reviewed the literature on depressive, anxiety, and eating disorders and found that roughly half the patients with these diagnoses also had a comorbid personality disorder.

The problem of coexisting disorders is particularly germane to the assessment of personality disorders. Clinicians may mistakenly assume that impairment or distress related to an Axis I disorder is evidence of an Axis II criterion. For instance, a perception of oneself as socially inept may be a manifestation of avoidant personality disorder, depression, or social phobia, to name just a few possibilities. Because depression is known to lead to negative biases both in current self-perception and in retrospective reporting (Clark & Beck, with Alford, 1999), it takes careful questioning and clinical sophistication to distinguish the diagnostic significance of this symptom. This problem may be most likely to occur when trying to differentiate symptoms of depression and anxiety from symptoms of personality disorders in the "anxious–fearful" cluster (Cluster C: avoidant, dependent, and obsessive–compulsive personality disorders; see Peselow, Sanfilipo, & Fieve, 1994). Similar complexities arise from the overlap of criteria among different personality disorders. For instance, paranoid ideation is a defining criterion for paranoid personality disorder, but it is also seen under stressful circumstances in borderline personality disorder (criterion 9).

Higher- versus Lower-Order Personality Dimensions

There is robust evidence of three to five higher-order dimensions of personality (e.g., neuroticism, extraversion, introversion, agreeableness, conscientiousness or openness to experience; Costa & McRae, 1992). However, these constructs are so broad and high in the hierarchy of personality traits that they may lack utility for many clinical purposes. Moreover, they were not derived with the purpose of explaining personality pathology, and attempts to map them onto the various personality disorders have been lacking in theoretical basis (Millon & Davis, 1996).

There have been numerous efforts to identify lower-order personality dimensions that are relevant to assessment of personality disorders. When researchers have used factor-analytic techniques to identify lower-order personality dimensions, they have typically found between 15 and 22 dimensions that are relevant to personality disorders. In many cases, these dimensions show replicability similar to that found with the higher-order dimensions. For instance, L. Clark (1999) found considerable convergent validity between three self-report questionnaires of lower-order personality traits: the Schedule for Nonadaptive and Adaptive Personality (SNAP; L. Clark, 1993), the Dimensional Assessment of Personality Pathology—Basic Questionnaire (DAPP-BQ; Livesley, 1990), and the Multiple Personality Questionnaire (MPQ; Tellegen, 1993). Personality disorder beliefs and schemas represent lower-order dimensions that are particularly useful in the cognitive therapy of personality disorders.

ASSESSMENT STRATEGIES

Self-Report Questionnaires

Self-report questionnaires represent the most practical strategy for efficiently gathering information relevant to personality disorders. Numerous questionnaires of personality pathology have been developed over the past two decades and most of these have been extensively reviewed elsewhere (Millon & Davis, 1996; J. Reich, 1987; Widiger & Frances, 1987). Some of these instruments were designed to assess personality disorders as defined on Axis II of DSM; two of the more commonly used ones being the Millon Clinical Multiaxial Inventory (MCMI-III; Millon, Millon, & Davis, 1994) and the Personality Diagnostic Questionnaire— Revised (PDQ-R; Hyler & Rieder, 1987). Others were developed to assess traits relevant to personality disorders. Prominent examples of such instruments include the DAPP-BQ (Livesley, 1990), the SNAP (L. Clark, 1993), and the Wisconsin Personality Disorders Inventory (WISPI; Klein et al., 1993). Still others were constructed specifically to assess cognitive dimensions relevant to personality disorders: the Personality Belief Questionnaire (PBQ; Beck & Beck, 1991) and the Schema Questionnaire (SQ; Young & Brown, 1994). These questionnaires are reviewed in detail later in this chapter.

When compared to other strategies (e.g., structured clinical interviews), self-report questionnaires require less training and demand less time from the clinician to administer. They also yield scores that can be compared with group norms and used in preparing profiles. Moreover, the commonly used questionnaires identified previously have generally been found to have good face validity, adequate-to-good internal consistency and test–retest reliability, and fair construct validity. Establishing criterion validity has been problematic as there is no "gold standard" for assessing personality disorders. However, this problem is equally true for all assessment strategies.

The issue of criterion validity is important and deserves some additional discussion. Recognizing that a gold standard was probably not realistic in the area of personality disorder assessment, Spitzer (1983) suggested a LEAD standard (referring to Longitudinal, Expert, All Data). The LEAD procedure formalizes the integration of expert clinical judgment, increased attention to reliability, the use of multiple sources of information (including previous treatment records, feedback from treating clinicians, and interviews with significant others), and monitoring of the patient's condition and diagnosis over time. Although others have noted practical problems with implementing the method (Loranger, 1991), use of the LEAD standard in research has produced some informative findings. Pilkonis et al. (1991) found that diagnoses arrived at through the LEAD procedure were less influenced by the symptomatic status of the patient than were diagnoses that depended solely on a structured clinical interview at intake. Currently, comparisons of self-report questionnaires against the LEAD standard are lacking. However, it is unlikely that they would fare better than structured interviews. Based on current findings, practicing clinicians are cautioned against sole reliance (or even primary reliance) on self-report questionnaires for diagnosis on Axis II.

Structured Clinical Interviews

Several structured clinical interviews have been developed for assessing personality disorders and related personality dimensions. As with self-report questionnaires, these have been reviewed in detail elsewhere (e.g., Millon & Davis, 1996; J. Reich, 1987; Widiger & Frances, 1987) and are summarized here. In particular, van Velzen and Emmelkamp (1996) provide a concise review of the most widely used and investigated structured interviews. These include the Structured Clinical Interview for DSM-IV (SCID-II; First, Spitzer, Gibbon, & Williams, 1995), the Personality Disorder Examination—Revised (PDE-R; Loranger, Susman, Oldham, & Russakoff, 1987), and the Structured Interview for DSM-IV Personality Disorders (SIDP-R; Pfohl, Blum, Zimmerman, & Stangl, 1989). All three interviews have shown generally adequate and in some cases excellent reliability when administered by adequately trained clinicians. The importance of clinician training and competence cannot be understated.

In terms of the end products of structured interviews, estimates of reliability have universally been higher for dimensional scores than for categorical diagnoses (L. Clark, 1999; Pilkonis et al., 1995). The PDE-R is particularly useful for deriving dimensional scores for each Axis II disorder, but it also requires the most time to administer. Although the SCID-II does not provide for dimensional scoring, it has the advantage of relatively shorter administration time (a mean of 36 minutes compared to 60–90 minutes for the SIDP-R and 2 hours and 20 minutes for the PDE-R; van Velzen & Emmelkamp, 1996). The SCID-II has been studied somewhat more than the other interviews. A recent study found interrater reliability coefficients on the SCID-II ranging from .48 to .98 for categorical diagnosis, and from .90 to .98 for dimensional judgments (Maffei et al., 1997). The impact of clinical experience and training on SCID-II diagnoses was recently investigated by Ventura, Liberman, Green, Shaner, and Mintz (1998). They found that clinically experienced interviewers tended to have better interrater reliability and overall diagnostic accuracy than neophyte interviewers, but both were able to achieve high interrater reliability and diagnostic accuracy after appropriate training.

Use of Informants

Both self-report questionnaires and structured clinical interview depend on patients being capable of and willing to report accurately on their own inner experiences and long-standing patterns of behavior. However, clinical experience, cognitive theory, and empirical findings all point to several possible forms of bias in self-reports. Part of this bias comes from the effect of psychiatric state on self-reports. For instance, depression has been shown to be associated with negatively biased perceptions of the self, one's personal world, and the future (Clark et al., 1999). Such distortions are likely to inflate self-reports of Axis II symptoms associated with these domains (e.g., avoidant and dependent; Loranger et al., 1991; Peselow et al., 1994). Patients with other personality features (e.g., obsessive–compulsive) may underreport dysfunctional behaviors due to social desirability concerns, or because they perceive disclosure is not in their best interest. The possibility of dissimulation must always be considered when obtaining self-report data from patients with antisocial tendencies and in forensic settings. Finally, it has been commonly noted that patients with or without significant personality pathology may exaggerate their distress or impairment because they are frantically seeking help or are dissatisfied with the attention or treatment they are receiving (Loranger, 1999).

Clinicians often have the opportunity to supplement a patient's self-report with information gathered from informants who know the patient well, such as family members, friends, or coworkers. Although informants do not have as much access to a patient's inner experience as the patient him- or herself, and their perceptions may be biased to some degree, they can often provide insight into behavioral patterns that the patient is not aware of or willing to report (Zimmerman, Pfohl, Stangl, & Corenthal, 1986).

Given the differences between patients' and informants' perspectives, and the aforementioned sources of bias in patients' self-reports, it is not surprising that some research has found only modest correlations between the two sources of personality information (Zimmerman, Pfohl, Coryell, Stangl, & Corenthal, 1988; however, see Peselow et al., 1994, who found strong correlations). Several studies have found that informants' reports of dysfunctional personality traits are greater than corresponding reports made by patients (Peselow et al., 1994; Zimmerman et al., 1986, 1988). When there are discrepancies between self-report and informant reports, clinicians may turn to other sources of data (clinical observation, treatment records, reports by previous providers) and use their own clinical judgment to reconcile these differences.

Nonstructured Clinical Interviews

In practice, many clinicians use a nonstructured interview to assess for personality pathology. It is important to note that research comparing structured and unstructured interviews has found poor agreement between diagnoses arrived at through the two processes (Steiner, Tebes, Sledge, & Walker, 1995). The clinical experience and sophistication of the interviewer is especially critical for accurate assessment without a structured interview.

Whether using a structured or unstructured clinical interview, it is essential to ascertain not only the current salience of personality disorder traits/criteria but also the pervasiveness, persistence, and level of impairment related to these features. The protocol for the SCID-II interview, for instance, requires that the interviewer ask for multiple examples of situations in which a criterion is evident. It is also important to ask questions that assess the presence of the personality feature in the absence of Axis I pathology (e.g., a current episode of major depression).

Some aspects of every assessment interview are atheoretical (e.g., identification of presenting problems and general psychosocial history), but other aspects are influenced by the theoretical orientation of the interviewer. For example, in schema-focused therapy the initial assessment includes a focused life history interview in which the clinician looks for periods of past schema activation and establishes thematic links between these experiences and presenting problems (Young, 1994). Standard cognitive therapy interviewing techniques can also be used when assessing personality disorder criteria or dimensions. Techniques for identifying patient's key beliefs and assumptions can be found in various cognitive therapy manuals (e.g., Beck, Rush, Shaw, & Emery, 1979; J. Beck, 1995). For instance, the clinician can ask about the patient's automatic thoughts related to current problem situations, identify the underlying meanings attached to these thoughts, and explore the developmental antecedents to cognitive themes that the patient reports as longstanding.

COGNITIVE MEASURES OF PERSONALITY PATHOLOGY

Cognitive theory of personality disorders emphasizes the importance of schemas and core beliefs as organizational structures and global mental representations that guide information processing and behavior. Hence, assessment of schemas and related beliefs and assumptions warrants particular attention in cognitive therapy. Indeed, it is crucial that multiple sources of data be considered when assessing patients' dysfunctional beliefs and that this process be ongoing throughout therapy. Patients' developmental histories, current problems and symptoms, and interview behaviors all provide clues to their dysfunctional beliefs. The therapeutic relationship itself provides an important context for assessing some personality disorder beliefs. In addition, two relevant self-report questionnaires have been developed and tested: the PBQ (Beck & Beck, 1991) and the SQ (Young & Brown, 1994). Each of these is reviewed in turn.

The Personality Belief Questionnaire

The PBQ is a natural outgrowth of the cognitive theory of personality disorders. Based on cognitive theory and clinical observations, Beck et al. (1990) proposed the prototypical schema content of most of the Axis II disorders. The appendix of Beck et al. (1990) listed the specific beliefs and assumptions thought to be associated with each disorder. This schema content was subsequently incorporated into the PBQ. The PBQ contains nine scales that can be administered separately or together and that correspond to nine of the personality disorders on Axis II of the DSM-III-R. The nine PBQ scales contain 14 items each for a total of 126 items. The scale contains the following instructions: "Please read the statements below and rate how much you believe each one. Try to judge how you feel about each statement most of the time." Response options range from 0 "I don't believe it at all" to 4 "I believe it totally." Since the mid-1990s the PBQ has been administered routinely in two outpatient cognitive therapy settings, the Center for Cognitive Therapy at the University of Pennsylvania, and the Beck Institute for Cognitive Therapy and Research in Greater Philadelphia. Table 3.1 shows the PBQ beliefs most frequently endorsed for each of six personality disorders.

An early version of the PBQ showed evidence of good internal consistency for the various subscales among college students (Trull, Goodwin, Schopp, Hillenbrand, & Schuster, 1993). Research on psychiatric outpatients has shown similarly good internal consistency reliability, with Cronbach's alpha coefficients ranging from .81 for Antisocial to .93 for Paranoid (Beck et al., 2001). Test–retest correlations for a subset of 15 patients over a period of 8 weeks ranged from .57 for the Avoidant scale to .93 for the Antisocial scale (Beck et al., 2001). Trull et al. (1993) found rather high intercorrelations between the subscales (median $r = .40$) and modest correlations between the PBQ and both the Personality Disorder Questionnaire—Revised (Hyler & Rieder, 1987) and the Minnesota Multiphasic Personality Inventory—Personality Disorder (MMPI-PD; Morey, Waugh, & Blashfield, 1985). Beck et al. (2001) also found unexpectedly high intercorrelations among many of

TABLE 3.1. PBQ Beliefs Most Strongly Associated with Specific Personality Disorders

Avoidant personality disorder

- "I am socially inept and socially undesirable in work or social situations."
- "If people get close to me, they will discover the 'real' me and reject me."
- "I should avoid situations in which I attract attention, or be as inconspicuous as possible."
- "Being exposed as inferior or inadequate will be intolerable."
- "Other people are potentially critical, indifferent, demeaning, or rejecting.

Dependent personality disorder

- "If I am not loved, I will always be unhappy."
- "The worst possible thing would be to be abandoned."
- "I am helpless when I'm left on my own."
- "I must maintain access to my supporter or helper at all times."
- "I am basically alone—unless I can attach myself to a stronger person.

Obsessive–compulsive personality disorder

- "Details are extremely important."
- "It is important to do a perfect job on everything."
- "People should do things my way."
- "I need order, systems, and rules in order to get the job done properly."
- "If I don't have systems, everything will fall apart.

Narcissistic personality disorder

- "I don't have to be bound by the rules that apply to other people."
- "I have every reason to expect grand things."
- "Because I am so superior, I am entitled to special treatment and privileges."
- "Other people don't deserve the admiration or riches they get."
- "Because I am so talented, people should go out of their way to promote my career."

Paranoid personality disorder

- "People will take advantage of me if I give them the chance."
- "Others will try to use me or manipulate me if I don't watch out."
- "I have to be on guard at all times."
- "If people act friendly, they may be trying to use or exploit me."
- "Other people will deliberately try to demean me."

Borderline personality disorder

- "Unpleasant feelings will escalate and get out of control."
- "I can't cope as other people can."
- "People often say one thing and mean something else."
- "If people get close to me, they will discover the 'real' me and reject me."
- "A person to whom I am close could be disloyal or unfaithful."
- "I am needy and weak."
- "I cannot trust other people."
- "I have to be on guard at all times."
- "I need somebody around available at all times to help me to carry out what I need to do or in case something bad happens."
- "People will take advantage of me if I give them the chance."
- "Any signs of tension in a relationship indicate the relationship has gone bad; therefore, I should cut it off."
- "I am helpless when left on my own."
- "People will pay attention only if I act in extreme ways."
- "People will get at me if I don't get them first."

Note. With the exception of borderline personality disorder (BPD), the five PBQ beliefs that most strongly discriminated the criterion personality disorder from other personality disorders are listed. All 14 beliefs that were found by Butler et al. (2002) to discriminate BPD from other personality disorders are listed.

the PBQ scales. There are several possibilities for these findings. Some of the belief sets may not be as conceptually distinct as proposed by cognitive theory. Alternatively, some shared variance between the belief sets may be due to a general distress factor. Also, these findings may reflect some degree of overlap in the Axis II diagnoses themselves (Beck et al., 1990).

The criterion validity of five PBQ scales was recently investigated by Beck et al. (2001). This study examined the validity of the PBQ Avoidant, Dependent, Obsessive–Compulsive, Narcissistic, and Paranoid scales among psychiatric outpatients with corresponding SCID-II-derived diagnoses. A set of between-subject analyses was conducted to test whether patients with a given Axis II diagnosis would score higher on the corresponding PBQ scale than patients with alternative Axis II diagnoses. Twenty of 25 (80%) of the study predictions were confirmed, and an additional three tests (12%) approached significance. A set of within-subject analyses was then conducted to test the hypothesis that patients with a given Axis II diagnosis would score higher on the corresponding PBQ scale than on other PBQ scales. Results were again highly supportive of the discriminative validity of these PBQ scales, with 19 of 20 (95%) of predictions being confirmed. The within-subject findings are particularly informative regarding the potential of the PBQ to provide meaningful patient profiles of Axis II beliefs. Figure 3.1 graphically displays the results. As can be seen, in each case, patients with a given personality disorder score the highest on the PBQ scale theoretically associated with that diagnosis.

The belief sets listed in the appendix of Beck et al. (1990) did not include a belief set for borderline personality disorder (BPD). At that time it was thought that these patients endorsed numerous beliefs associated with many different personality disorders. Hence, an empirical investigation was conducted and 14 PBQ beliefs were identified that discriminated between patients with BPD and patients with other personality disorders (Butler, Brown, Beck, & Grisham, 2002; all 14 BPD beliefs are listed in Table 3.1). These findings were cross-validated in two independent samples with 42 BPD patients in each. The empirically keyed BDP beliefs were subsequently incorporated into a borderline belief scale. Figure 3.1 graphically displays the mean scores for various personality disorders on this scale.

Evidence of the predictive validity of the PBQ was obtained by Kuyken, Kurzer, DeRubeis, Beck, and Brown (2001). These researchers found that the PBQ Avoidant and Paranoid scales predicted outcome in cognitive therapy of depressed patients, with higher scores on these scales being associated with poorer outcome. More recently, the PBQ has been split into two parallel forms of 63 items each. Preliminary results indicate generally good internal consistency and adequate test–retest reliability for subscales of both parallel versions (Butler & Beck, 2002).

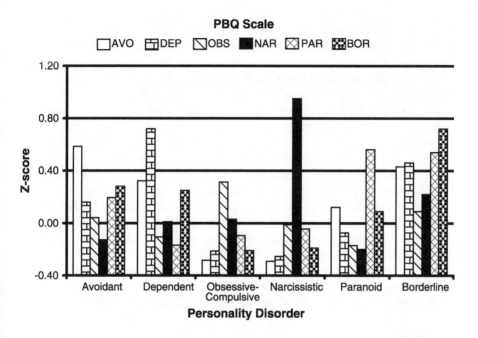

FIGURE 3.1. Mean PBQ scale scores for six personality disorders. PBQ, Personality Belief Questionnaire; AVO, avoidant; DEP, dependent; OBS, obsessive–compulsive; NAR, narcissistic; PAR, paranoid; BOR, borderline.

The PBQ can be used clinically in two ways: to provide a cognitive profile and to identify specific dysfunctional beliefs that can be addressed in treatment. Standardized PBQ scores can be plotted to produce idiographic patient profiles of personality disorder beliefs. Figure 3.2 shows the PBQ profiles for two patients, each of whom has diagnoses of avoidant personality disorder on Axis II and major depressive disorder on Axis I. Patient A is a 32-year-old divorced man who lives alone and works as a computer technician. He spends much of his free time reading and watching TV. When not depressed he spends some of this time working on personal projects at home. He became depressed after moving across country to take a new job in large city. He had gradually made a couple of friends at his former job. However, he has not kept in touch with these people and has made no effort to make new friends since relocating. He was divorced 5 years ago and has not dated since that time. Patient B is a 23-year-old engaged woman who lives with her parents and works in a flower shop. She has no close friendships. Her depressive episode was precipitated by an on-again-off-again relationship with her fiancé, and conflicts with her mother, whom she describes as controlling, and her older brother, who also lives at home and has a long history of unemployment, alcohol abuse, and domineering behavior. The family as a whole is overinvolved and isolated.

An examination of the two PBQ profiles in Figure 3.2 shows similar elevations on the avoidant scale but important differences on several other scales. Patient A shows relatively strong endorsements of beliefs associated with obsessive–compulsive and schizoid personality disorders whereas patient B endorses beliefs characteristic of dependent, borderline, and paranoid personality disorders. Thus, although both patients are timid and chronically reclusive and see themselves as socially inept and others as potentially critical and rejecting, patient B depends on a small group (her family and fiancé) for support and tends to be distrustful and significantly distressed when this support is absent, whereas patient A tends to disavow needs for attachment, emphasizes details, orderliness and rules, and has adopted a solitary lifestyle.

Figure 3.2 shows the value of using a dimensional (profile) approach rather than just a categorical approach to assessment of personality pathology. Much more clinical information is revealed about each

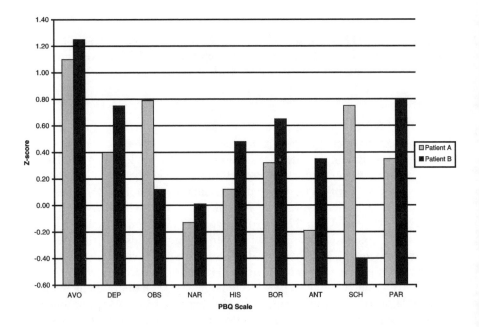

FIGURE 3.2. PBQ profiles of two patients with avoidant personality disorder. PBQ, Personality Belief Questionnaire; AVO, avoidant; DEP, dependent; OBS, obsessive–compulsive; NAR, narcissistic; HIS, histrionic; BOR, borderline; ANT, antisocial; SCH, schizoid; PAR, paranoid.

patient. Moreover, this information is highly relevant for case conceptualization and clinical decision making. In the examples of patients A and B, the cognitive aspects of the two personality structures suggest that different approaches may be needed to treat both the avoidant personality disorder and the coexisting depression.

The Schema Questionnaire

In contrast to the PBQ, which is designed to map directly on to Axis II disorders, the SQ is an example of a personality construct–dimension approach that is conceptually independent of the Axis II nosology. Rather, the SQ (sometimes referred to as the Young Schema Questionnaire (YSQ; Young & Brown, 1994) was designed to measure early maladaptive schemas (EMSs) that cut cross DSM categories. EMSs are defined by Young (1994) as "extremely broad, pervasive themes regarding oneself and one's relationships with others, developed during childhood and elaborated throughout one's lifetime, and dysfunctional to a significant degree" (Young, 1994, p. 9). EMSs are described as deeply entrenched patterns that are central to one's sense of self. Young (1994) identified 16 schemas organized under five headings:

> *Disconnection and rejection* (abandonment/instability, mistrust/abuse, emotional deprivation, defectiveness/shame, and social isolation/alienation)
> *Impaired autonomy and performance* (dependence/incompetence, vulnerability to "random" events, enmeshment/underdeveloped self, and failure)
> *Impaired limits* (entitlement/domination, and insufficient self-control/self-discipline)
> *Other-directedness* (subjugation, self-sacrifice, and approval-seeking)
> *Overvigilance and inhibition* (vulnerability to "controllable" events/negativity, overcontrol, unrelenting standards, and punitiveness)

The SQ is a 205-item self-report questionnaire developed to measure these 16 schemas. More recently, Young (2002a) has increased the number of clinically observed EMSs to 18.

Schmidt, Joiner, Young, and Telch (1995) assessed the psychometric properties of the SQ. They found support for 13 schemas in a factor analysis using a college student sample. Among psychiatric inpatients, evidence of factorial validity was found for 15 of the schemas proposed by Young. Three higher-order factors were also found which capture some elements of the superordinate themes proposed by Young: Disconnection, Overconnection, and Exaggerated Standards. A subsequent factor analysis of the SQ in a larger clinical sample largely replicated these findings (Lee, Taylor, & Dunn, 1999), finding the same proposed 15 factors plus a 16th factor related to a fear of losing control.

Recently, a shortened version of the SQ has been developed and tested. The Schema Questionnaire—Short Form (SQ-SF) contains 75 items selected from the SQ to tap the early maladaptive schemas that had been found in factorial studies of the original measure. For each of the 15 factors that had been replicated, the 5 SQ items with the highest loadings were selected for inclusion in the SQ-SF. A subsequent factor analysis of the SQ-SF with a sample of psychiatric patients in day treatment found 15 factors closely resembling the 15 schemas proposed by Young (Wellburn, Coristine, Dagg, Pontefract, & Jordan, 2002). The internal consistency of the corresponding subscales was moderate to good (Cronbach's alpha coefficients ranged from .76 to .93). Most of the scales showed significant positive correlations with measures of current psychiatric distress. In multiple regression analyses, five subscales accounted for unique variance in anxiety: abandonment, vulnerability to harm, failure, self-sacrifice, and emotional inhibition. Such findings linking schemas with current psychiatric state are consistent with schema theory (Young, 1994). Of course, being correlational and cross-sectional, they do not establish a direction of causality. As with all self-report measures of personality, scores on the SQ-SF are likely to be influenced by both trait and state effects. However, a recent study suggests that a significant portion of the variance in SQ-SF scores may be related to relatively stable (trait-like) schemas (Wellburn, Dagg, Coristine, & Pontefract, 2000). In this study, the SQ-SF and the Brief Symptom Inventory (BSI) were administered to 84 psychiatric patients before and after completion of a 12-week intensive group therapy in a day treatment program. These patients showed significant improvements on psychiatric symptoms by the end of treatment. Their scores on 12 of the 15 SQ-SF scales did not change over the same interval. These findings suggest that the associated schema are relatively enduring trait-like constructs and are not simply epiphenomena related to current distress.

Young and Brown (1994) have provided a scaling format for producing patient SQ profiles. Schema theory also emphasizes the role of coping styles and schema modes (Young, 2002a). According to schema theory, people cope with their schemas in different ways at different times. Young and colleagues have proposed three maladaptive coping styles that are found in mild form among nonclinical populations and in extreme and rigid forms in clinical populations: overcompensation, surrender, and avoidance. Schema modes are defined as moment-to-moment emotional states and coping responses that are currently active for an individual. Activation of a dysfunctional mode leads to strong emotions or rigid coping styles that then take over and control an individual's functioning. Modes are categorized under headings as follows:

child modes (vulnerable child, angry child, impulsive/undisciplined child, and happy child), *maladaptive coping modes* (compliant surrenderer, detached protector, and overcompensator), *maladaptive parent modes* (punitive parent, demanding parent), and *healthy adult mode*. Self-report questionnaires designed to assess the coping styles and modes proposed by schema theory have been developed and are available online (Young, 2002b), but there is currently no published psychometric data on them.

It is noteworthy that Young proposes that individuals may shift from one schema mode into another and that, as such shifts occur, different schemas or coping responses that were previously dormant may become active. To the degree this is true it would suggest that scores on the SQ or SQ-SF might be relatively unstable. However, as mentioned earlier, research has shown many of the SQ-SF scales have proven to be stable in a clinical population even when measures of immediate psychiatric state have shown significant improvement over the same period (Wellburn et al., 2000).

CONCLUSION

Treatment planning starts with accurate assessment and case conceptualization. When assessing personality pathology there are some key points to keep in mind. First, thorough familiarity with both the general and specific criteria for personality disorders is a prerequisite. Second, clinicians should be careful to assess the pervasiveness, persistence, and degree of impairment associated with specific criteria, traits, or cognitive correlates of personality pathology (e.g., dysfunctional beliefs and schemas). Differentiating episodic or transient psychiatric states from enduring personality traits is especially important given the relatively high rates of comorbidity between Axis I and Axis II disorders. Third, due to the more inferential nature of Axis II diagnosis as compared with Axis I diagnosis, the inexperienced clinician should be especially sensitive to the possibility of overpathologizing.

One's choice of assessment strategies depends on several factors. Dimensional approaches to conceptualizing and measuring personality pathology have gained increasing favor over the past decade due to the amount of clinical information they provide and to conceptual and empirical problems with the categorical approach. One common dimensional approach is to quantify the degree to which different Axis II disorders are present (or absent). Measurement methods for this approach include summing the number of criteria met for a disorder as assessed by a structured interview (e.g., the PDE-R; Loranger et al., 1987), using a self-report inventory with items worded to assess specific DSM criteria directly (e.g., the PDQ-R; Hyler & Rieder, 1987) or items that assess disorder-specific pathology across multiple domains (e.g., the MCMI-III; Millon et al., 1994), or using a self-report inventory that targets a single key domain such as dysfunctional beliefs (e.g., the PBQ; Beck & Beck, 1991).

An alternative dimensional approach involves assessment of personality traits or trait-like constructs (e.g., early maladaptive schemas) that are relevant to personality disorders. Self-report questionnaires are the principle measurement method for this type of dimensional model. Psychometrically sound questionnaires that assess comprehensive arrays of relevant personality traits include the SNAP (L. Clark, 1993), DAPP-BQ (Livesley, 1990), and WIPSI (Klein et al., 1993). For clinicians using a schema-focused approach, the SQ and SQ-SF both do a good job of assessing early maladaptive schemas. Therapists who want to assess more of the nuances of each schema will generally prefer the SQ (Young, 2002b).

There are some advantages to a categorical approach to assessment including conceptual clarity, ease in communication, and familiarity to clinicians. In addition, many clinical settings require a diagnostic impression be documented on Axis II for an assessment report, and research on personality disorders depends on reliable and valid diagnoses. Compared to nonstructured interviews, structured clinical interviews such as the SCID-II can significantly enhance the accuracy and reliability of personality disorder diagnoses with relatively low time demands for patients and clinicians. Appropriate training and quality assurance oversight are important for obtaining reliable and valid diagnoses using any of the structured interviews.

Clinicians may wish to integrate categorical and dimensional approaches to assessment. A structured interview can assist categorical decisions about the presence or absence of personality disorders. Self-report questionnaires can provide idiographic profiles that "fill in" the clinical picture, facilitating case conceptualization and treatment planning. For the purpose of cognitive conceptualization, measures such as the PBQ and SQ or SQ-SF yield personality profiles that cognitive therapists may find particularly useful.

Key cognitive elements to consider when assessing personality disorders include characteristic views of self and others, dysfunctional beliefs, main strategies and affects, and specific styles of processing information. Being cognizant of the prototypical cognitive profile of each personality disorder can help guide clinicians as they conceptualize individual cases. However, it is important to keep in mind that many patients with personality pathology vary from the prototypical pattern, and care should be taken to expose variations as well as consistencies in order to make a complete evaluation.

CHAPTER 4

General Principles and Specialized Techniques

Patients with Axis I disorders return to their premorbid cognitive mode after the disorder subsides. For example, most patients who have recovered from depression no longer blame themselves for every mishap, are less prone to think that they are inadequate or inferior, and stop making negative predictions about the future. Some patients, however, continue to show these characteristics and acknowledge that they have "always" thought this way. Nonetheless, they are no longer clinically depressed.

The Axis II mode differs from the Axis I mode in a variety of ways. The frequency and intensity of dysfunctional automatic thoughts observed during the acute disorder level off when the patients return to their regular cognitive functioning. Although the patients may readily identify and test their dysfunctional automatic thoughts during their "normal neurotic period," these exaggerated or distorted interpretations and the associated disruptive affect continue to occur in specific situations. A highly intelligent and competent woman, for example, would automatically have the thought "I can't do it" whenever she was offered a position requiring a higher level of intellectual functioning.

The most plausible explanation for the difference between Axis I and the personality disorders is that the extreme faulty beliefs and interpretations characteristic of the symptomatic disorders are relatively plastic—and, indeed, become more moderate as the depression subsides even without any therapeutic intervention. However, the more persistent dysfunctional beliefs of the personality disorder are "structuralized"; that is, they are built into the "normal" cognitive organization. Hence, considerably more time and effort are required to produce the kind of structural change necessary to change a personality disorder than to change the dysfunctional thinking of, say, the affective disorders.

The therapist generally uses "standard" cognitive therapy techniques to relieve acute Axis I episodes (American Psychiatric Association, 2000) such as depression (Beck, Rush, Shaw, & Emery, 1979) or generalized anxiety disorder (GAD; Beck & Emery, with Greenberg, 1985). This approach is effective in dealing with the dysfunctional automatic thoughts and helps to produce the cognitive shift from the depressive (or GAD) mode of processing back to the "normal" mode. The testing of automatic thoughts and beliefs during the depressive or anxious episode is good practice for dealing with these cognitive processes during the relatively quiescent period. The patients observed during this quiescent period have been described in earlier psychiatric and colloquial terminology as "neurotic." The characteristics of the "neurotic personality" have generally been described in terms of labels such as "immature" or "childish": emotional lability, exaggerated responses to rejection or failure, unrealistically low or high concept of self, and—above all—intense egocentricity.

The dysfunctional beliefs are still operative because they form the substrate for patients' orientation to reality. Because people rely on their beliefs to interpret events, they cannot relinquish these beliefs until they have incorporated new adaptive beliefs and strategies to take their place. When patients return to their premorbid level of functioning, they rely once again on the strategies they customarily use. The underlying beliefs are generally less dysfunctional in this phase than during the depression or GAD, but they are less amenable to further modification than during the acute phase.

Both patient and therapist need to acknowledge that these hardcore residual beliefs (schemas) are deeply ingrained and do not yield readily to the techniques used in the standard antidepressant or antianxiety treatment. Even when patients are convinced that their basic beliefs are dysfunctional or even irrational, they cannot make them disappear simply by questioning them or "wishing" them away.

A long, sometimes tedious process is necessary to effect change in these patients' character structure. The "characterological phase" of treatment tends to be prolonged and much less punctuated by dramatic spurts of improvement.

CONCEPTUALIZATION OF THE CASE

Specific conceptualization of each case is crucial to provide a framework for understanding the patient's maladaptive behavior and modifying dysfunctional attitudes. Consequently, the therapist should formulate the case early, preferably during the evaluation process. Of course, as new data are collected, the therapist modifies the formulation accordingly. Some hypotheses are confirmed, others are modified or dropped, and still others are entered into the formulation.

Sharing this conceptualization with the patient can help the data-gathering process; it provides a guide to the patient as to what experiences to focus on, and what interpretations and underlying beliefs to identify. Patient and therapist can then test fresh material for "fit" into the preliminary formulation. As new data are collected, the therapist reformulates the case on the basis of these new data.

Drawing diagrams for patients can show them how to fit subsequent experiences into this overall formulation. It often helps for the patients to take the diagrams home with them. Some therapists use a blackboard or flip cards to demonstrate to the patients how their misconstruction of reality is derived from their beliefs. The dependent personality who tells the therapist "I need help" when confronting a new challenge, for example, needs to see the connection between this notion and the core belief "I am not capable of doing anything without help" or "I am helpless." Repeated, systematic disconfirmations through devising and carrying out "behavioral experiments" can eventually erode these dysfunctional beliefs and lay the groundwork for more adaptive attitudes, such as "I can carry out a wide range of tasks without help" and "I am competent in many ways."

Table 4.1 presents a structural formulation of the problems of a couple who had somewhat similar sets of beliefs but who differed in crucial ways. The presenting problems of this couple have been presented in detail elsewhere (Beck, 1988). In brief, Gary, who had a narcissistic personality disorder, had periodic violent outbursts against Beverly, whom he accused of needling him all the time for not attending to specific chores. Gary believed the only way he could control Beverly, who had a dependent personality disorder, was to strike out at her to make her "shut up." Beverly, on the other hand, believed that she had to control Gary's continuous defaulting on his role as husband and father by "reminding" him in a reproachful way of his derelictions. She believed that this was the only way she could carry out her responsibility as housewife and mother. Beneath this view was her firm belief that she could not function at all unless she had somebody to lean on.

TABLE 4.1. Cognitive Processing from Core Schemas: An Example

	Beverly's beliefs	Gary's beliefs
Should	"Gary should help when I ask."	"Beverly should show more respect."
Must	"I must control others' behavior."	"I must control others' behavior."
Special conditional belief	"If Gary doesn't help, I won't be able to function."	"If I give them a chance, people will dump on me."
Fear	"I will be abandoned."	"I will be dumped on."
Core schema	"I am a helpless baby."	"I am a wimp."

Gary had been brought up in a household in which "might makes right." His father and older brother had intimidated him into believing he was a "wimp." He compensated for this image of himself by adopting their interpersonal strategy: In essence, the best way to control other people's inclination to dominate or demean one is to intimidate them—if necessary, through threat of force. The initial formulation, which was borne out by subsequent conjoint and individual interviews, was as follows: Gary's core schema was "I am a wimp." This self-concept threatened to surface whenever he regarded himself as vulnerable to being demeaned. To protect himself, he consolidated the belief "I have to control other people" that was inherent in his father's behavior. Later, we will return to the methods used to deal with these beliefs. In essence, the therapist was able to trace Gary's behavior to these beliefs.

Beverly similarly believed that "I need to control Gary." Her imperative was derived from a fear of being incapable of performing her duties without help. Her core schema was "I am a helpless child." Note that Gary's behavior ("not helping") was processed by her core schema ("Without help from somebody, I am helpless"), which led to a limp feeling in Beverly. She reacted to this debilitating feeling by blaming Gary and becoming enraged.

Through imagery and reliving past experiences of helplessness, the therapist was able to activate the core schema and help Beverly to recognize that her profound involvement in getting Gary to help out was derived from her image of herself as a helpless child. Consequently, her nonadaptive "nagging" was an attempt to stave off her profound sense of helplessness. The interaction of Gary and Beverly demonstrates how partners' personality structures can aggravate each other's problems and illustrates the importance of viewing personality problems as they are expressed in a particular context, such as a marital situation.

IDENTIFICATION OF SCHEMAS

The therapist should use the data that he or she is collecting to extract patients' self-concept and the rules and formulas by which they live. Often, the therapist has to determine the patients' self-concept from its manifestations in their descriptions across a variety of situations.

For example, a patient makes statements such as the following: "I made a fool of myself when I gave the conductor the wrong change," "I don't know how I got through college or even through law school. I always seem to be fouling up," and "I don't think that I can describe situations properly to you." The therapist can pick up a thread that suggests that at a basic level the patient perceives him- or herself as inadequate or defective. The therapist also makes a quick judgment as to whether there is any validity to the patient's self-description. Of course, when the patient is depressed, this broad global generalization (core belief) comes out full-blown: After the patient has described a problematic situation, he or she concludes with a remark such as "That shows how worthless, inadequate, and unlikable I am."

The therapist can elicit the *conditional* assumptions through statements that specify the conditions under which the negative self-concept will express itself. For example, if the person has thoughts such as "Bob or Linda doesn't like me any more" under circumstances in which another individual shows less than the usual friendly response, the therapist can derive the underlying formula, such as "If other people do not show a strong expression of affection or interest, it means they don't care for me." Of course, for some people under some circumstances there may be truth in this formula, and they may require special attention to deficiencies in social skills or abrasive interpersonal style. Individuals with personality problems, however, tend to apply the formula arbitrarily, willy-nilly, in an all-or-nothing fashion across all relevant situations, even when there are alternative explanations or compelling evidence that is contradictory to this belief.

Similarly, the therapist tries to elicit the patient's views of other people. Certain statements of a paranoid personality, for example, may indicate that the basic schema is that other people are devious, manipulative, prejudiced, and the like. This schema would be manifested in statements such as "The doctor smiled at me. I know it's a phony professional smile that he uses with everybody because he is anxious to have a lot of patients," or "The clerk counted my change very slowly because he doesn't trust me," or "My wife is acting extra nice to me tonight. I wonder what she wants to get out of me." Such patients often reach these conclusions without any evidence to support them or when there is strong contradictory evidence.

When such persons are in an acute paranoid state, the global thoughts run through their minds, such as "He's trying to put something over on me" or "They are all out to get me." The core schemas are, "People can't be trusted" and "Everybody has devious motives." A consequent pattern of arbitrary conclusions reflects a cognitive bias and is said to be "schema driven."

SPECIFICATION OF UNDERLYING GOALS

People generally have broad goals that are very important to them but may not be completely in their awareness. The therapist has the job of translating the patient's stated aspirations and ambitions into the underlying goal. For instance, a patient may say, "When I got to the party, I felt bad because only a few people came up to say hello to me," or "I had a great time because a lot of people crowded around me and wanted to know how my trip went." From a wide range of descriptions across a number of diverse situations, the therapist can infer that the underlying goal is something like "It is very important for me to be liked by everybody." Goals are derived from the core schema; in this case it would be phrased, "If I'm not liked, I'm worthless."

Another patient, for example, stated that he felt bad because he did not get a perfect grade on an exam. He also felt a little put out when he was unable to recall the name of a particular scientist during a conversation with a friend. In addition, he became so excited that he had a sleepless night after being told that he was going to get a full scholarship into graduate school. His goal, which he did not articulate until he was questioned about his experiences, was "to be famous." Associated with this goal was this conditional assumption: "If I do not become famous, then my whole life will be wasted."

Other kinds of goals may be inferred in much the same way. Take an individual who rejects any offer of help, insists on having complete freedom to move around, and is reluctant to become involved in any type of "relationship." Once the therapist extracts the common theme, "I need to have space," he or she can test this striving by observing the patient's reaction in therapy and in other situations. If the patient, for example, tends to seek physical distance during the interview, terminates the interview promptly, and expresses the desire to work on his or her problems alone, these are indicators of an underlying goal for autonomy. The conditional assumption may well be, "If I get too dependent on anybody or too intimate, then I can no longer be free," Associated with this notion is the belief that "I am helpless unless I have complete freedom of action."

After the therapist has all the data and has extracted the core assumptions, conditional beliefs, and goals, he or she can then formulate the case according to the cognitive model (e.g., the formulation of Gary and Beverly's case previously discussed).

EMPHASIS ON THE THERAPIST–PATIENT RELATIONSHIP

Collaboration

One of the cardinal principles of cognitive therapy is instilling a sense of collaboration and trust in the patient. The building of the relationship is probably more important in the chronic personality disorder than in the acute symptomatic phase. In the period of acute distress (usually depression and/or anxiety), the patient can usually be motivated to try out the therapist's suggestions and is rewarded by the fairly prompt reduction of suffering. In the chronic personality disorder, the changes take place much more slowly and the payoff is much less perceptible. Hence, therapist and patient have considerable work to do on the long-term project of personality change.

Patients frequently need to be motivated to do homework assignments. The patients' motivation often declines after the acute episode has subsided, as the unpleasant feelings (anxiety, sadness, anger) that acted as a spur to action subside. Further, the personality disorder itself frequently interferes with carrying out assignments. The avoidant personality may think, "Writing down my thoughts is too painful"; the narcissistic, "I'm too good for this sort of thing"; the paranoid, "My notes can be used against me" or "The therapist is trying to manipulate me."

The therapist should regard these forms of "resistance" as "grist for the mill" and should subject them to the same kind of analysis as that used for other forms of material or data.

Guided Discovery

Part of the artistry of cognitive therapy consists of conveying a sense of adventure—in unraveling and ferreting out the origins of patients' beliefs, exploring the meanings of traumatic events, and tapping into the rich imagery. Otherwise, therapy can decline into a repetitive process that becomes increasingly tedious in time. In fact, varying the way hypotheses are presented, using different phrases and words, and illustrating points with metaphors and anecdotes all help to make the relationship into a human educational experience. A certain lightness and judicious use of humor can also add spice to the experience.

In the chronic phase, the therapist spends more time with patients on unraveling the *meaning* of experiences, in order to determine the patients' specific sensitivities and vulnerabilities and to ascertain why they overreact to specific situations. As indicated in Chapter 2, the meanings are determined to a large extent by the underlying beliefs ("If somebody criticizes me, it means that person doesn't like me"). To determine the meaning, the therapist may have to proceed gradually through a number of steps.

Use of "Transference" Reactions

The patient's emotional reactions to the process of therapy and the therapist are of central concern. Always alert but not provoking, the therapist is ready to explore these reactions for more information about the patient's system of thoughts and beliefs. If not explored, possible distorted interpretations will persist and may interfere with collaboration. If brought out into the open, they often provide rich material for understanding the meanings and beliefs behind the patient's idiosyncratic or repetitious reactions. In terms of countertransference, it is extremely important to remain nonjudgmental and sympathetic, yet objective in responding to the patient's maladaptive patterns. Work with personality disorders typically requires significant effort, planning, and stress management on the part of the therapist. Chapter 5 details more fully strategies for conceptualizing issues of noncollaboration and managing emotional reactions to therapy by both patient and therapist.

SPECIALIZED TECHNIQUES

The planning and application of specific strategies and techniques need to take into account not only the specific pathology of the patients but also their unique methods for integrating and using information about themselves. Different patients learn in different ways. Furthermore, methods that are successful at a particular time with a given patient may be ineffective at another time. Therapists must use their best judgment in designing treatment plans and selecting the most useful techniques from the wide variety available, or improvising new ones. A certain amount of trial and error may be necessary. At times, introspection may be most successful; at other times, ventilation or skills training may be the appropriate choice.

The most effective application of techniques depends not only on a clear conceptualization of the case and the formation of a friendly working relationship but also on the artistry of the therapist. The *art of therapy* involves the judicious use of humor, anecdotes, metaphors, and self-disclosure of the therapist's experiences, as well as the standard cognitive and behavioral techniques. Skillful therapists know when to draw out sensitive material, draw back when necessary, and confront avoidances.

They can heat up a monotonous rendition or cool off an overly heated flow. They vary their words, style, and mode of expression.

Flexibility within a given session is important: The therapist may vary his or her approach from active listening to focusing and probing to modeling new behavioral styles. It is expected that therapists reading this volume will have mastered the basic principles of cognitive-behavioral psychotherapy. Many of these have been covered in volumes such as that by Beck et al. (1979). We have arbitrarily divided techniques into those that are primarily "cognitive" and those that are "behavioral." We need to keep in mind that no techniques are purely either cognitive or behavioral. Further, cognitive strategies can produce behavioral change, and behavioral methods generally instigate some cognitive restructuring.

Among the most effective tools in treating personality disorders are the so-called *experiential techniques,* such as reliving childhood events and imagery. Such dramatic techniques seem to open up the sluices for new learning—or unlearning. A rule of thumb is that cognitive change depends on a certain level of affective experience.

Cognitive and behavioral techniques play complementary roles in the treatment of personality disorders. The main thrust is to develop new schemas and modify old ones. Ultimately, of course, the cognitive techniques probably account for most of the change that occurs. The cognitive work, like the behavioral, requires more precision and persistence than usual when patients have personality disorders. Because specific cognitive schemas of these patients continue to be dysfunctional, even after more adaptive behaviors have been developed, a larger variety and longer duration of cognitive reworking are typically required.

COGNITIVE STRATEGIES AND TECHNIQUES

Following is a list of cognitive techniques from which therapists can draw in treating Axis II disorders. Given that several methods have been described elsewhere in the treatment of depression (Beck et al., 1979), we do not discuss them in detail here. We do, however, expand on specific techniques for Axis II problems. This list is representative and by no means exhaustive.

Some of the cognitive techniques that are helpful in dealing with personality disorders include (1) guided discovery, which enables the patient to recognize stereotyped dysfunctional patterns of interpretation; (2) searches for idiosyncratic meaning, given that these patients often interpret their experiences in unusual or extreme ways; (3) labeling of inaccurate inferences or distortions, to make the patient aware of bias or unreasonableness of particular automatic patterns of thought; (4) collaborative empiricism—working with the patient to test the validity of the patient's beliefs, interpretations, and expectations; (5) examining explanations for other people's behavior; (6) scaling—translating extreme interpretations into dimensional terms to counteract typical dichotomous thinking; (7) reattribution—reassigning responsibility for actions and outcomes; (8) deliberate exaggeration—taking an idea to its extreme, which places a situation in high relief and facilitates reevaluation of a dysfunctional conclusion; (9) examining the advantages and disadvantages of maintaining or changing beliefs or behaviors, and clarifying primary and secondary gains; (10) decatastrophizing—enabling the patient to recognize and counter the tendency to think exclusively in terms of the worst possible outcome of a situation.

The "Cognitive Probes"

The same techniques used in eliciting and evaluating automatic thoughts during depression or GAD (Beck et al., 1979; Beck et al., 1985) are useful when dealing with personality problems. Specifically, the therapist and patient identify incidents that illuminate the personality problems, and focus on the cognitive underpinnings of these incidents. Let us say that an avoidant patient, Lois, becomes upset when the other workers at her place of work appear to ignore her. The first cognitive probe should attempt to recover her automatic thoughts (Beck, 1967). If the patient is well trained at identifying automatic thoughts, she might say, for example, "I thought 'They don't like me.' "

If the patient fails to recover the automatic thought, she might then be encouraged to *imagine* the experience "as though it is happening right now." As the experience is brought to life, as it were, she is likely to experience the automatic thoughts just as she would in the actual situation. Of course, she would have many opportunities in future encounters to ascertain the automatic thoughts as they occur without priming. If a patient can anticipate a particular "traumatic" experience, it is useful for her to prepare herself in advance by starting to tune in to her train of thought prior to entering the aversive situation ("I wonder whether Linda will snub me at lunch today"). Our patient, Lois, thus is primed to catch the relevant thought of rejection. Noting that Linda seems to be aloof, she can pick up the negative thoughts: "She doesn't like me." "There is something wrong with me." Of course, automatic thoughts are not necessarily dysfunctional or unrealistic and, as we shall see, need to be tested.

Of most importance is the ultimate meaning of the event. For example, Lois could shrug off Linda's seeming rejection with the thought, "So what? I don't like her either," or "She's not one of my friends." However, when the patient has a specific vulnerability to rejection, a chain reaction is started that may culminate in a prolonged feeling of sadness.

Sometimes the patient is able to discern the chain reaction through introspection. Often, through skillful questioning, the therapist can arrive at the salient starting point (core schema). He or she can also use this exercise as a way of demonstrating the particular fallacy or flaw in the patient's process of making inferences and drawing conclusions. Take the following interchange between the therapist and Lois, who has become upset because Linda, her friend, has been absorbed in a conversation with a fellow worker at lunch:

THERAPIST: What thought went through your mind at lunch?

LOIS: Linda is ignoring me. [Selective focus, personalization]

THERAPIST: What did that mean?

LOIS: I can't get along with people. [Self-attribution, overgeneralization]

THERAPIST: What does that mean?

LOIS: I will never have any friends. [Absolute prediction]

THERAPIST: What does it mean "not to have friends"?

LOIS: I am all alone. [Core schema]

THERAPIST: What does it mean to be *all alone*?

LOIS: That I will always be unhappy. (*Starts to cry.*)

Because the patient starts to cry, the therapist stops the line of questioning because he believes he has come to the bedrock, the core schema ("I will always be unhappy"). The arousal of a strong feeling suggests not only that a core schema has been exposed but also that the dysfunctional thinking is more accessible to modification. This type of questioning, attempting to probe for deeper meanings and access to the core schema, has been called the "downward arrow" technique (Beck et al., 1985). At a later date, therapist and patient will want to explore further to ascertain whether there are other core schemas.

In this particular case, Lois's problem stems from her beliefs: "If people are not responsive to me, it means they don't like me" and "If one person doesn't like me, it means I'm unlikable." When she goes into the cafeteria in the office building in which she works, she is very sensitive to how receptive the other workers are—whether they seem eager to have her sit next to them, whether they include her in the conversation, whether they are responsive to her remarks. Because she has an avoidant personality disorder and tends to avoid entering situations of possible rejection, she is inclined not to sit at a table with people she knows, particularly Linda. One way to deal with this is to confront the issue head on, as illustrated in the following dialogue.

Lois has become upset after sitting down at a table where a group of women have been carrying on an animated conversation. The therapist probes for the meaning of this event.

THERAPIST: Suppose the people don't welcome you with open arms, then what?

LOIS: I don't know. I suppose I would feel they don't like me.

THERAPIST: If they showed they liked you, then what?

LOIS: I'm not sure. I really don't have much in common with them. I'm not really interested in the kind of things they are.

THERAPIST: Would you choose to have any of them as your close friends?

LOIS: I guess not.

THERAPIST: You really aren't interested in being friendly with any of them. So it's the meaning, the importance you attach to "being liked" or "not liked" rather than the practical importance that throws you. Is that right?

LOIS: I guess it is.

Because of her core schemas revolving around the issue of being likable, almost every encounter Lois has with other people involves a test of her acceptability, becoming almost a matter of life and death. By exposing the core schema through the downward-arrow technique, the therapist is able to bring the underlying meanings of "being ignored" to the surface and demonstrate that the belief about the necessity of being liked by everyone is dysfunctional.

Once the underlying beliefs are made accessible (conscious), the patient can then apply realistic, logical reasoning to modify them. Thus, Lois is able to counter the automatic thought, "They don't care for me," with the rational response, "It doesn't matter if they don't care for me. I don't have anything in common with them anyhow." Patients tend to attach absolutistic meanings to events and to view them in all-or-nothing terms. The therapist's role is to show the patient that the importance of events or people can be placed on a continuum. Thus, Lois can see that when she ranks her acquaintances on a continuum of "how important" they are to her, they rank much lower than her real friends. Once she has made this objective rating, she may no longer be so concerned about being liked by her acquaintances.

Of course, in most situations casual acquaintances usually are neutral rather than rejecting, but because patients are prone to interpret neutrality as rejection, they need to articulate the core beliefs and experience the associated affect in order to change this dysfunctional way of thinking. Techniques for dealing with negative automatic thoughts and the underlying beliefs are dealt with elsewhere (Beck et al., 1979; Freeman, Pretzer, Fleming, & Simon, 1990).

Confronting the Schemas

In discussing or elucidating the schemas with the patient, the diagnostic labels of paranoid, histrionic, narcissistic, or borderline may induce a bias in the therapist's view of the patient. The patient's style can be translated into operational terms. The schizoid style, for example, can be described and discussed as the patient's being "very individualistic" or not being "dependent on other people." The dependent personality disorder can be discussed in terms of "having a strong belief in the value of attachment to others," or of "placing a large emphasis on the importance of being a more social person." In every case, a nonjudgmental description modified to fit the particular belief system can be offered to the patient.

A comprehensive therapeutic program addresses all cognitive, behavioral, and affective schemas. The density, breadth, activity, and valence of the targeted schemas (Chapter 2) are all factors in determining the therapeutic mix. Using the patient's cognitive biases or distortions as the signposts that point to the schemas, the therapist first helps the patient to identify the dysfunctional rules that dominate his or her life, then works with the patient to make the modifications or alterations necessary for more adaptive functioning. The therapist has several options in working with the schemas. The choice of a particular option is based on the goals and the conceptualization of the case.

The first option we will call "schematic restructuring." This may be likened to urban renewal. When a conclusion is reached that a particular structure or complex of structures is unsound, a decision is made to tear down the old structures in a stepwise fashion and build new structures in their place. This has been the goal of many therapeutic approaches for many years (especially psychoanalysis and the dynamic derivatives of the psychodynamic schools). Not all dysfunctional schemas can be restructured, nor is doing so always a reasonable goal, given the time, energy, or available patient (or therapist) skills.

An example of total schematic restructuring would be the transformation of an individual with a paranoid personality disorder into a fully trusting individual. The particular schemas about the potential and imminent danger from others would be eliminated, and in their place would be other beliefs about the general trustworthiness of people, the unlikely possibility of being attacked and hurt, and the belief that generally there will be others available to offer help and succor. Obviously, this is a most difficult and time-consuming treatment option, and a compromise must be reached between the overactive schemas relevant to distrust and more benevolent schemas. In other words, the restructuring consists of attenuating the dysfunctional schemas and developing more adaptive schemas.

Many patients have never formed adequate schemas to incorporate experiences that contradict their dysfunctional basic beliefs. Hence, they are unable to integrate new positive experiences and, consequently, continue to filter events through their preexisting schemas. As a result, their life experiences are shaped in such a way that they confirm the patients' dysfunctional—usually negative—beliefs about themselves and other people. More severely impaired patients, especially those with borderline personality disorder, may have one or more areas in which adaptive schemas are simply not available. Hence, they have to build up adaptive structures to store new constructive experiences.

A variety of techniques may be used to build new schemas or shore up defective ones. Diaries can be used creatively to accomplish the goal of organizing and storing new observations. For example, a person who believes "I'm inadequate" could keep a notebook with several sections labeled "work," "social," "parenting," "alone." Every day small examples of adequacy could be recorded in each area. The therapist can help the patient identify adequacy examples and monitor that they are recorded regularly. The patient can also review this log to help counter his or her absolute belief in the negative schema in times of stress or "failure" when the more familiar negative schema is strongly activated.

A different type of diary can be used to weaken the negative schemas and support the need for alternative schemas. In predictive diaries, patients write down predictions of what will happen in certain situations if their negative schemas are true. Later, they write what actually happened and compare this to the predictions.

For example, one woman with obsessive–compulsive personality disorder believed that terrible catastrophes awaited her each day and that she was totally inadequate to cope with these. She made a diary in which she listed each predicted catastrophe in the first column. In the second column she listed whether or not the catastrophe happened and also any unforeseen catastrophes that actually occurred. In a third column she rated her coping with any actual "catastrophes." After 1 month, this woman reviewed her diary and found that of five predicted catastrophes, only one actually happened and that she was able to handle this one with 70% adequacy.

A third type of diary more actively analyzes daily experiences in terms of old and new schemas. Patients who have begun to believe somewhat in their new, more adaptive schemas can evaluate critical incidents during their week. For example, a patient who believed she was unlovable if she displeased others analyzed her daily experiences in which this old belief was activated. In one incident she criticized an employee for poor work performance. In her diary she wrote, "H seemed annoyed at me that I criticized his work. With my old schema, I would feel this is terrible and shows I am unlovable. Now I can see that it is my responsibility to correct my work and, if he is mad at me, that is OK. I don't need everyone to be happy with me all the time to be lovable."

In these ways "schema diaries" can help build up adaptive schemas, ensure that subsequent experiences reinforce the new schemas, and help counteract the old nonadaptive schemas in the processing of new events and reformulating of old events. The types of "functional schemas" to be developed vary, of course, according to the nature of the patient's problems and the diagnostic category.

Although transforming an individual with a personality disorder into a fully mature person, functioning at the peak of his or her capacity, would seem to be an ideal, it is rarely achieved during therapy. However, most patients do continue to mature after therapy is completed and may ultimately approximate this ideal.

The second possibility on the change continuum is "schematic modification." This process involves smaller relative changes in the basic manner of responding to the world than reconstruction. A relevant metaphor would be renovating an old home. A clinical example would be changing a paranoid personality's relevant schemas regarding trust into less mistrusting and suspicious beliefs and experimenting by inducing the patient to trust *some* people in *some* situations and to evaluate the results.

The third possibility on the continuum is "schematic reinterpretation." This involves helping patients to understand and reinterpret their lifestyles and their schemas in more functional ways. For example, a histrionic person could recognize the dysfunctionality of the belief that being loved or admired is an absolute necessity. However, the person could still receive affection as a source of gratification—for example, by choosing to teach preschool children who kiss and hug the teacher. If a narcissistic person wants to be looked up to and respected, by earning a title (e.g., Professor or Doctor), he or she could meet the desire for status without being driven by compulsive beliefs regarding the value of prestige.

Mary, a 23-year-old computer programmer (mentioned briefly in Chapter 1), came to therapy because of "tremendous work pressure, inability to enjoy life, a perfectionistic approach to virtually all tasks, and a general isolation from others" (Freeman & Leaf, 1989, pp. 405–406), as well as sleep difficulty and suicidal ideation. Not only was she getting very little satisfaction from her work; she was constantly late in getting it completed. Her obsessive–compulsive personality traits had been rewarded in school and at home. Without the school structure in her life, work took all her time, and she was no longer rewarded for her perfectionism. She reported that if she needed extra time to complete an assignment, the teachers always gave it to her, knowing that the finished product would be well worth waiting for.

She thought it was essential to keep her "high standards." Attempts to alter these hypervalent schemas were met with great resistance. She wanted surcease from the stress she felt but did not want to give up rules and standards that she considered important. One choice discussed in therapy was her finding a new position that would allow her to use her "high standards." After a brief job search, she found a position at a university research center, where a requirement of the job was that she work "slowly and carefully" without regard to time. Her coworkers found her style compatible with the aims of their project. Continued therapy worked toward modification of her rules in social situations and in the vocational arena.

Given that anxiety is likely to be aroused as schemas are changed, patients must be apprised of this possibility so that they will not be disturbed when it surfaces. A depressed patient diagnosed at intake as having borderline personality disorder asked, "Why are you trying to teach me to control my anxiety? I'm depressed; I'm not anxious at all." At that point, the therapist told the patient of the need to master anxiety reduction skills. These skills, it was pointed out, would be an essential factor in successful therapy. One patient, as noted in Chapter 1, responded to this explanation by stating, "It's good to have that safety and I don't understand why I should ever give it up." Unless patients are able to cope with anxiety, they may slide back into the old dysfunctional patterns and leave therapy. (See Beck et al., 1985, for detailed discussions of anxiety treatment.)

Making Decisions

One of the areas in which therapists often enter into the "outside lives" of patients with personality disorders is helping them to make decisions. While the personality problems are being treated, joint work is required to help patients learn how to make certain important decisions that have been postponed initially. During the acute phase of depressive or anxiety disorders, the therapist focuses on getting patients mobilized and back into the pattern of confronting *immediate problems*, which may seem insoluble during the depression (indeed, this feeling may be a byproduct of the depression): "Should I get out of bed today?" "How can I get the children off to school?" "What should I buy at the supermarket?" A depressed attorney, for instance, could not decide which cases she should attend to first when she got to the office. She needed help in setting priorities and then listing what needed to be done for each case. The symptoms of depression may interfere with making even the simplest routine decisions. Important long-range decisions—for example, regarding marital problems, childrearing, or career changes—may need to be put off until the depression has subsided.

When the acute symptoms have subsided, the therapist can focus on the more chronic or long-range problems regarding marriage, career, and so on. Decisions that seem to tie patients in knots—especially in the area of interpersonal relations—need to be tackled. Some patients are paralyzed into inaction, and others make impulsive decisions when faced with questions regarding choice of career, dating, marriage or divorce, and having children (as well as more mundane issues). Helping the personality problems can promote solving the realistic problems and making decisions. The calculated procedures involved in making decisions are often blocked by the patients' personality problems. The avoidant and passive–aggressive personalities tend to procrastinate; the histrionic is more likely to be impulsive; the obsessive–compulsive gets caught up in perfectionism; the dependent looks for somebody else to make the decision; the narcissistic focuses on how the decision will make him or her look; the antisocial focuses on immediate personal gain.

It is clear that the therapist cannot treat the personality problems in a vacuum. The cognitive problems encroach on the way the individual is able to cope with "real-life situations." Conversely, by helping the patient to learn and integrate new coping strategies, the therapist is able to neutralize some of the maladaptive strategies that are manifestations of the personality disorder. Incorporating a new strategy of decision making can increase the self-reliance of the dependent, improve the decisiveness of the avoidant, make the histrionic more reflective, and increase the flexibility of the obsessive–compulsive. Thus, new decision-making patterns can modify the personality styles of each disorder.

Therapists can draw on the practical techniques described in various writings on making decisions. One method used successfully by D'Zurilla and Goldfried (1971), for example, consists of a series of steps such as defining the problem, setting the goals, brainstorming to generate ideas, and so forth.

A method that elicits the unreasonable meanings that influence people when they are confronted with an either-or choice is to list the pros and cons for each option in separate columns. With the therapist's assistance, the patient lists the advantages and disadvantages of each alternative and attempts to assign weights to each of these items.

For example, Tom, who tended to obsess about making decisions, had decided to drop out of law school because of the discomfort he felt in taking exams and his fear of not living up to expectations. His habit of obsessing about his performance generated a significant amount of tension. He was prompted to consider dropping out by his belief that this was the only way he could relieve the stress. As a way of helping him to make an objective decision, the therapist and Tom set up four columns and filled them in together as shown in Table 4.2. The first column listed the reasons for dropping out or staying. In the second column, he gauged the importance of these reasons. The third column contained rebuttals and the fourth the value or importance of the rebuttals.

After Tom went down the list with his therapist, he was able to view the question of dropping out more objectively. He experienced some relief when he realized that his perfectionism and obsessing were the real sources of distress rather than the difficulties of law school per se and that he could get help from his therapist with this distressing personality problem that had plagued him most of his life.

It should be noted that decisions that may be relatively simple for one patient become momentous for another because they touch on specific personality sensitivities. Thus, Agnes, a dependent personality, had no difficulty in deciding to have a dinner party but agonized over making a decision whether to take a trip alone. Phil, an autonomous person, on the other hand, was able to plan trips alone but was stymied when he had to call a friend for directions.

BEHAVIORAL TECHNIQUES

The goals of using behavioral techniques are threefold. First, the therapist may need to work directly to alter self-defeating behaviors. Second, patients may be deficient in skills, and the therapy must include a skill-building component. Third, the behavioral assignments can be used as homework to help to test out cognitions. Behavioral techniques that can be helpful (although we do not discuss all of them in detail here) include (1) activity monitoring and scheduling, which permit retrospective identification and prospective planning of changes; (2) scheduling mastery and pleasure activities, to enhance personal efficacy and validate the successfulness of and pleasure derived from changed experiences (or lack thereof); (3) behavioral rehearsal, modeling, assertiveness training, and role playing for skill development prior to early efforts to respond more effectively, either in old problematic situations or in new ones; (4) relaxation training and behavioral distraction techniques, for use when anxiety becomes an imminent problem during efforts to change; (5) *in vivo* exposure, by arranging for the therapist to go with the client to a problematic setting, so that the therapist can help the client deal with dysfunctional schemas and actions that have (for whatever reason) not been tractable in the ordinary consultation setting; and (6) graded task assign-

TABLE 4.2. Tom's Decision-Making Process

In favor of dropping out	Value	Rebuttal	Value
"I won't have to worry so much."	60%	"I'm in therapy to get me over my *perfectionism*, which is what's making me miserable."	40%
"I can find out whether I want to be a lawyer."	10%	"I don't need to make an irreversible decision to find this out . . . I can play it by ear as I continue in school."	30%
"It will be a big relief. I can take time out and knock around for a while."	40%	"I will feel relieved at first, but I may feel really sad about it later."	30%

In favor of staying	Value	Rebuttal	Value
"I've prepared myself for going to law school and have only 1½ more years to go."	40%	None	—
"I might really like the practice of law. (It's the exams that are getting me down.)"	30%	None	
"Even if I don't like the practice of law, it's a good jumping-off point for a number of different jobs (even a college presidency!)."	30%	None	—
"Some of the courses turn me on."	20%	None	—
"My perfectionism might work well for me in the law."	20%	None	

ment, so that the patient can experience changes as an incremental step-by-step process, during which the difficulty of each component can be adjusted and mastery achieved in stages.

Role play may be used for skill development and overcoming inhibitions, as in "assertiveness training." When the role play involves an emotionally charged topic, dysfunctional cognitions usually are aroused. These can be "worked through" just like any other automatic thoughts can be.

In reverse role playing, the therapist can "model" appropriate behavior. Also, the therapist can more readily visualize the perspective of another person. Such reverse role playing is a crucial component of empathy training.

An 18-year-old woman was in a continuous state of anger toward her father, whom she regarded as "critical, mean, and controlling." She claimed, "He tries to run my life for me and disapproves of everything I do." Initially, after proper briefing, the therapist played the father role in a recent scenario in which the father had questioned her about taking drugs and the patient had flared up. During the role play, she had these thoughts: "You don't like me!" "You're trying to run all over me!" "You have no right to do this!" Subsequently, they reversed roles. The patient made a strong effort to do a good job—to see the situation through her father's eyes. She was moved to tears during the role play and explained, "I can see that he really is concerned about me and is genuinely worried about me." She had been so locked into her own perspective that she had been unable to see his.

RELIVING CHILDHOOD EXPERIENCES

Use of childhood material is not crucial in treating the acute phase of depression or anxiety but is important in treating the chronic personality disorder. Reviewing childhood material opens up windows for understanding the origins of nonadaptive patterns. This approach can increase perspective and objectivity. One patient who kept criticizing herself, despite consistent demonstration of the unreasonableness and dysfunctionality of her beliefs, was able to attenuate her self-criticisms when she reexperienced childhood scenes of criticism. "I criticize myself now not because it's right to do so, but because my mother always criticized me and I took this over from her."

Role playing and reverse role playing of key interactions from the past can mobilize affect and produce "mutation" of the schemas or core beliefs. Recreating "pathogenic" situations of the developmental period often provides an opportunity to restructure attitudes that were formed during this period. Cases like this are similar to "combat neurosis": The patients need to experience an emotional catharsis in order to change their strong beliefs (Beck et al., 1985).

By role playing a figure from the past, patients can see a "bad" parent (or sibling) in more benign terms. They can start to feel empathy or compassion for the parents who traumatized them. They can see that they themselves were not and are not "bad," but that they developed a fixed image of badness because their parents were upset and vented their anger on them. They can also see that their parents had rigid unrealistic standards that they arbitrarily imposed. Consequently, the patients can soften their own attitudes toward themselves.

Their parents' behavior becomes more understandable, and they can see that their own views of themselves were not based on logic or reasoning but were products of the parents' unreasoning reactions. A parent's statement, "You are worthless," is taken as valid and incorporated into a patient's system of beliefs—even though the patient him- or herself may not actually believe the label is justified. The rationale for "reliving" specific episodes from childhood may be fitted into the more general concept of state-dependent learning. To "reality-test" the validity of childhood-originated schemas, these beliefs have to be brought to the surface. Reexperiencing the episode facilitates the emergence of the dominant structures (the "hot schemas") and makes them more accessible. Thus, the patient can correct them.

USE OF IMAGERY

The use of imagery in anxiety disorders has been described at length elsewhere (Beck et al., 1985). The same methods can be used in personality disorders—to enable the patient to "relive" past traumatic events and thus to restructure the experience and consequently the derivative attitudes.

The rationale for this procedure requires some consideration: simply talking about a traumatic event may give intellectual insight about why the patient has a negative self-image, for instance, but it does not actually change the image. To modify the image, it is necessary to go back in time, as it were, and recreate the situation. When the interactions are brought to life, the misconstruction is activated—along with the affect—and cognitive restructuring can occur.

A 28-year-old single woman was treated successfully for panic disorder over 12 visits. It was apparent, however, that this symptomatic condition existed in the context of an avoidant personality. The patient decided that she wanted to get further treatment for her personality disorder after the panic disorder subsided.

The patient gave a typical avoidant history. She would tend to avoid social situations and consequently had few contacts with either sex—although she was eager to get married. Further, she was overqualified for the various jobs she held but was hesitant to do anything that would enable her to take on a job requiring more responsibility.

During the first few sessions with the therapist, she received the standard cognitive therapy for personality problems. In one visit, after she had been given a homework assignment that she failed to follow through with, she told her therapist that she was feeling particularly upset over not having done the homework. The therapist asked her where the feeling was localized. The patient responded that she felt it somewhere in her "stomach." The therapist then asked her whether she had an image in reference to what was upsetting her. She then said the following: "I see myself coming into the session. You are larger than life; you are critical and demeaning; you are like a big authority."

The therapist then asked when this had occurred previously. The patient responded that she had experienced this many times during childhood when she had unpleasant encounters with her mother. Her mother drank a good deal and was frequently irritable toward the child when she had been drinking. One day the child came home from school early, and her mother "blasted" her for waking her up.

The therapist asked her to re-create this experience in image form. The patient then had the following fantasy or image: "I came home and rang the doorbell. My mother came to the door. She looked at me. She was larger than life. She looked down on me and screamed at me for waking her up. She said, 'How dare you interrupt my sleep!' She said I was bad, wrong."

The patient extracted from this experience (and many other similar experiences) the following: "I am a bad kid," and "I am wrong because I upset my mother."

The therapist tried to elicit explanations for the mother's behavior other than that the patient was a bad kid. The patient volunteered that the mother did drink a lot, was irritable, and flew off the handle easily; nevertheless, the patient could not get away from holding herself accountable for her mother's behavior.

The therapist attempted to bring to bear the patient's "adult part" in dealing with this powerful memory. She "modeled" for the patient what would be an appropriate response to the mother if the child had all the maturity and skills of an adult. The patient practiced these rejoinders, with the therapist playing the role of the mother. Each time that she practiced, she became less uncertain about it until she was finally able to say it with some degree of conviction: "It's not my fault—you are being unreasonable, picking on me for no good reason. I haven't done anything wrong."

The patient then attempted to relive the situation in fantasy, again ringing the doorbell, but this time—instead of cowering and feeling helpless—she answered her mother back (in the image) in an assertive way, making the statements cited previously.

The "working through," using role plays, fantasy inductions, and testing and assessment of beliefs, was carried on for somewhat more than a year. In the course of time, the patient's degree of conviction in her beliefs shifted substantially. Concomitantly, she expressed a pronounced symptomatic change. She became much less self-critical and ultimately was able to leave her job for which she was overqualified and obtain a much higher-level position that matched her qualifications.

Imagery was also used successfully with an avoidant personality who worked in his wife's family's business. The problem he presented was that his in-laws were fed up with him because he did not attend to things he was supposed to. He stated to the therapist: "My father-in-law [who was also his boss] doesn't like me. I know he will be critical of me, so I just don't do things. I'm always afraid that he will be critical." The therapist then asked him to have an image of his last encounter with his boss, and to describe it in detail. The patient had a picture of the boss towering over him saying, "I'm so disappointed in you. Don't you see the trouble you've caused?" The emotions this scene elicited—shame, sadness, and the desire to withdraw—were the same as those he had experienced as a child when his mother berated him for his poor performance in school. As a child, he had received no help with his schoolwork; when he would fail, his mother would say to him: "You're the only child who did miserably. Now I'll have to go to that school and talk to the teacher."

The patient was able to discriminate the past from the present; that is, he was able to "see" at an experiential level that although he was reacting to his boss as he once had to his mother, they were obviously different people, and he was no longer a child. It would not have been possible for him to have achieved this degree of "emotional insight" simply by making verbal comparisons between his present and his past experiences, between his reactions to his boss and his reactions to his mother.

The strategies described in this chapter are elaborated in subsequent chapters in the context of specific personality disorders.

CHAPTER 5

The Cognitive Therapy Relationship with Personality-Disordered Patients

EXPANDING THE INTERPERSONAL DOMAIN

With most personality-disordered patients, the therapeutic relationship requires more attention than an acute (Axis I) disorder such as anxiety or depression in which the patient has a stable and adaptive premorbid personality adjustment. In the uncomplicated acute disorder, the therapist usually takes on the role of an authority who knows the necessary procedures to help the patient release the painful symptoms. The patient usually accepts and welcomes this influence and direction, without undue authority conflicts. Trust is readily established, and relatively uncomplicated by strong doubts or concerns about the therapist's acceptance or rejection. The patient understands his or her portion of responsibility and, with the therapist's guidance, makes appropriate efforts toward improvement. In response to the therapist's guidance, the patient often feels warmth and gratitude toward the expert helper, first in anticipation of relief and then in recognition of rapid improvement in the clinical state. This interpersonal exchange reflects functional expectations and skills of both parties. Relatively little explicit planning or discussion is needed to establish and maintain this working relationship.

In dealing with the more persistent and pervasive personality disorder, the role of the therapist subtly shifts. More specific effort is needed to foster acceptance of the therapist's influence, and understanding of barriers to the patients' efforts. A larger portion of the therapy time is devoted to becoming familiar with the patient's total life—children, spouse, job, personal history, interests. Such involvement by the therapist, provided it is kept within reasonable bounds, casts him or her in the role of friendly advisor. In fact, much of the therapist's role consists of drawing on his or her own life experiences and observations of others to propose possible solutions to problems, as well as to educate the patient regarding the nature of interpersonal relationships. This process of education and skill building is particularly important in treating patients with borderline personality disorder, whose own personality deficits or negative experiences may have prevented them from acquiring and consolidating basic skills and functional beliefs of self-control, stress tolerance, and stable relations with others.

In the course of time, the therapist ideally becomes a role model for the patient—someone the patient can emulate in showing consideration, tact, gratitude and understanding toward his or her own circle of intimates and friends. Many patients have remarked how they have learned to be cool and relaxed under stress, not to overreact to disappointment, to think before talking or acting on the basis of observing the therapist's example. On rare occasions, patients may go too far and incorporate their therapists' entire persona, but this too can be dealt with cognitively. For example, the therapist may want to explore the patient's reasons for discarding his or her own identity.

Establishing and maintaining this friendly working relationship, however, is often quite difficult and emotionally challenging. More of the therapist's energy is devoted to conceptualizing and working with the direct interaction between patient and therapist, as the interpersonal psychopathology is typically present in characteristic form during and between sessions. The therapist's expectations regarding the amount of effort needed, the relevance of immediate interpersonal exchanges, the target of an expanded interpersonal domain, and attributions regarding causes of difficulty in cooperation or progress may all require adjustment.

It can be quite useful to include collateral contacts with significant others in the patient's life to gain further information about the patient's difficulties and work directly on interpersonal problems. With some Axis II disorders, especially Cluster B, significant others may experience the greater distress and motivation for treatment. With adult patients, it is typically most constructive and consistent with boundaries of confidentiality to encourage the patient to invite the significant other to participate in a conjoint session, where the goals are either to work on a specific problem or to gather more information. With adolescent patients, a similar approach is advisable to maintain therapeutic rapport and share information with parents in a way that supports the growing autonomy of the teen.

Although the role of the therapist may shift in treating the personality disorder patient, basic therapeutic boundaries should be maintained at all times. Therapists strive to remain objective and responsible for ensuring that protective limits are kept intact, especially when the patient's skill deficits are taxed or impaired beliefs are highly activated (Newman, 1997). As in any professional psychotherapy, dual relationships and sexual involvements are explicitly prohibited (American Psychological Association, 2002; Koocher & Keith-Spiegel, 1998).

NONCOLLABORATION

Difficulties in collaboration can occur with any patient. The chronic and pervasive nature of personality disorders, however, makes the Axis II patient more prone to be noncollaborative or noncompliant than the Axis I patient. We have chosen the terms "noncollaboration" and "noncompliance" to distinguish a cognitive conceptualization from more traditional views of resistance as an expected and unconscious response. A number of behaviorally oriented volumes have addressed this important issue (A. Ellis, 1985; Shelton & Levy, 1981; Wachtel, 1982).

The schemas regarding change, view of self, and view of others can be extreme and highly exaggerated. This exaggerated view may then be expressed in a number of ways. The noncollaboration may be manifested directly through behavior that does not comply with agreed plans (e.g., tardiness or missing appointments) or more subtly through omissions in the material reported in the sessions. Passive noncollaboration that stems from a patient schema of low self-efficacy may be different from active avoidance triggered by negative, personalized meanings (Davis & Hollon, 1999). The most common themes of noncollaboration involve distrust of the therapist, unrealistic expectations, personal shame, externalized blame and grievances against others (either persons or institutions), deprecation of self or others, or fear of rejection and failure.

Occasionally, patients may show extreme forms of noncollaborative behaviors that cross the line into harassment, emotional abuse, or potential physical abuse of the therapist. In any extreme case, the therapist can conceptualize the possible reasons for the behavior and, at the same time, clearly label the behavior as a therapy-interfering process that cannot be allowed if therapy is to proceed (see Newman, 1997). Consultation with colleagues in instances of extreme patient behaviors is typically helpful for developing one's conceptualization of the noncompliance, generating ideas for effective contingencies that may redirect the therapy into a productive direction, and obtaining emotional support and appropriate self-protection.

There are many reasons for noncompliant behavior other than the patient's "not wanting to change" or "a pitched battle taking place between the patient's intra-psychic structures." These reasons can appear in any combination or permutation, and the relative strength of any noncompliant action may change with the patient's life circumstances, with progress in therapy, with the therapist's skill in addressing beliefs that interfere with collaboration, and so forth.

CONCEPTUAL UNDERSTANDING OF NONCOLLABORATION

Various causes of noncollaboration can be conceptualized in terms of skills, beliefs, and setting conditions. With an accurate conceptualization, an appropriate remedial plan can be targeted to the specific causes, using the technology of the cognitive model. Although these causes are described one at a time, multiple causes may apply to any given problem or any given patient across time.

To explore causes of noncollaboration, therapists may find a series of questions useful as follows. First, are there skill deficits contributing to this noncollaboration, either mine or the patient's? Are there interfering beliefs, either mine or the patient's? Are there setting conditions or contingencies interfering with progress? In what ways are these problems possibly blended? And finally, what can we do about this?

1. *The patient may lack the skill to collaborate.* Individual skill deficits may impair the patient's ability to work effectively with the therapist. For many patients, difficulty complying with the therapeutic regimen may parallel their problems in performing particular actions in their lives. Both areas of difficulty stem from inadequately developed skills. Although their skills may be adequate for "getting by" in certain areas, their skills may not be adequate for more complex tasks. For example, an Axis II patient may have well-developed academic or intellectual skills but lack practical life or social skills. The therapist may need to break tasks down by specific skills and teach or practice particular behaviors to help the patient collaborate and move along in therapy and thereby in life.

Clinical Example: Alan was a 39-year-old lawyer, diagnosed as having avoidant personality disorder. He entered therapy during his divorce because of thoughts that he could never find another woman, he would always be hurt, and therefore life was not worth living. He saw the goals of getting over his hurt and developing a social life as unrealistic for him. "It's not me," he would repeat over and over. A homework assignment over several sessions involved his calling a woman whose number was given to him by a colleague. During the eighth session, the therapist questioned Alan as to why the call was so difficult to make. Alan replied that he had virtually no experience in calling women for dates. The therapist asked Alan to role-play the phone call to the woman and discovered that Alan had no idea of what to say to her. After practicing several different approaches, Alan attempted the call in the office and was successful in setting a date.

His limited experience, combined with his characteristic avoidance, made it difficult for Alan to comply with the homework. If the therapist had not discovered this, Alan might never have complied. That failure could possibly have been interpreted as further evidence to support his beliefs about the hopelessness of ever having a mate again.

2. *The therapist may lack the skill to develop collaboration.* As we recognize the individual differences in our patients, we must also acknowledge that there are differences in therapists' skills. A therapist may not have the skill to work with a particular patient because of limited experience with a particular problem (e.g., trauma), a particular population (e.g., the elderly), or the level of severity of a problem (e.g., severely disturbed). Working within the context of an agency or hospital may facilitate consultation or supervision for the therapist on a particular case or problem. In some situations, however, consultative services may not be available. If the therapist's skills are not adequately developed to cope effectively with a problem, then transfer to another therapist is the ethical requirement. If, however, another therapist is not available, it is incumbent upon therapists to seek an upgrade in their skills through additional training. Continuing education through postgraduate courses, seminars, workshops, institutes, and self-study should be part of the ongoing professional growth of all therapists, no matter what their training or background.

Clinical Example: Maureen, a postdoctoral psychology fellow, was referred an 18-year-old female student, identified as having obsessive–compulsive personality disorder, with a presenting complaint of psychogenic urinary retention. The urinary retention was not only unhealthy and painful but socially problematic, as the student lived in a university dormitory with shared toilet facilities. Lacking experience with the problem of urinary retention, the therapist promptly brought this issue to her supervision meeting. However, the supervisor also had limited experience in treating female urinary retention. The two were unable to find any other therapist in their local community with experience in treating this problem, so they contacted colleagues from around the country to gather more data on treatment of this disorder. In addition, Maureen searched the literature for further technical information.

Given the unusual nature of the problem, the therapist needed to develop strategies and interventions so that she and her supervisor could work effectively with the patient. Maureen's research into female anatomy, exercise, and muscle control led her to the solution in a women's physical workout book: Kegel exercises. The patient was instructed in how to carry out these exercises and, through practice on her own, was able to gain greater control over her bladder. The behavioral therapy was done concurrently with the cognitive work of identifying and responding to the dysfunctional thoughts about urinating in a public toilet. This led in turn to the work of modifying the schema related to cleanliness, goodness, and perfectionism.

3. *The therapist underestimates the role of the patient's culture.* By definition, the problematic behavior or inner experience of the patient must markedly deviate from the expectations of the *individual's* culture (American Psychiatric Association, 2000), not the *therapist's* culture, to meet the criteria for personality disorder. An ethnocentric bias must be checked in making assumptions about the functional or dysfunctional elements of a patient's situation. Failure to do so can lead to a mismatch in the therapy goals, overpathologizing the patient, and patient feelings of being misunderstood or disrespected.

Clinical Example: Vidya, an Asian Indian graduate student, sought therapy for test anxiety as she was approaching major graduate examinations. Upon completion of her degree, she planned to return to her family home and proceed with a marriage arranged by her parents. She was distressed and perplexed by her therapist's formulation of a dependent personality disorder, and she did not agree with proposed therapeutic goals of increasing her assertiveness and ability to separate from her family.

4. *Beliefs of significant others may preclude change or reinforce dysfunctional behavior.* There may be circumstances or individuals in the patient's life that maintain the dysfunctional schema and the associated dysfunctional behaviors. The beliefs of significant others may be subtle or obvious deterrents to the patient's participation in therapy. These interfering beliefs may reflect some stigma about the use of therapy for change, discomfort with the predicted direction of that change, or distorted ideas about positive affect (sinful, undeserved, risky) or negative affect (saintly, justified). The message "Do not change" may be communicated either overtly or covertly. Overtly, a patient may be physically assaulted for talking of "private family matters with a stranger " or teased and verbally abused for being a "psycho," "needing to get your head shrunk," and wasting time and money on problems that are "just a crock of s——." Covertly, the message may be sent by the withdrawal of significant others, withholding of attention or affection, or spiteful actions that provoke the patient's distress. Even when contact with significant others is very limited or no longer active, significant beliefs about

the dangerousness or inappropriateness of allowing oneself to feel good may persist, arousing anxiety whenever self-enhancing efforts are pursued. The patient's experiences with significant others have led him or her to the conclusion that attempting to feel good will inevitably provoke ridicule, rejection, or some form of deflating event, with a net result of feeling worse for having taken the risk.

Clinical Example: Bob was a 30-year-old single male who lived at home with his parents. He was a college graduate, successfully employed as a customer service representative for a large corporation. Although his income was ample enough for him to be self-supporting, his parents insisted that he continue to live at home. Their genuine concern was that he could not manage his weight while living on his own, and he would relapse to his previous morbidly obese weight exceeding 300 pounds. Although he presently weighed 225 pounds, was in therapy, and attended weight management support group, their concern was overtly and covertly obvious. Bob felt torn when his mother wondered whether the therapy was putting unrealistic and dangerous ideas in his head if it led him to think about living on his own. He was frightened by their belief that he would fail in his weight management without their structure and guidance. His thoughts of disappointing them and doubts about his own role in his success kept him from attempting to live on his own. He stayed at home to allay their concern, to remain dependent and continue to be their little boy, and to cope with his own fears of a loss of control over food. He continued to believe, as did his parents, that worry was necessary to cope, and that feeling confident about his self-management was dangerous and unjustified.

5. Patients' ideas and beliefs regarding their potential failure in therapy may contribute to noncollaboration. The patient's thoughts about his or her personal success in the endeavor of therapy are important to address in any cognitive therapy. Detecting thoughts about potential failure and examining and learning to respond to these negative and self-deprecatory cognitions can be highly salient short-term objectives. Success can be cast as a dimensional, progressive effort rather than an all-or-nothing single outcome. Through the use of graded task assignments, small sequential steps, evaluation of responses and reactions to attempted changes, stress and anxiety inoculation, and therapeutic support for persistence, frustration tolerance, and the experimental process of discovery, the patient may become less focused on potential failure and more willing to attempt changes.

Clinical Example: Mitch, a 20-year-old college junior diagnosed with avoidant personality disorder, had very little social or dating experience. After living in a dorm for 2 years, he moved off campus to get away from having to see the active social lives of other men and women in his dorm as they dated, went to parties, and had numerous informal social contacts such as phone calls and casual conversations. Entering therapy, Mitch intellectually accepted the importance of a social life during his college years, but he also recognized his lack of skill, anxiety, and reluctance. His thoughts about therapy were similar to his thoughts about dating. In both situations, he saw himself as wanting to invest himself and succeed but predicted that he would be rejected because of his lack of skill or competence. Once the inevitable rejection occurred, he anticipated feeling even worse because of failure. His automatic thoughts about therapy (and dating) were as follows: "I'm better off not even trying. I'll just end up being ridiculed and feeling foolish. In fact, I'm better off dead. No one would even miss me. Any social life for me is doomed to failure, even this therapy."

6. *Patients resist collaboration because of beliefs that their changes will be detrimental to the well-being of others.* Another set of interfering beliefs involves the patient's magnified view of the detrimental consequences of his or her attempts to change on the lives of significant others. The patient may catastrophize his or her impact on others, thinking "something terrible will happen," even though related details about what would happen are vague and unspecified. In some instances, the significant other makes threats that the patient accepts without question.

Clinical Example: Marta, a 42-year-old never-married woman diagnosed with obsessive–compulsive personality disorder, lived with her mother, who was demanding and chronically preoccupied with her own physical health. Though quite healthy, she constantly visited doctors at Marta's expense. Marta feared that limiting her financial support of these unnecessary medical visits and saying no to other demands from her mother for time and attention would literally cause her mother to become sick and die. In addition, she believed that by remaining at home and sacrificing any personal life separate from her mother would have the effect of extending her mother's life. Her mother reinforced the idea that her health, her ability to cope, and her very reason for living depended on the constant caretaking of her daughter and that she "just knew something terrible would happen" if things were any different.

7. *The patient believes that therapy collaboration will destroy his or her personality or sense of self.* Axis II patients may perceive alterations in ideas, beliefs, or behaviors as a direct threat to their personal identity. Although this may seem paradoxical, in that their thinking makes them anxious, depressed, suicidal, or generally dysfunctional, these patients fear becoming unknown to themselves. They often choose the familiarity of their discomfort, no matter how destructive, to the discomfort and uncertainty of a new mode of thought or behavior.

Clinical Example: Mary had been chronically depressed and suicidal for 3 years, diagnosed with histrionic personality disorder in addition. She had been hospitalized four times for suicidal ideation, though she had never made an attempt. Her ideas about suicide were very dramatic. When confronted by her therapist with her style of thinking, she would state, "This is how I am. I've never been different. I can't imagine being any other way." She realized that her suicidal thinking was painful not only to herself but to significant others; she had great difficulty changing her perspective because of her strong disposition to believe that "This is me."

8. *The patient's and therapist's dysfunctional beliefs may be harmoniously blended.* A therapist's blind spot may be an impediment to progress with a particular patient when both share a particular dysfunctional idea (e.g., "Things are hopeless"). This sharing of belief, based on congruent underlying schemas, can result in the therapist's "buying into" the patient's hopeless ideas and beliefs.

Clinical Example: Dr. M's work was very careful and precise. She was prone to become obsessive when stressed. Her general belief was that extreme care and extra effort would help to reduce stress. Her thorough work was a major factor in her obtaining a 4.0 grade point average in her studies at a major university. When she selected a difficult patient to discuss in supervision, she described "a perfectionistic, obsessive, internally demanding man" whom she was trying to help "completely eliminate all of the perfectionism that makes him feel so hopeless." Rather than trying to modify the patient's perfectionism, she saw the total removal of the perfectionism as the therapeutic goal. The supervisor raised the idea that such a goal might actually reinforce the patient's problems. In reply, Dr. M tried to develop an argument in favor of perfectionist striving to always do one's best and not to settle for less than complete results.

9. *Poor socialization to the model may be a factor in noncompliance.* Patients who do not understand what is expected of them in therapy will typically have difficulty complying with homework instructions or recommendations. Socialization to the basics of cognitive therapy is a process that begins in the first session, perhaps even prior to that at a point of referral, and continues throughout the therapy work. Effective collaboration demands that the therapist prioritize time as much as necessary to explain terminology, concepts, the importance of the patient's active participation, and the objectives of skill building and self-help. Further, the therapist needs to elicit feedback to check the patient's level of understanding on an ongoing basis. Although it is important to demonstrate respect for the patient's effort and accomplishment in having read books on cognitive therapy or done research on the Internet, one cannot assume that this guarantees adequate socialization to cognitive therapy. Even prior cognitive therapy may not guarantee adequate socialization to the model. There may also be proactive interference because of involvement in previous therapy, particularly if the therapy was based on a different theoretical approach. In addition, the patient's ability to listen and understand may be impaired by hopelessness, impulsivity, selective abstraction, personalizing, or frustration with the effort of establishing yet another therapy relationship.

Clinical Example: Ed was a 42-year-old physician referred for cognitive therapy subsequent to the death of his psychoanalyst. Ed had been in psychoanalysis for 15 years, three sessions per week for most of that time, due to chronic depression and periodic suicidal thinking. After his analyst died, he attempted to continue analysis with another analyst but terminated after several months by mutual consent. He then entered cognitive therapy specifically to address his depression. At the beginning of each session, Ed began immediately to speak of his free associations. The therapist struggled to get a word in edgewise and felt quite frustrated with trying to establish an agenda as Ed pursued dreams, fantasies, and whatever came into his mind in the moment. Persistent but patient redirection and a scheduling of 10–15 minutes of free association at the beginning of the session helped to keep the rest of the session directed and focused. The therapist explicitly discussed the differences between cognitive therapy and analysis, validated Ed's feelings of disorientation with a new model, and asked for his participation in an experimental test of the usefulness a problem-focused session agenda. The 10 minutes of free association was then added to the agenda as part of Ed's collaborative contribution. After trying this for several sessions and evaluating the productivity of the session, both felt more satisfied with their work together.

10. *A patient may experience secondary gain from maintaining the dysfunctional pattern.* A patient may have great difficulty initiating or affecting change because his or her current condition has some significant benefit or payoff. Family members may treat the patient with "kid gloves," avoid any pressure or confrontation, and generally allow the patient to do whatever he or she wishes so as to decrease acting-out potential. Secondary gain may be obtained from family, friends, employers, or other individuals or systems with whom the patient interacts. This includes the interaction between the patient and the therapist. One potential way to address this secondary gain cognitively is to assess the "primary loss" that goes into achieving the secondary gain.

Clinical Example: Sid was a 38-year-old unemployed carpenter, diagnosed as having both passive–aggressive personality disorder and dependent personality disorder. He had not worked regularly in 5 years. His time was spent at home, watching television. His wife worked full-time and he collected disability support from government social security. He reported that when he exerted himself in any way, he was concerned about having a heart attack or even stroke. Even though he had never had either problem or, indeed, any major illness or family history of cardiovascular disease, his wife and two children were so concerned about his health that they never asked him to do anything at home. If pressed to find work, Sid would consider suicide rather than expose himself to the excruciating pain of the anxiety. A local community mental health center had been giving him letters that allowed him not to be pressured into working. Both Sid and his therapist believed, for reasons unspecified, that he simply "couldn't work." Sid's day involved getting up at 11:00 A.M., reading the newspaper until noon, and then watching television. When his children came home from school, he would take a nap and get up in time for dinner. After dinner, he would watch television or listen to music until it was time for bed. It was very difficult to initiate any change in this highly comfortable early "retirement."

11. *Poor timing of interventions may be a factor in noncompliance.* When interventions are rushed or untimely, the patient may appear to be noncompliant because the importance or relevance of the therapeutic work has not been sufficiently communicated. If the therapist, because of his or her anxiety, tries to push or rush the Axis II patient, the result may be the loss of collaboration, the missing of sessions, a misunderstanding of therapeutic issues, or a premature termination. Sometimes, therapists misunderstand the cognitive model as a "cookbook" approach and push the use of techniques in a rapid fashion to demonstrate their own expertise at the expense of sufficiently engaging the client in a learning and discovery process.

Clinical Example: Marie, a predoctoral intern, was learning to conduct cognitive therapy. As a result of her anxiety and internal pressure to succeed, she tended to attempt to interpret schemas without gathering enough data to support her interpretations or interventions. As a result, patients often responded by telling her that she was not understanding them, which further increased her anxiety and often caused her to make more grandiose leaps of interpretation and mistiming.

12. *Time limits of managed care may provoke reactance and alter collaboration.* There are many times when access to treatment is affected by insurance reimbursement with contract limits of a specified number of sessions. This can lead to collaboration problems when the therapist makes a pressured effort to complete treatment within these time limits, or when the patient becomes hopeless and focuses prematurely on the looming separation and end of treatment. Adjustment of the treatment goals and generating options for additional "courses" of therapy work can maximize the productive opportunity in any length of treatment contact.

Clinical Example: Dr. R was a participating provider of services on more than three dozen different insurance panels, and through these contracts typically had between 6 and 25 sessions of treatment that would be reimbursed per patient. For many patients, this was adequate for meeting specific treatment goals. However, Dr. R noted that his Axis II patients were more difficult to "get going" on specific homework assignments, and he felt frustrated when his patients failed to progress at the rate needed to complete treatment within the allotted time limits. He believed that his livelihood and the patient's continued insurability depended on completing treatment within these preset limits, no matter what the complications. To cope, he became increasingly directive, dominating sessions with advice, lectures, and demanding homework, allowing for little input from his Axis II patients. His rate of patient dropout after three or four sessions was quite high, which he believed was evidence that Axis II patients only wanted quick relief but did not want to make personal effort to change.

13. *The goals of therapy may be unstated.* There are times at which the goals of therapy may appear implicit in the initial presentation of the problem list. For example, implicit in "marital discord" may be relationship skill deficits, communication deficits, sexual skill deficits, parenting skill deficits, financial skill deficits, depression, or many other problems. The goals of therapy need to be made explicit in the context of the problem list. This list can, of course, be modified as the therapy progresses. Without baseline information about what the targets of therapy are, it becomes difficult to assess the progress of the therapy.

Clinical Example: Maryann, age 51, entered therapy for anxiety. It was clear after several sessions that the anxiety was part of a clinical picture that included obsessive–compulsive personality disorder. The therapist, working on helping Maryann to be more flexible, found that she became more agitated as the sessions progressed. At the sixth session, she announced she was leaving therapy because of her increased anxiety: "I thought therapy was supposed to help, not make me worse." The therapist had assumed that Maryann would be willing to change her rigid personality pattern, without ever discussing that pattern as a focus of the therapy.

14. *The goals of therapy may be vague and amorphous.* Patients typically present with vague statements about "getting my act together," "getting my head on straight," "dealing with my family issues," or "finding a happy life." The therapist must guide the patient to restate these goals as workable, observable, and operationally defined goals.

Clinical Example: Seth, age 19, was referred by his resident dormitory counselor because of his constant fighting. Seth had seen a counselor at the college counseling center and worked on "anger" and "problems in my background." After eight sessions, the counselor terminated the counseling with the note that Seth now had sufficient insight to allow change. The present referral was based on this insight not resulting in behavioral change. This time, the goals of the therapy were made clear and specific, with criteria for change, a graded task approach to relating to dormmates, and a discrete focus on his impulse control, use of nonoffensive language, and skills for respectful, assertive communication.

15. *The goals of therapy may be unrealistic.* This issue can come either from the patient or from the therapist. Goals that are unrealistically high or unrealistically low may establish a very negative set in the ther-

apy. If the patient wants to be a totally new person—that is, exactly opposite to the way he or she has been for the past 40 years—the therapist may have to help the patient set more realistic and graded goals. Change is possible, but setting out the goal of total change may set the patient up for failure. If the therapist has unrealistically high or low goals for the patient, the patient may feel either overwhelmed or demeaned by these expectations. Therapists may be less diligent or creative if they hold negative expectations about the patient's ability to change, a particular risk when working with Axis II patients.

Clinical Example: Nick, age 52, diagnosed with avoidant personality disorder, came for therapy because of his depression and isolation. He stated in the first session that he wanted to change his whole life. He had never been married, had not dated until he was 31, and had only dated a few times in his life. He saw the world as passing him by. He saw himself as aging and being alone in his old age. He reported crying when he watched television shows about families. His goal was to start dating immediately and be married within the year, as he wasn't getting any younger. This unrealistic goal would likely have set up a failure situation and sabotaged the therapy. Nick's therapist, on the other hand, believed that the chronicity of his problems predicted little chance for appreciable change. He focused primarily on reducing Nick's distress over being alone, and did little to help Nick expand his social network.

16. *There may have been no agreement between therapist and patient about the treatment goals.* Given that the goals of therapy are explicit and operationally defined, the patient and therapist need to check their agreement on the therapeutic goals. Developing a treatment plan and having the patient read and sign the plan are parts of informed consent procedure for treatment that is required in many mental health settings. Stating the goals for a set period (e.g., for 3 months), discussing the rationale for the goals, accepting patient input, negotiating changes, checking patient understanding, and getting and giving feedback are intrinsic to the cognitive therapy model. A review and reference back to treatment goals to check ongoing agreement as therapy proceeds is also crucial to maintaining collaboration across time.

17. *The patient feels forced into treatment and lacks motivation.* Many patients are sent to therapy against their will, under some outside pressure. Significant others may have threatened them to seek therapy or else suffer some great consequence. Other patients may have been referred against their will by the court. Because of a tendency to view themselves as victims of some other person or circumstance, such patients will be reluctant to shift their attention away from complaints about others toward possible constructive actions. The therapy work in such cases must focus initially on building a relationship, reducing per-

ceptions that therapy is an aggressive, forceful process that the patient has to fight against, and exploring the patient's interest in a range of options.

Clinical Example: Sam was a 59-year-old jeweler who was chronically depressed and intermittently suicidal because of his failing business. His perception was that his business difficulty was not his fault but had to do with the jewelers in large malls undercutting his prices. He saw no way to regain the lost income, customers, and status that he had once had and refused to "waste" money on advertising. Although he went to work daily, he allowed the store to become cluttered with boxes of "junk," sought no new business, and was surly and unpleasant when the occasional customer wandered in. He approached therapy in the same way. He did not want to come to therapy, saw no benefit in coming, complained about the time and cost involved, and agreed to come only to quiet his wife and daughter.

18. *The patient believes therapy is a passive or magical process.* As part of the clinical picture, some Axis II patients see both problems and solutions as external to themselves. They may appear to be highly motivated, but their motivation is to simply absorb some curative effect from being around the therapist. Some believe that it is the therapist's job to do all the work, with little or no input from them, and they hope to gain both insight and behavioral change from the remarkable observations and directions that the therapist will provide. They may idealize or flatter the therapist initially but easily become defensive or disenchanted with the expectations of productive therapy.

Clinical Example: Carolyn, a 40-year-old housewife with no children, entered therapy to "figure herself out" after a friend recommended cognitive therapy as a productive alternative to psychoanalysis. She had a history of recurrent depression and a personality disorder combining narcissistic and dependent features. After thorough explanation of the parameters of cognitive therapy and the importance of patient involvement, Carolyn remained vague about pinpointing any problems or goals, telling the therapist, "I expect you to figure that out." The homework of planning one or two items for the session agenda was explicitly assigned several times, and each time Carolyn returned for the following session without anything for the agenda but a pleasantly stated redirection of the session agenda to the therapist. When gently prompted for greater participation in the session structure, Carolyn became defensive and scolded the therapist for not meeting her expectations for advice and instructions.

19. *The patient's rigidity may foil compliance.* In many cases, the very problems that bring patients to therapy may be the major contributor to the noncompliance. With patients who are obsessive–compulsive or paranoid, among others, the rigidity of these patterns makes the patient obdurate and nonaccepting of influence. Such patients may, in fact,

question the therapist's motives or goals. More frequently, they find themselves unable to break out of the rigid position that they believe they must maintain to stay safe.

Clinical Example: Elena, a 28-year-old nurse diagnosed with paranoid personality disorder, saw the therapy (and the therapist) as extensions of her mother's need to control her. By maintaining her right to do whatever she wanted, including killing herself, she saw herself as being able to overcome her mother's power. The therapist had to take great care not to feed the distortion and in any way try to control the patient, as it might have meant Elena's making an attempt to die.

20. *The patient may have poor impulse control.* For patients with poor impulse control, the constraints of weekly sessions, a structured therapeutic approach, a set time for the session, or the time limit of the therapeutic hour may create anxiety or anger. The schemas of "doing what one wants when one wants" may fly in the face of the therapy. These patients often require the therapist to do what we term "brushfire therapy"—that is, constantly working at putting out the small brushfires and dealing with the crisis of the moment, rather than working on broader goals.

Clinical Example: Therapy with Alice was chaotic. At 23 years of age, she was in constant motion. She met criteria for borderline personality disorder. Her crises were related to her frequent job changes, frequent changes in friends and love relationships, frequent changes in residence, and frequent changes in therapists. Already, she had been married and divorced seven times. Within the session, she was quite labile, and any attempts to focus her either in the session or in her life were met with the familiar refrain, "It's just not me." Her missing of sessions, lateness, and inability to pay the fee because of her impulsive spending and erratic employment all served to sabotage the therapy interaction and therapeutic goal of reducing her impulsivity.

21. *The patient or therapist may be frustrated because of a lack of progress in therapy.* Given the long-term nature of Axis II problems, their generalized effect throughout the patient's life, and the long-term nature of the therapy, either patient or therapist, or both, can become frustrated. In either case, the result may be negative reactions to further therapy, thoughts about failure (either the therapist's or patient's), and anger toward the source of the perceived frustration (either therapist or patient).

Clinical Example 1: Pamela, a psychologist in supervision, was "thoroughly frustrated" by Lara, a patient with borderline personality disorder: "She doesn't change; she just keeps getting angry at the drop of the hat, usually at me.

I really dread the day when she is scheduled to come in, and am happy when she has to cancel." Having been quite successful in her work as a cognitive therapist working with more typical, uncomplicated depression, Pamela was not used to patients' taking so long in treatment or being oppositional: "I've read about borderline patients, heard about them, but never thought I would have this kind of trouble." The focus of supervision was on helping Pamela deal with her dysfunctional thoughts and expectations regarding therapy, the treatment of complex and difficult cases, and therapist emotional reactions.

Clinical Example 2: Marla had originally come to therapy to relieve her depression. The depression was superimposed on an obsessive–compulsive personality disorder. She chose cognitive therapy after reading of its short-term nature and demonstrated effectiveness, as described in several mass media publications. After 25 sessions, she demanded to know why she was not "cured" yet. The therapist had neglected to differentiate the symptom versus schema focus of the therapy.

22. *Issues involving the patient's perception of lowered status and self-esteem preclude compliance.* For many people, becoming "patients" implies that there is something fundamentally wrong with them. This means that they are "weak" persons, unable to cope with things that are normally expected. In addition, they may be stigmatized by others as "psychos," "nut cases," or "crazy."

Clinical Example: Roy, age 60, a successful businessman, was referred by his family physician because of his depression. His first statement in therapy was this: "I do not want to be here. Coming here has actually made me more depressed. I've never been a psycho patient before, and I don't want to be one now. This is not how a man of my generation was raised. I sneaked out of the house to come here, and parked down the street. Never call me at the office or at my home. No one can know that I am coming to a shrink."

The therapist must be aware of the myriad reasons for a patient's lack of collaboration or noncompliance with the therapeutic effort. These include, among others, lack of patient skill; lack of therapist skill; environmental stressors that preclude compliance; insufficient understanding of the patient's culture; patient cognitions regarding failure in therapy; patient cognitions regarding the effects on both self and others of the patient's changing; distorted congruence of patient and therapist; incomplete socialization to the cognitive model; secondary gain; poor timing of interventions; reactance to time limits of managed care; the goals of therapy being unstated, vague, or unrealistic; patient's lack of motivation or passive expectations; rigidity or poor impulse control; patient or therapist frustration; and issues revolving around the patient's lowered self-esteem.

Every effort is made in cognitive therapy to turn adversity to advantage. When a patient shows signs of noncollaboration, this is an opportunity to identify and explore beliefs and attitudes. The beliefs and attitudes that appear to interfere with the process of therapy are often the very beliefs and attitudes that complicate the pursuit of larger life goals. Once identified, these interfering beliefs can be explored within the collaborative framework of the cognitive model. Given the complexity of the personality disorder itself, combined often with acute Axis I problems that spark the referral for therapy, it is quite likely that there will be challenges to a smooth collaboration. Armed with the theoretical and practical skills of case conceptualization, the therapist can thoughtfully respond to the unique needs of different patient personalities. We consider it essential that therapists master the conceptual model of cognitive therapy and consistently follow the general and specific treatment guidelines offered in the earlier chapters. Reduction of the noncollaborative barriers to treatment will create both a stronger working alliance, and a more productive therapeutic interaction.

EMOTIONS IN THE THERAPEUTIC RELATIONSHIP: COGNITIVE CONCEPTUALIZATION OF TRANSFERENCE AND COUNTERTRANSFERENCE

Both patient and therapist are likely to experience strong emotional reactions to one another and the process of therapy in the course of treating an Axis II disorder. Traditionally, these reactions have been termed "transference," and "countertransference." To avoid confusion with psychodynamic assumptions and remain focused within the cognitive model, we refer to these simply as emotional reactions within the therapy process. Attention to emotional reactions of both patient and therapist is a fundamental component cognitive therapy with the Axis II patient.

Patient Emotions

The therapist should allow negative or positive reactions to him or her to arise but should not deliberately provoke or ignore them. He or she should be vigilant for signs of anger, disappointment, and frustration experienced by the patient in the therapeutic relationship. Similarly, the therapist should be alert to excessive praise, idealization, or attempts to divert the attention of therapy onto the therapist. These reactions open windows into the patient's private world. However, therapists cannot view the meanings or beliefs beyond these windows if the arousal of their own affective responses is viewed as a distraction to be controlled, avoided, or suppressed. One of the more common errors in cognitive therapy is moving too quickly away from emotions being expressed about the therapist or the therapy, and failing to sufficiently attend to this rich opportunity for further understanding of the patient.

There are many telltale signs of the patient's emotional response to the therapy and the associated cognitions. These are the same signs that suggest the presence of any automatic thoughts during the session. For instance, there may be a sudden change in the patient's nonverbal behavior—pauses in the middle of a train of statements, sudden change in expression, clenching fists, slumping posture, or a kicking or tapping foot. Or, the patient may abruptly switch to a new topic, stammer, block, and so on. One of the most revealing signs is a shift in the patient's gaze, especially if he or she has had a thought but prefers not to reveal it. When questioned, the patient may say, "It's not important. It's nothing." The therapist should press the patient nonetheless, gently, as it might be important. Some patients may have automatic thoughts throughout the interview, and it is not practical to report more than a few. However, they can keep track of the automatic thoughts and record them on paper.

Therapist Emotions

To effectively guide patients in discovering their thoughts and expressing their feelings, therapists need to have a foundation of skills for recognizing, labeling, understanding, and expressing their own emotions. Rather than having no feelings, or being an expert at repression, the cognitive therapist is attuned to personal emotions that might affect the therapy environment. Just as the therapist would encourage a client to do, cognitive therapists use awareness of their own physical sensations and subtle mood shifts as cues, suggesting the presence of automatic thoughts. Any changes in the therapist's typical behavior might also signal an emotional reaction and associated automatic thoughts, such as talking in a commanding (or hesitating) tone of voice, increased frequency of thoughts about a client outside sessions, or perhaps avoidance of returning a client's phone call or tardiness in starting or ending a session. The therapist can also use a self-directed inquiry of thoughts about a session or a situation or working with a particular client or Axis II problem and log these thoughts into a dysfunctional thought record.

The way the therapist views or deals with therapy-related thoughts and emotions may need some cognitive restructuring to reduce intensity of negative affect or to maintain adequate focus on therapy goals and objectives. First, it may be useful to confront any fears about therapist emotions being "mistakes" or indications of failure in therapy and instead focus on ways of understanding the emotional antecedents. Therapist emotions may stem from a number of sources, including the therapist's view of his or her professional role, cultural or value-related beliefs, and unique learning history, as well as from the interactions with the patient's problematic behaviors (Kimmerling, Zeiss, & Zeiss, 2000).

In preparing to work professionally with personality disorders, the therapist needs to be especially careful to be nonjudgmental. The very terms that we use to describe these disorders (narcissistic, compulsive, dependent, etc.) carry a pejorative taint. It is difficult to take the "personal" out of "personality," when we refer to the nature of the disorder. Once the therapist has made the diagnosis, it is much better to avoid labels and think in terms of beliefs, predictable reactions, meanings, behaviors, and so forth. It is valuable for the therapist to be sympathetic with the patient. By trying to put him- or herself in the patient's shoes—perhaps imagining him- or herself with the same set of sensitivities, sense of helplessness, and vulnerability—the therapist can better understand the patient. At the same time, the therapist has to be on guard not to become so involved with the patient's problems that objectivity is lost. Patient, persistent, and problem-focused in a nonjudgmental context describe the desired therapist demeanor.

Sheer willpower and good intentions, however, may not be sufficient for enacting this desired demeanor, given the many challenges in treating personality disorders. Emotional reactions of the therapist can be bridges to change rather than barriers to progress, if the therapist takes advantage of the cognitive technology. The therapist can guide him- or herself, perhaps with the help of supervision or consultation, to discover the meaning or judgment being applied to any given trigger situation. For example, consider the Dysfunctional Thought Record completed by a therapist regarding a difficult session with a patient with histrionic personality disorder (Figure 5.1).

Other forms of self-care and coping skills for stress management can be extremely useful as well. These may include options such as using self-statements of encouragement and acceptance (covertly) during sessions, targeting specific emotional or relationship objectives for a session and rating the degree one's mastery after the session, rehearsing calming images of working productively with a difficult patient, and improving the rate of positive comments in the session by recognizing and praising the client's strengths. Outside the therapy setting, it is important to make regular opportunities for pleasant activities, exercise, social contacts, and time away from work.

Although there is little doubt that therapist emotions play a significant role in treatment implementation and effectiveness, research endeavors are only beginning to adequately address the complexity of this topic. During the course of over 40 years of psychotherapy research,

Situation	Emotion	Automatic thought(s)	Rational response
Patient arrives late; persists with dramatic storytelling; breaks into sobs when therapist redirects to agenda setting.	Frustrated Disappointed Uncertain Embarrassed	This patient will never get it! We are making no progress using cognitive therapy. I don't know what to do next. I must be ineffective with this approach.	Contempt on my part will not help, so I could avoid such eternalized judgments and be more sympathetic. She is showing more skill in labeling affect, and identifying thoughts. Also, I'm focusing on the importance of making a list when her obvious priority is interpersonal support. I need to respect her values, help her learn to define problems, and not give up. Just because I feel uncertain does not mean I am ineffective, or have committed any shameful action. My discomfort comes from believing all patients must change quickly, and if they don't, it's my fault. Does it make sense that an effective therapist "never" feels uncertain? I can brainstorm some options to try next.

FIGURE 5.1. Therapist's Dysfunctional Thought Record.

therapist emotions have been placed at the classic split between practice and research, with therapist emotions emphasized as crucial to practice across a variety of theories, yet essentially no sophisticated empirical development has occurred (Najavits, 2000). In the absence of clarification, it is best to proceed with caution and be sensitive to the possibilities inherent in the emotional responses of both patient and therapist.

SUMMARY

In cognitive therapy with the Axis II patient, therapists are alert to the need for expanding the interpersonal domain and spending more time on developing their overall knowledge of the patient, as well as crafting an extended series of interactions to address the patient's skill deficits and impaired beliefs. A persistent, patient, problem-focused, nonjudgmental stance toward the patient and the process of therapy is essential. At the same time, sufficient boundaries for professional practice are never compromised. Difficulties in collaboration are conceptualized in terms of skills, beliefs, and possible setting conditions, as well as possible solutions targeted to this conceptualization. Strong emotional responses are accepted as vital to fully understanding the patient and engaging in active, productive therapy. When needed, cognitive tools can be used by the therapist as well as the patient to understand and potentially adjust these emotional responses.

PART II

CLINICAL APPLICATIONS

CHAPTER 6

Paranoid Personality Disorder

Individuals with paranoid personality disorder (PPD) are characterized by a persistent, unrealistic tendency to interpret the intentions and actions of others as demeaning or threatening, but they are free of persistent psychotic symptoms such as delusions or hallucinations. For example, Ann was a married secretary in her mid-30s who sought help due to problems with tension, fatigue, insomnia, and being short-tempered. She attributed these problems to job stress and when asked to describe the main sources of stress at work she reported, "People at work are constantly dropping things and making noise just to get me," and "They keep trying to turn my supervisor against me."

Ann described a long-standing tendency to ascribe malicious intentions to others, and she was unwilling to consider alternative explanations for the actions of her coworkers. She portrayed herself as typically sensitive, jealous, easily offended, and quick to anger. However, despite her unrealistic suspicions, there was no evidence of thought disorder, persistent delusions, or other symptoms of psychosis.

In Ann's case, her paranoia was obvious from the beginning of treatment. However, the disorder often is much less apparent initially and can easily be missed. For example, Gary was a single radiologist in his late 20s and had a steady girlfriend but was living with his parents while working full time and going to graduate school part time. He described himself as being chronically nervous and reported problems with worry, anxiety attacks, and insomnia. He said he was seeking therapy because his symptoms had intensified due to school pressures. During the interview he talked openly and seemed forthright. The initial interview was remarkable only for his not wanting his family to know he was in therapy "because they don't believe in it" and his not wanting to use his health insurance because of concerns about confidentiality. He explained that "at the hospital I see how much confidential information is just laying around."

Cognitive therapy, focused both on learning skills for coping more effectively with stress and anxiety and on examining his fears, continued unremarkably and effectively for six sessions. At the beginning of the seventh session Gary described a number of occasions on which progressive relaxation techniques "didn't work." In discussing these episodes he made comments including "It's like I don't want to relax," "Maybe I'm afraid of people just taking from me," "I don't want him stealing my idea," and "Every little thing you say is used against you." Finally he described people in general as "out to take you for what they can get."

Further discussion made it clear that a suspicious, defensive approach to interpersonal situations was characteristic of Gary's long-term functioning and played a central role both in his problems with stress and anxiety and in his difficulty using relaxation techniques. However, this had not been obvious through the first six sessions of therapy.

HISTORICAL PERSPECTIVES

The general topic of paranoia has been discussed since ancient times when the term was used freely to refer to all forms of serious mental disorder. Paranoia in its more modern meaning has received extensive attention from psychodynamic writers from Freud to the present. A typical view was presented by Shapiro (1965) who argued that the disorder is a result of "projection" of unacceptable feelings and impulses onto others. In theory, attributing unacceptable impulses to others rather than to oneself reduces or eliminates guilt over these impulses and thus serves as a defense against internal conflict. The psychoanalytic view, in essence, is that the individual inaccurately perceives in others that which is actually true of him- or herself and, as a result, experiences less distress than would result from a more realistic view of self and others.

A cognitive-behavioral model of paranoia that is similar to this traditional view has been presented by Colby and his colleagues (Colby, 1981; Colby, Faught, & Parkinson, 1979). These investigators developed a computer simulation of a paranoid client's responses in a psychiatric interview that is sufficiently realistic that experienced interviewers are unable to distinguish between the responses of the computer and the responses of a paranoid client as long as the interview is narrow in scope (Kochen, 1981). Colby's model is based on the assumption that paranoia is actually a set of strategies directed toward minimizing or forestalling shame and humiliation. The paranoid individual is assumed to believe strongly that he or she is inadequate, imperfect, and insufficient. This assumption is believed to result in intolerable levels of shame and humiliation in situations such as being the object of ridicule, being falsely accused, or developing a physical disability. Colby hypothesized that when a "humiliating" situation occurs, the individual can avoid accepting the blame and the consequent feelings of shame and humiliation by blaming someone else for the event and asserting that he or she was mistreated.

PPD per se has received attention from a number of authors. Cameron (1963, 1974) saw the disorder as stemming from a basic lack of trust that results from parental mistreatment and a lack of consistent parental love. The child learns to expect sadistic treatment from others, to be vigilant for signs of danger, and to act quickly to defend him- or herself. The individual's vigilance results in him or her detecting subtle cues of negative reactions in others and then reacting strongly to them, at the same time having little awareness of the impact of his or her own hostile attitudes on others.

Like Cameron, Millon (1996) described the paranoid individual's lack of trust as playing a central role in PPD. The lack of trust is hypothesized to give rise to a strong fear of being coerced and controlled by others and as playing an important role in the individual's interpersonal problems. In addition, the lack of trust and fear of being coerced or controlled by others results in interpersonal isolation which deprives the paranoid individual of "reality checks" that might restrain his or her suspicions and fantasies. However, Millon (1996, p. 701) argues that there is no consistent set of attributes which is the "essence" of PPD. Instead he discusses five subtypes rather than providing an overall conceptualization of this disorder.

Turkat (1985, 1986, 1987, 1990; Turkat & Banks, 1987; Turkat & Maisto, 1985) has presented a cognitive-behavioral model of the development and maintenance of PPD that is based on detailed examination of clinical cases. Turkat's view was that early interactions with parents teach the child, "You must be careful about making mistakes" and "You are different from others." These two beliefs are hypothesized to result in the individual's being quite concerned about the evaluations of others but also being constrained to conform to parental expectations which interfere with acceptance by peers. This results in the individual's eventually being ostracized and humiliated by peers but lacking the interpersonal skills needed to overcome the ostracism. Consequently, the individual spends much time ruminating about his or her isolation and mistreatment by peers and eventually concludes that he or she is being persecuted because he or she is special and the others are jealous. This "rational" explanation is hypothesized to reduce the individual's distress over the social isolation. It is argued that the resulting paranoid view of others perpetuates the individual's isolation both because the individual's anticipation of rejection results in considerable anxiety regarding social interactions and because acceptance by others would threaten this explanatory system.

RESEARCH AND EMPIRICAL DATA

Limited research has been conducted on PPD, perhaps in part because of the difficulty of assembling a pool of subjects. Much of the available data come from studies in which PPD was one of many personality disorders that were examined. Research to date provides evidence that genetics play a role in this disorder. For example Coolidge, Thede, and Jang (2001) obtained a heritability coefficient of .50 for paranoid features in a study of 112 twins, ages 4 to 15. Other studies provide evidence that early experience plays a role as well demonstrating that verbal abuse (Johnson et al., 2001), conflict with parents (Klonsky, Oltmanns, Turkheimer, & Fiedler, 2000), and both emotional neglect and supervision neglect (Johnson, Smailes, Cohen, Brown, & Bernstein, 2000) are implicated. There is also empirical support for the proposition that both dysfunctional cognitions (Beck et al., 2001) and dysfunctional coping strategies (Bijettebier & Vertommen, 1999) play a role in this disorder as well as other personality disorders. Unfortunately, the available evidence is not adequate to test the conceptualization of PPD presented in this chapter or to provide grounds for conclusions regarding the efficacy of the treatment approach which is proposed.

DIFFERENTIAL DIAGNOSIS

As can be seen from reviewing the diagnostic criteria presented in Table 6.1, PPD is characterized by a persistent paranoid outlook which is not accompanied by thought disorder, hallucinations, or persistent delusions. Despite the clear diagnostic criteria provided in DSM-IV-TR (American Psychiatric Association, 2000), diagnosis of PPD is not always easy because these clients rarely enter therapy saying, "Doc, my problem is that I'm paranoid."

Paranoid individuals have a strong tendency to blame others for interpersonal problems, usually can cite many experiences which seem to justify their convictions about others, are quick to deny or minimize their own problems, and often have little recognition of the ways in which their behavior contributes to their problems. Thus, when an assessment is based on the client's self-report, it can easily appear that the

TABLE 6.1. DSM-IV-TR Diagnostic Criteria for Paranoid Personality Disorder

A. A pervasive distrust and suspiciousness of others such that their motives are misinterpreted as malevolent, beginning in early adulthood and present in a variety of contexts, as indicated by four (or more) of the following:

  (1) suspects, without sufficient basis, that others are exploiting, harming, or deceiving him or her
  (2) is preoccupied with unjustified doubts about the loyalty or trustworthiness of friends or associates
  (3) is reluctant to confide in others because of unwarranted fear that the information will be used maliciously against him or her
  (4) reads hidden demeaning or threatening meanings into benign remarks or events
  (5) persistently bears grudges, i.e., is unforgiving of insults, injuries, or slights
  (6) perceives attacks on his or her character or reputation that are not apparent to others and is quick to react angrily or to counterattack
  (7) has recurrent suspicions, without justification, regarding the fidelity of spouse or sexual partner

B. Does not occur exclusively during the course of Schizophrenia, a Mood Disorder With Psychotic Features, or another Psychotic Disorder and is not due to the direct physiological effects of a general medical condition.

Note. From American Psychiatric Association (2000, p. 694). Copyright 2000 by the American Psychiatric Association. Reprinted by permission.

client's suspicions are justified or that the problems are due to inappropriate actions by others. In addition, because the characteristics of paranoia are understood to some extent by most laymen, paranoid individuals are likely to recognize that others consider them to be paranoid, and to realize that it is prudent to keep their thoughts to themselves. When this is the case, indications of paranoia tend to emerge only gradually over the course of therapy and may easily be missed.

Often it is easiest to identify paranoid individuals by watching for characteristics other than blatantly unrealistic suspicions. Table 6.2 presents a number of possible signs of a paranoid personality style which may be early indications of PPD. Individuals with PPD are typically quite vigilant, tend to interpret ambiguous situations as threatening, and are quick to take precautions against perceived threats. They frequently are perceived by others as argumentative, stubborn, defensive, and unwilling to compromise. They also may manifest some of the characteristics they perceive in others, being seen by others as devious, deceptive, disloyal, hostile, and malicious.

Several distinct disorders are characterized by "paranoid" thinking. In addition to PPD, these are schizophrenia, paranoid type (formerly paranoid schizophrenia), delusional disorder, persecutory type (formerly paranoid disorder), and possibly mood disorder with psychotic features. Each of these other disorders is characterized by persistent paranoid de-

TABLE 6.2. Possible Indications of Paranoid Personality Disorder

Constant vigilance, possibly manifested as a tendency to scan the therapist's office during the interview and/or to glance frequently out the window.

Greater than normal concern about confidentiality, possibly including reluctance to allow the therapist to maintain progress notes and/or requests that the therapist take special steps to assure confidentiality when returning telephone calls from the client.

A tendency to attribute all blame for problems to others and to see him- or herself as being mistreated and abused.

Recurrent conflict with authority figures.

Unusually strong convictions regarding the motives of others and difficulty considering alternative explanations for their actions.

A tendency to interpret small events as having great significance and thus react strongly, apparently "making mountains out of molehills."

A tendency to counterattack quickly in response to a perceived threat or slight, or a tendency to be contentious and litigious.

A tendency to receive more than his or her share of bad treatment from others or to provoke hostility from others.

A tendency to search intensely and narrowly for evidence which confirms his or her negative expectations regarding others, ignoring the context and reading (plausible) special meanings and hidden motives into ordinary events.

Inability to relax, particularly when in the presence of others, possibly including unwillingness or inability to close his or her eyes in the presence of the therapist for relaxation training.

Inability to see the humor in situations.

An unusually strong need for self-sufficiency and independence.

Disdain for those he or she sees as weak, soft, sickly, or defective.

Difficulty expressing warm, tender feelings or expressing doubts and insecurities.

Pathological jealousy, persistent attempts to control partner's behavior and interpersonal relationships in order to prevent infidelity.

---

lusions and other psychotic symptoms. In contrast, PPD is characterized by an unwarranted tendency to perceive the actions of others as intentionally threatening or demeaning but is free of persistent psychotic features (American Psychiatric Association, 2000). An individual with PPD may experience transient periods of delusional thinking during periods of stress but does not manifest persistent delusional thinking.

Schizophrenia, paranoid type and delusional disorder have been the subject of much theoretical attention and empirical research; however, there is no clear consensus regarding the relationship between PPD and these two psychoses (Turkat, 1985). Thus, it is not clear whether the findings of research conducted on psychotic samples can be generalized to PPD or not. However, it is clearly important to differentiate between PPD and the psychoses that are characterized by paranoid thinking because the presence of psychosis would call for major adjustments in the treatment approach. See Perris and McGorry (1998) for an overview of current approaches to applying cognitive therapy in the treatment of psychosis.

CONCEPTUALIZATION

A number of the aforementioned theoretical perspectives on PPD share the view that the individual's suspicions regarding others and his or her ruminations about persecution and mistreatment at the hands of others are not central to the disorder but are rationalizations used to reduce the individual's subjective distress. A different view of the role of these cognitions in PPD is presented in the cognitive analysis developed by the author (Beck, Freeman, & Associates, 1990; Freeman, Pretzer, Fleming, & Simon, 1990; Pretzer, 1985, 1988; Pretzer & Beck, 1996). Figure 6.1 summarizes the cognitive and interpersonal components of the paranoid approach to life manifested by Gary, the tense radiologist discussed earlier. Gary held three basic assumptions: "People are malevolent and deceptive," "They'll attack you if they get the chance," and "You can be OK only if you stay on your toes." These assumptions led him to expect deception, trickery, and harm in interpersonal interactions and led him to conclude that vigilance for signs of deception, trickery, and malicious intentions was constantly necessary. However, this vigilance for signs of malicious intentions produced an unintended side effect. If one is vigilant for subtle indications that others are deceptive and malicious (and not equally vigilant for signs of trustworthiness and good intentions), one quickly observes many actions on the part of others that seem to support the view that people cannot be trusted. This happens both because people are not universally benevolent and trustworthy and because many interpersonal interactions are sufficiently ambiguous that

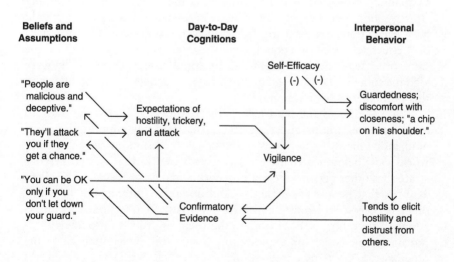

FIGURE 6.1. Cognitive conceptualization of paranoid personality disorder.

they can appear to reveal malicious intentions even if the individual's actual intentions are benign. Thus, as is shown in Figure 6.1, Gary's vigilance produced substantial evidence to support his assumptions about human nature and tended to perpetuate his paranoid approach to life.

In addition, Gary's expectations regarding the actions of others had an important effect on his interactions with colleagues and acquaintances. He avoided closeness for fear that the emotional involvement and openness involved in close relationships would increase his vulnerability. In addition, he was generally guarded and defensive while interacting with others, tended to overreact to small slights, and was quick to counterattack when he believed he had been mistreated. These actions did not encourage others to be kind and generous towards him but rather tended to provoke distrust and hostility from others. Thus, Gary's expectations led him to interact with others in a way that provoked the type of behavior that he anticipated and provided him with the repeated experience of being treated badly by others. These experiences, of course, supported his negative expectations of others and also perpetuated his paranoid approach to life.

The third factor shown in Figure 6.1 is self-efficacy, a construct which Bandura (1977) has defined as the individual's subjective estimate of his or her ability to cope effectively with specific problems or situations as they arise. If Gary had been confident that he could easily see through the deceptions of others and thwart their attacks, he would have felt less need to be constantly on guard and thus would have been both less vigilant and less defensive. If he had been convinced that he could not cope effectively despite his efforts, he would have been likely to abandon his vigilance and defensiveness and adopt some other coping strategy. In either case, the cycles that perpetuated his paranoia would have been attenuated or disrupted. However, Gary doubted his ability to deal effectively with others unless he was constantly vigilant and, at the same time, was fairly confident that he could at least survive if he were vigilant enough. Thus, he maintained his guardedness and vigilance and this perpetuated his paranoia.

In addition to the tendency of the two cycles discussed earlier to generate observations and experiences that strongly support the paranoid individual's assumptions, another factor results in the paranoid's world view being nearly impervious to experiences that should demonstrate that other persons are not universally malicious. Because the client assumes that people are malicious and deceptive, interactions in which other people seem benign or helpful can easily be interpreted as an attempt to trick him or her into trusting them in order to provide an opportunity for attack or exploitation. Once this interpretation of the other person's acts as deceptive occurs, the "fact" that the person has tried to deceive the client by acting nice or trustworthy seems to prove that their intentions are malicious. This leads to the commonly observed tendency of paranoid individuals to reject "obvious" interpretations of the actions of others and to search for the "real" underlying meaning. Usually, this search continues until an interpretation consistent with the paranoid individual's preconceptions is found.

The paranoid's conviction that he or she faces dangerous situations in which vigilance is needed to remain safe accounts for many of the characteristics of PPD. Vigilant for signs of danger, the individual acts cautiously and purposefully, avoiding carelessness and unnecessary risks. Because the most important danger is seen as coming from others, the paranoid is alert for signs of danger or deception during interactions, constantly scanning for subtle cues of the individual's true intentions. In such a "dog eat dog" world, to show any weakness is to court attack; thus the paranoid carefully conceals his or her insecurities, shortcomings, and problems through deception, denial, excuses, or blaming others. Assuming that anything others know about an individual may be used against him or her, the paranoid carefully guards his or her privacy, striving to suppress even trivial information and, in particular, suppressing signs of his or her own emotions and intentions. In a dangerous situation, any restrictions on one's freedom can leave one trapped or increase one's vulnerability; thus the paranoid tends to resist rules and regulations. The more powerful another individual is, the more of a threat he or she poses. Thus the paranoid is keenly aware of power hierarchies, both admiring and fearing persons in positions of authority, hoping for a powerful ally but fearing betrayal or attack. Typically the paranoid individual is unwilling to "give in" even on unimportant issues, because compromise is seen as a sign of weakness and the appearance of weakness might encourage attack. However, he or she is reluctant to directly challenge powerful individuals and risk provoking attack. As a result, covert or passive resistance is common.

When one is vigilant for signs of threat or attack and presumes malicious intentions, it follows that any slights or mistreatments are intentional and malicious and deserve retaliation. When others protest that their actions were unintentional, accidental, or justified, their protestations are seen as evidence of deception and as proof of their malicious intentions. Given that attention is focused on mistreatment by others, yet any apparently good treatment by others is discounted, situations constantly seem unfair and unjust. Because the individual believes that he or she has been treated unfairly and is convinced that he or she will be treated badly in the future, there is little incentive to treat others well except for fear of their retaliation. Thus, when the paranoid individual feels powerful enough to resist retaliation from others or believes that he or she can escape detection, that individual is likely to engage in the malicious, deceptive, hostile acts which he or she expects from others.

There are a number of differences between this view of PPD (also see Freeman et al., 1990; Pretzer, 1985, 1988; Pretzer & Beck, 1996) and those presented by Colby (1981; Colby et al., 1979) and Turkat (1985). First, in this conceptualization, the individual's attribution of malicious intentions to others is seen as being central to the disorder rather than as a complex side effect of other problems. Thus, there is no need to assume that these suspicions of others are due to "projection" of unacceptable impulses, are attempts to avoid shame and humiliation by blaming others (Colby et al., 1979), or are a rationalization used to cope with social isolation (Turkat, 1985). Second, although the fear of making mistakes emphasized by Turkat is commonly observed in these clients, it is seen as secondary to the assumption that others are dangerous and malicious rather than as central to the disorder. Finally, the importance of the individual's sense of self-efficacy is emphasized in this model. At this point the empirical evidence needed to determine which model of PPD is most valid is not available.

In discussing PPD, Turkat (1985) presented his ideas about the development of the disorder at length. This author has not developed an equally detailed perspective on the etiology of PPD because it is difficult to determine the accuracy of historical information obtained from paranoid clients. In clinical practice, paranoid clients' views of others and their recollections of previous events are frequently found to be distorted in a paranoia-congruent way. This observation raises the possibility that their reports of childhood experiences may be distorted as well. However, it is interesting to note that a paranoid stance would be adaptive if one were faced by a truly dangerous situation where others were likely to prove to be overtly or covertly hostile. Many paranoid clients describe growing up in families they experienced as quite dangerous. For example, Gary described a long history of being ridiculed for any sign of sensitivity or weakness, of being lied to and cheated by parents and siblings, and of verbal and physical assaults by family members. In addition, he reported being explicitly taught by his parents that the world was a "dog eat dog" place where one must be tough to survive. Such accounts give the impression that growing up in a generally hostile or paranoid family where vigilance is truly necessary could contribute substantially to the development of PPD. Such a hypothesis is appealing, but it will remain speculative until it is possible to obtain more objective data regarding the histories of these individuals. A comprehensive theoretical treatment of the etiology of PPD would also need to account for studies which find an unusually high incidence of "schizophrenic spectrum" disorders among relatives of individuals diagnosed with PPD (Kendler & Gruenberg, 1982). Such findings raise the possibility of a genetic contribution to the etiology of the disorder, but the mechanisms through which such a link could occur are not yet understood.

TREATMENT APPROACH

At first glance, the conceptualization summarized in Figure 6.1 may appear to provide little opportunity for effective intervention. One goal of intervention would be to modify the individual's basic assumptions because these are the foundation of the disorder. However, how can one hope to challenge these assumptions effectively when the client's vigilance and paranoid approach to interactions constantly produce experiences that seem to confirm the assumptions? If it were possible to get the client to relax his or her vigilance and defensiveness, it would simplify the task of modifying assumptions. But how can the therapist hope to induce the client to relax his or her vigilance or to treat others more nicely as long as the client is convinced that they have malicious intentions? If these two self-perpetuating cycles were the whole of the cognitive model there would be little prospect for effective cognitive-behavioral intervention with these clients. However, the client's sense of self-efficacy plays an important role in the model as well.

The paranoid individual's intense vigilance and defensiveness is a product of the belief that this is necessary to preserve his or her safety. If it is possible to increase the client's sense of self efficacy regarding problem situations so that he or she is reasonably confident of being able to handle problems as they arise, then the intense vigilance and defensiveness seem less necessary. This should result in some decrease in vigilance and defensiveness that could substantially reduce the intensity of the client's symptomatology, making it much easier to address the client's cognitions through conventional cognitive therapy techniques and making it more possible to persuade the client to try alternative ways of handling interpersonal conflicts. Therefore, the primary strategy in the cognitive treatment of PPD is to increase the client's sense of self-efficacy before attempting to modify other aspects of the client's automatic thoughts, interpersonal behavior, and basic assumptions.

Collaboration Strategy

Establishing a collaborative relationship is obviously no simple task, considering that one is working with someone who assumes others are likely to prove malevolent and deceptive. Direct attempts to convince the client to trust the therapist are apt be perceived by the client as deceptive, provoking the client's suspicions. The approach that proves most effective is for the therapist to openly accept the client's distrust once it has become apparent and to gradually demonstrate trustworthiness through action rather than pressing the client to trust him or her immediately. For example, once it was clear that Gary, the radiologist, was generally distrustful of others, the issue was addressed as follows:

GARY: I guess that's what I do all the time, expect the worst of people. Then I'm not surprised.

THERAPIST: You know, it strikes me that this tendency to be skeptical about others and to be slow to trust them seems like something that would be likely to come up in therapy from time to time.

GARY: Umm . . . (*pause*).

THERAPIST: After all, how are you to know if it's safe to trust me or not? People tell me I have an honest face but what does that prove? I've got a degree after my name, but you know that doesn't prove I'm a saint. Hopefully the things I'm saying make sense, but you're not dumb enough to trust someone just because he's a good talker. It seems like it could be hard for a person to decide whether to trust a therapist or not, and that puts you in a tough situation. It's hard to get help without trusting at least a little but it's hard to tell if it's safe to trust . . . How's that sound so far?

GARY: You've got it about right.

THERAPIST: One way out of that dilemma is to take your time and see how well I follow through on what I say. It's a lot easier to trust actions than words.

GARY: That makes sense.

THERAPIST: Now if we're going to take that approach we'll need to figure out what to work on first . . .

It is then incumbent upon the therapist to make a point of proving trustworthy, and ideally this is not difficult. It includes being careful only to make offers he or she is willing and able to follow through on, making an effort to be clear and consistent, actively correcting the client's misunderstandings and misperceptions as they occur, and openly acknowledging any lapses that do occur. It is important for the therapist to remember that it takes time to establish trust and to refrain from pressing the client to talk about sensitive thoughts or feelings until sufficient trust has gradually been established. Standard cognitive techniques such as the use of the Dysfunctional Thought Record may require too much self-disclosure for the client to be willing to comply with them early in therapy. Thus, it may be useful to select a problem that can be addressed primarily through behavioral interventions as the initial focus of therapy.

Collaboration is always important in cognitive therapy, but it is especially important in working with paranoid individuals, because they are likely to become intensely anxious and/or angry if they feel coerced, treated unfairly, or placed in a "one-down" position. It is important to focus on understanding and working toward accomplishing the client's goals for therapy. Some therapists fear that in focusing on the client's stress, marital problems, and so on, the "real problem" of their paranoia might be missed. However, by using a problem-solving approach in pursuing the client's goals, the ways in which his or her paranoia contributes to the other problems will quickly become apparent. This creates a situation in which it is possible to engage the client in working collaboratively on his or her distrust of others, feelings of vulnerability, defensiveness, and so on because doing so is an important step toward attaining the client's goals for therapy.

The initial phase of therapy can be quite stressful to paranoid clients even when it seems to the therapist that the focus is on superficial topics that should not be at all threatening. Simply participating in therapy requires the client to engage in a number of activities that paranoid individuals experience as being very dangerous. These include disclosing one's thoughts and feelings, acknowledging weakness, and trusting another person. This stress can be reduced somewhat by focusing initially on the least sensitive topics, by starting with more behavioral interventions, and by discussing issues indirectly (i.e., through the use of analogies or through talking about how "some people" react in such situations) rather than pressing for direct self-disclosure. One of the more effective ways to increase a paranoid client's comfort with therapy is to give him or her even more than the usual amount of control over the content of sessions, homework assignments, and especially the frequency of sessions. The client may be more comfortable and may progress more quickly if sessions are scheduled less frequently than the usual once per week.

Specific Interventions

In beginning work on the client's initial goals, it is most productive to focus on increasing the client's sense of self-efficacy regarding problem situations, or to increase the client's conviction that he or she can cope with any problems that arise. There are two main ways this can be done. First, if the client is capable of handling the situation but overestimates the threat posed by the situation or underestimates his or her capacity for handling the threat, interventions that result in a more realistic appraisal of the individual's ability to cope will increase self-efficacy. Second, if the client is not capable of handling the situation, or if there is room for improvement in his or her coping skills, interventions that improve coping skills will increase self-efficacy. In practice, it often works best to use the two approaches in combination.

With Ann (the secretary mentioned earlier), the therapist's initial attempts to directly challenge her paranoid ideation ("They are making noise just to get me") were ineffective. However, efforts to help her re-

evaluate the extent of danger posed by the actions of her provoking coworkers and reevaluate her capacity for coping with the situation were
quite effective. For example:

THERAPIST: You're reacting as though this is a very dangerous situation.
    What are the risks you see?

ANN: They'll keep dropping things and making noise to annoy me.

THERAPIST: Are you sure nothing worse is a risk?

ANN: Yeah.

THERAPIST: So you don't think there's much chance of them attacking
    you or anything?

ANN: Nah, they wouldn't do that.

THERAPIST: If they do keep dropping things and making noises how bad
    will that be?

ANN: Like I told you it's real aggravating. It really bugs me.

THERAPIST: So it would continue pretty much as it has been going for
    years now.

ANN: Yeah, it bugs me, but I can take it.

THERAPIST: And you know that if it keeps happening, at the very least
    you can keep handling it the way you have been—holding the ag-
    gravation in, then taking it out on your husband when you get
    home. . . . Suppose we could come up with some ways to handle the
    aggravation even better or to have them get to you less—is that
    something you'd be interested in?

ANN: Yeah, that sounds good.

THERAPIST: Another risk you mentioned earlier was that they might talk
    to your supervisor and turn her against you. As you see it, how long
    have they been trying to do this?

ANN: Ever since I've been there.

THERAPIST: How much luck have they had so far in doing that?

ANN: Not much.

THERAPIST: Do you see any indications that they're going to have any
    more success now than they have so far?

ANN: No, I don't guess so.

THERAPIST: So your gut reaction is as though the situation at work is re-
    ally dangerous. But when you stop and think it through, you con-
    clude that the worst they're going to do is to be really aggravating
    and that, even if we don't come up with anything new, you can han-
    dle it well enough to get by. Does that sound right?

ANN: (*smiling*) Yeah, I guess so.

THERAPIST: And if we can come up with some ways to handle the stress better or handle them better, there will be even less they can do to you.

Clearly, this interchange alone did not transform Ann dramatically, but following this session she reported a noticeable decrease in vigilance and stress at work that apparently was due to her perceiving the work situation as much less threatening. This resulted in her noticing fewer apparent provocations and consequently experiencing less anger and frustration. Further rapid improvement was achieved by reevaluating perceived threats and improving stress management, assertion, and marital communication. According to her husband's report as well as her own, Ann continued to be somewhat guarded and vigilant but no longer overreacted to minor provocations. In addition, she was able to be assertive rather than hostile, no longer exploded at her husband as a result of aggravations at work, and was significantly more comfortable visiting her in-laws.

With Gary, the young radiologist, by the time that his PPD was recognized, the successful stress-management interventions described previously had already raised his sense of self-efficacy substantially. However, he still felt that vigilance was necessary in many innocuous situations because he doubted his ability to cope if he was not constantly vigilant. It became clear that he had strict standards for competence in work and in social interactions. Further, his dichotomous view of competence held that either one was fully competent or totally incompetent. The "continuum technique" was used to help Gary reevaluate his view of competence:

THERAPIST: It sounds like a lot of your tension and your spending so much time double-checking your work is because you see yourself as basically incompetent and think "I've got to be careful or I'll really screw up."

GARY: Sure. But it's not just screwing up something little; someone's life could depend on what I do.

THERAPIST: Hmm. We've talked about your competence in terms of how you were evaluated while you were in training and how well you've done since then without making much headway. It occurs to me that I'm not sure exactly what "competence" means for you. What does it take for somebody to really qualify as competent? For example, if a Martian came down knowing nothing of humans and he wanted to know how to tell who was truly competent, what would you tell him to look for?

GARY: It's someone who does a good job at whatever he's doing

THERAPIST: Does it matter what the person is doing? If someone does well at something easy, do they qualify as competent in your eyes?

GARY: No, to really be competent they can't be doing something easy.

THERAPIST: So it sounds like they've got to be doing something hard and getting good results to qualify as competent.

GARY: Yeah.

THERAPIST: Is that all there is to it? You've been doing something hard and doing well at it, but you don't feel competent.

GARY: But I'm tense all the time and I worry about work.

THERAPIST: Are you saying that a truly competent person isn't tense and doesn't worry?

GARY: Yeah. They're confident. They relax while they're doing it and they don't worry about it afterward.

THERAPIST: So a competent person is someone who takes on difficult tasks and does them well, is relaxed while he's doing them, and doesn't worry about it afterwards. Does that cover it or is there more to competence?

GARY: Well, he doesn't have to be perfect as long as he catches his mistakes and knows his limits.

THERAPIST: What I've gotten down so far [the therapist has been taking notes] is that a truly competent person is doing hard tasks well and getting good results, he's relaxed while he does this and doesn't worry about it afterward, he catches any mistakes he makes and corrects them, and he knows his limits. Does that capture what you have in mind when you use the word competent?

GARY: Yeah, I guess it does.

THERAPIST: From the way you've talked before, I've gotten the impression that you see competence as pretty black and white, either you're competent or you aren't.

GARY: Of course. That's the way it is.

THERAPIST: What would be a good label for the people who aren't competent? Does incompetent capture it?

GARY: Yeah, that's fine.

THERAPIST: What would characterize incompetent people? What would you look for to spot them?

GARY: They screw everything up. They don't do things right. They don't even care whether it's right or how they look or feel. You can't expect results from them.

THERAPIST: Does that cover it?

GARY: Yeah, I think so.

THERAPIST: Well, let's look at how you measure up to these standards. One characteristic of an incompetent person is that he screws everything up. Do you screw everything up?

GARY: Well, no. Most things I do come out OK but I'm real tense while I do them.

THERAPIST: And you said that an incompetent person doesn't care whether it comes out right or how they look to others, so your being tense and worrying doesn't fit with the idea that you're incompetent. If you don't qualify as incompetent, does that mean that you're completely competent?

GARY: I don't feel competent.

THERAPIST: And by these standards you aren't. You do well with a difficult job and you've been successful at catching the mistakes you do make, but you aren't relaxed and you do worry. By these standards you don't qualify as completely incompetent or totally competent. How does that fit with the idea that a person's either competent or incompetent?

GARY: I guess maybe it's not just one or the other.

THERAPIST: While you were describing how you saw competence and incompetence I wrote the criteria here in my notes. Suppose we draw a scale from 0 to 10 here where 0 is absolutely, completely incompetent and 10 is completely competent, all the time [see Figure 6.2]. How would you rate your competence in grad school?

Incompetence	Competence
0 1 2 3 4 5 6 7 8 9 10	
Screws everything up.	Doing hard tasks well
Doesn't do anything right.	and getting good
Doesn't care whether it is	results.
right.	Being relaxed while doing
Doesn't care how he looks to	tasks.
others.	Not worrying about tasks
You can't expect results.	afterwards.
	Catching and correcting
	mistakes.
	Knowing his limits.

FIGURE 6.2. Continuum of competence developed from Gary's dichotomous view of competence.

GARY: At first I was going to say 3 but, as I think about it, I'd say a 7 or 8 except for my writing, and I've never worked at that until now.

THERAPIST: How would you rate your competence on the job?

GARY: I guess it would be an 8 or 9 in terms of results, but I'm not relaxed, that would be about a 3. I do a good job of catching my mistakes as long as I'm not worrying too much, so that would be an 8, and I'd say a 9 or 10 on knowing my limits.

THERAPIST: How would you rate your skiing?

GARY: That would be a 6 but it doesn't matter—I just do it for fun.

THERAPIST: So I hear several important points. First, when you think it over, competence turns out not to be all-or-nothing. Someone who's not perfect isn't necessarily incompetent. Second, the characteristics you see as being signs of competence don't necessarily hang together real well. You rate an 8 or 9 in terms of the quality of your work but a 3 in being relaxed and not worrying. Finally, there are times, such as when you're at work, when being competent is very important to you and other times, like skiing, when it is not very important.

GARY: Yeah, I guess I don't have to be at my peak all the time.

THERAPIST: What do you think of this idea that if a person's competent they'll be relaxed, and if they're tense that means they're not competent?

GARY: I don't know.

THERAPIST: It certainly seems that if a person's sure they can handle the situation they're likely to be less tense about it. But I don't know about the flip side, the idea that if you're tense, that proves you're incompetent. When you're tense and worried does that make it easier for you to do well or harder for you to do well?

GARY: It makes it a lot harder for me to do well. I have trouble concentrating and keep forgetting things.

THERAPIST: So if someone does well despite being tense and worried, they're overcoming an obstacle.

GARY: Yeah, they are.

THERAPIST: Some people would argue that doing well despite having to overcome obstacles shows greater capabilities than doing well when things are easy. What do you think of that idea?

GARY: It makes sense to me.

THERAPIST: Now, you've been doing a good job at work despite being real tense and worried. Up to this point you've been taking your tenseness as proof that you're really incompetent and have just been getting by because you're real careful. This other way of looking at it would say that being able to do well despite being anxious shows that you really are competent, not that you're incompetent. Which do you think is closer to the truth?

GARY: I guess maybe I'm pretty capable after all, but I still hate being so tense.

THERAPIST: Of course, and we'll keep working on that, but the key point is that being tense doesn't necessarily mean you're incompetent. Now, another place where you feel tense and think you're incompetent is in social situations. Let's see if you're as incompetent as you feel there. . . .

Once Gary decided that his ability to handle stressful situations well despite his stress and anxiety was actually a sign of his capabilities rather than being a sign of incompetence, his sense of self-efficacy increased substantially. Following this increase in self efficacy he was substantially less defensive and thus was more willing to disclose thoughts and feelings, to look critically at his beliefs and assumptions, and to test new approaches to problem situations. This made it possible to use standard cognitive techniques with greater effectiveness.

Another series of interventions with particular impact was using the continuum technique to challenge his dichotomous view of trustworthiness, then introducing the idea that he could learn which persons were likely to prove trustworthy by noticing how well they followed through when trusted on trivial issues and raising the question of whether his truly malevolent family was typical of people in general or not. After this, he was able to gradually test his negative view of others' intentions by trusting colleagues and acquaintances in small things and observing their performance. He was pleasantly surprised to discover that the world at large was much less malevolent than he had assumed, that it contained benevolent and indifferent people as well as malevolent ones, and that when he was treated badly he could deal with the situation effectively.

When testing the client's perceptions of others as malevolent, it is important not to presume that the client's views are necessarily distorted. Paranoid individuals often turn out to have some malevolent associates or to have seriously alienated a number of acquaintances or colleagues. The goal is to enable the client to differentiate between persons who are generally safe to trust, persons who can be trusted to some extent, and persons who are malevolent or unreliable rather than simply presuming that all persons are malevolent. It also can be important to consider the impact of significant others on the client's beliefs. It is not unusual for paranoid individuals to marry persons who are also paranoid. When this is the case, the spouse may actively oppose the changes the therapist is working toward and couple sessions may be needed.

Concurrently with the primarily cognitive interventions, it is important to modify dysfunctional interpersonal interactions so that the client no longer provokes hostile reactions from others that support his or her paranoid views. In Gary's case, this required focusing on specific problem situations as they arose. It proved important to address cognitions that blocked appropriate assertion, including, "It won't do any good," "They'll just get mad," and "If they know what I want, they'll use that against me." It was also necessary to improve his skills in assertion and clear communication. When this resulted in improvements in his relationships with colleagues and with his girlfriend, it was fairly easy to use guided discovery to help him recognize the ways in which his previous interaction style had inadvertently provoked hostility from others.

THERAPIST: So it sounds like directly speaking up for yourself has been working out pretty well. How do the other people seem to feel about it?

GARY: Pretty good, I guess. Sue and I have been getting along fine and things have been less tense at work.

THERAPIST: That's interesting. I remember that one of your concerns was that people might get mad if you spoke up for yourself. It sounds as though it might be helping things go better instead.

GARY: Well, I've had a few run-ins, but they've blown over pretty quickly.

THERAPIST: That's a change from the way things used to be right there. Before, if you had a run-in with somebody it would bug you for a long time. Do you have any idea what's made the difference?

GARY: Not really. It just doesn't seem to stay on my mind as long.

THERAPIST: Could you fill me in on one of the run-ins you had this week? [A detailed discussion of a disagreement with Gary's boss ensued.] It sounds like two things were different from the old way of handling this sort of situation. You stuck with the discussion rather than leaving angry and you let him know what was bugging you. Do you think that had anything to do with it blowing over more quickly than usual?

GARY: It might.

THERAPIST: It works that way for a lot of people. If it turns out to work that way for you, that would be another payoff to speaking up directly. If they go along with what you want there's no problem and if they don't, at least it blows over more quickly. Do you remember how you used to feel after leaving a disagreement unresolved?

GARY: I'd think about it for days. I'd be tense and jumpy and little things would bug me a lot.

THERAPIST: How do you think it was for the people at work?

GARY: They'd be pretty tense and jumpy too. Nobody would want to talk to each other for a while.

THERAPIST: That makes it sound like it would be easy for a little mistake or misunderstanding to set off another disagreement.

GARY: I think you're right.

THERAPIST: You know, it seems pretty reasonable for a person to assume that the way to have as little conflict and tension as possible is to avoid speaking up about things that bug him and to try not to let his aggravation show, but it doesn't seem to work that way for you. So far it sounds like when you speak up about things that bug you, there are fewer conflicts and those conflicts blow over more quickly.

GARY: Yeah.

THERAPIST: Do you think that your attempts to keep from aggravating people may have actually made things more tense?

GARY: It sounds like it.

Toward the close of therapy, it is possible to "fine-tune" the client's new perspective on people and new interpersonal skills by helping him or her develop an increased ability to understand the perspectives of others and to empathize with them. This can be done through asking questions that require the client to anticipate the impact of his or her actions on others, to consider how it would feel if the roles were reversed, or to infer the thoughts and feelings of the other person from their actions and then to examine the correspondence between these conclusions and the available data. Initially the client is likely to find these questions difficult to answer and his or her responses are likely to be off the mark, but as he or she receives feedback both from the therapist and from subsequent interactions, his or her ability to accurately understand the other person's perspective is likely to steadily increase. The client discovers that aggravating actions by others are not necessarily motivated by malicious intentions, and that these actions are less aggravating if one can understand the other person's point of view.

At the close of therapy, Gary was noticeably more relaxed and was only bothered by symptoms of stress and anxiety at times when it is common to experience mild symptoms, such as immediately before major examinations. He reported being much more comfortable with friends and colleagues, was socializing more actively, and seemed to feel no particular need to be vigilant. When he and his girlfriend began having difficulties, due in part to her discomfort with the increasing closeness in their relationship, he was able to suspend his initial feelings of rejection and his desire to retaliate long enough to consider her point of view. He then was able to take a major role in resolving their difficulties by communicating his understanding of her concerns ("I know that after all you've been through it's pretty scary when we start talking about marriage"), acknowledging his own fears and doubts ("I get pretty nervous about this too"), and expressing his commitment to their relationship ("I don't want this to tear us apart").

MAINTAINING PROGRESS

The process of terminating treatment with individuals with PPD typically is much more straightforward than is the case with many of the personality disorders. Paranoid individuals usually prefer being self-reliant and often look forward to the conclusion of treatment. In fact, the therapist may need to be alert for the client's tendency to want to terminate therapy prematurely and may need to persuade the client to persist with treatment until there has been a chance to work explicitly on relapse prevention. Often it is easiest to persuade the client to agree to this if the interval between sessions is increased as the client is doing better.

In working on relapse prevention, it is particularly important to anticipate situations in which the client's suspiciousness, guardedness, and defensiveness will seem justified and to plan how to handle those situations effectively. Obviously, it is not safe to presume that the client will only encounter benevolent individuals in the future. Rather, it is important for therapist and client to recognize that the client will encounter malicious or deceptive individuals from time to time and to plan how to deal with such situations. It is very useful for the client to have the opportunity to practice dealing with situations in which he or she feels mistreated before the conclusion of treatment.

Paranoid individuals may be unwilling to return for "booster sessions" when needed if they see returning to treatment as a sign of weakness or of failure. It can be useful to present the idea that returning to consult the therapist as needed is a form of "preventive maintenance" and is a sign of the client's good judgment. Gary returned to treatment briefly on two occasions. Approximately 1½ years following termination of his initial treatment he returned because his girlfriend had developed a serious drinking problem which eventually resulted in his ending his relationship with her. Several years after that he returned for help in deciding whether to make a major career change. On both of these occasions he experienced considerable stress and his anxiety symptoms returned to some extent. However, he was able to cope with both situations without reverting to his initial suspiciousness and guardedness, and it was possible to alleviate his anxiety within a half-dozen sessions.

CONCLUSION

To a large extent, the client's paranoid views are not the main focus of the proposed intervention approach. Instead, standard cognitive-behavioral interventions are used to address the client's other problems, and his or her paranoid views are addressed when doing so is relevant to achieving the client's goals. The points that distinguish the approach presented in this chapter from the cognitive-behavioral approaches proposed by Colby et al. (1979) or by Turkat (1985; Turkat & Maisto, 1985) are the explicit attention paid to developing the therapist–client relationship, the emphasis on intentionally working to increase the client's sense of self-efficacy early in therapy, and the use of cognitive techniques and behavioral experiments to directly challenge the client's remaining paranoid beliefs later in therapy. The author's experience has been that this strategy typically facilitates the other interventions and produces improvement in paranoid symptomatology early in therapy as increases in self-efficacy reduce the need for vigilance.

Although no specific empirical data on the effectiveness of cognitive therapy with PPD are available, both the authors' clinical experience and the cases reported by Turkat and his colleagues are quite encouraging. The interventions recommended include increasing the client's sense of self-efficacy, improving his or her skills in coping with anxiety and interpersonal problems, developing more realistic perceptions of the intentions and actions of others, and developing an increased awareness of the other person's point of view. These all lead to changes which would be expected to have broad intrapersonal and interpersonal impacts. It appears that major "personality change" can occur as a result of cognitive therapy with these clients, but at this point no data are available regarding the extent to which the improvements achieved in therapy generalize and persist.

CHAPTER 7

Schizoid and Schizotypal Personality Disorders

SCHIZOID PERSONALITY DISORDER

The main feature seen in individuals with schizoid personality disorder is a lack of, and indifference to, interpersonal relationships. There is a pervasive pattern of detachment from social relationships across all contexts. Such individuals often present as withdrawn and solitary, seeking little contact with others and gaining little or no satisfaction from any contact they do have, irrespective of its focus. They spend the majority of time alone and choose to opt out of any activities involving contact with others.

Individuals with schizoid personality disorder also present with marked restriction in their displayed affect. They may appear slow and lethargic. Speech, when present, is frequently slow and monotonic, with little expression. They rarely show changes in their mood, despite external events. The mood they do present is generally moderately negative, with neither marked positive nor negative shifts. On questioning, these individuals rarely report strong emotions such as anger and joy. Such individuals, if functioning well, are likely to choose occupations with limited contact with the public or colleagues. Any social occupations are solitary. Schizoid persons are not given to the development of close relationships of either a sexual or platonic nature. Because of the schizoid person's slow and disengaging style of interaction, others tend to withdraw or ignore him or her. Over time, this leads to degeneration of the individual's already minimal social skills due to a lack of practice.

However, it is important to stress that such symptomatology lies on a continuum of experience, as do the beliefs behind such presenting features. It is vital when using a label such as "personality disorder" to remember that this should be held by the therapist and shared both to the client and others working with the individual, to allow the normalization of distressing experience and difficulties.

The DSM-IV-TR (American Psychiatric Association, 2000) diagnostic criteria for schizoid personality disorder are presented in Table 7.1.

Historical Perspectives

The diagnosis of schizoid personality disorder is arguably one of the most confusing of the Axis II diagnoses and as a diagnostic category has been in transition for about 100 years. The use of the term "schizoid" can be traced back to Manfred Bleuler of the Swiss Burgolzi Clinic (Siever, 1981). It is composed of the prefix "schizo" meaning "splitting" and "oid" meaning "representing or like." Campbell (1981) uses the traditional definition when he states that schizoid personality disorder re-

---

TABLE 7.1. DSM-IV Diagnostic Criteria for Schizoid Personality Disorder

A. A pervasive pattern of detachment from social relationships and a restricted range of expression of emotions in interpersonal settings, beginning by early adulthood and present in a variety of contexts, as indicated by four (or more) of the following:

  (1) neither desires nor enjoys close relationships, including being part of a family
  (2) almost always chooses solitary activities
  (3) has little, if any, interest in having sexual experiences with another person
  (4) takes pleasure in few, if any, activities
  (5) lacks close friends or confidants other than first-degree relatives
  (6) appears indifferent to the praise or criticism of others
  (7) shows emotional coldness, detachment, or flattened affectivity

B. Does not occur exclusively during the course of Schizophrenia, a Mood Disorder with Psychotic Features, another Psychotic Disorder, or a Pervasive Developmental Disorder and is not due to the direct psychological effects of a general medical condition.

Note. From American Psychiatric Assocation (2000, p. 67). Copyright 2000 by the American Psychiatric Assocation. Reprinted by permission.

sembles "the division, separation, or split of the personality that is characteristic of schizophrenia" (p. 563). Traditionally, Kraeplin (1913) viewed individuals with schizoid personality disorder as quiet, shy and reserved and "schizophrenic-like." This pattern of behavior was seen by many authors of this period as part of the schizophrenic process and indeed as a precursor to schizophrenia. Others such as Campbell (1981) argue that schizoid behavior can represent either a genetically determined chronic vulnerability to schizophrenia or present in those who are in partial recovery from schizophrenia.

The view of individuals with schizoid personality disorder presented in the past four editions of *Diagnostic and Statistical Manual of Mental Disorders* (DSM; American Psychiatric Association) differs markedly from this traditional view (Freeman, 1990). The individual with schizoid personality disorder is seen not as someone with prodromal or partial symptoms of psychosis, but rather as an individual whose beliefs maintain a chronically socially reclusive and isolated existence. Some authors have speculated as to a number of subtypes of schizoid personality disorder. Kretschmer (1936) postulated three subtypes, the first being stiff, formal and correct in social situations, showing a keen awareness of social requirements. The second subtype is the isolated and eccentric individual, one who is either unconcerned about or unaware of social conventions. Finally, the third subtype appears fragile, delicate, and hypersensitive. Alternatively, Millon and Davis (1996) propose four subtypes:

1. *Affectless,* in which the individual is passionless, unresponsive, unaffectionate, chilly, uncaring, unstirred, spiritless, lackluster, unexcitable, unperturbed, and cold and has all emotions diminished.
2. *Remote,* in which the individual is distant and removed, inaccessible, solitary, isolated, homeless, disconnected, secluded, aimlessly drifting, and peripherally occupied.
3. *Languid,* in which the individual presents with marked inertia and a deficient activation level and is intrinsically phlegmatic, lethargic, weary, leaden, lackadaisical, exhausted, and enfeebled.
4. *Depersonalized,* in which the individual is disengaged from others and the self, sees the self as disembodied or a distant object, and perceives body and mind as sundered, cleaved, dissociated, disjoined, and eliminated.

These hypothesized subtypes are used by Millon (1996) to propose a differential path of therapy for each of the subtypes. However, as yet there are insufficient empirical data to support these, and therefore this chapter is not guided by these subtypes.

Research and Empirical Data

Literature searches on research and empirical data appear to yield little for schizoid personality disorder. Some research carried out by Scrimali and Grimaldi (1996) found some specific, different patterns between a group with a diagnosis of schizophrenia, a group with diagnoses of Cluster A personality disorders, and a control group concerning arousal, human information processing, and attachment. The authors discuss these data in light of their implications for cognitive therapy and use the data to give different guidelines for cognitive therapy for individuals with a diagnosis of schizophrenia and individuals with a diagnosis of a Cluster A personality disorder. They speculated that the data gleaned from the study could be hypothesized to predict that the cognitive approach with patients affected by Cluster A personality disorders can be profitably applied through verbal communication by using cognitive restructuring techniques (Beck, Freeman, & Associates, 1990; Freeman, 1988; Freeman & Datillio, 1992). However, they added that this treatment should also include techniques such as socialization and bodily expression (Breier & Strauss, 1983; Dowrick, 1991).

Differential Diagnosis

Schizoid Personality Disorder and Delusional Disorder, Schizophrenia and Mood Disorders with Psychotic Features

When such diagnoses are present, in order to give an additional diagnosis of schizoid personality disorder, the personality disorder must have been present before the onset of psychotic symptoms and must persist when the psychotic symptoms are in remission (DSM-IV-TR, American Psychiatric Association, 2000).

Schizoid Personality Disorder and Avoidant Personality Disorder

On initial presentation it may appear that individuals with these two diagnoses appear similar. Both display a lack of close interpersonal relationships and engage in many solitary activities. However, the difference can be elicited by questioning their desire for such relationships. Individuals with avoidant personality disorder will avoid such relationships due to their fear of rejection and criticism. Those with schizoid may also fear such criticism or rejection but will not desire these relationships, and, thus, this self-enforced solitude appears less problematic.

Schizoid Personality Disorder and Those with Milder Forms of Autistic Disorder and Asperger's Disorder

There may be great difficulty in distinguishing between these two diagnoses, as both display severely impaired social interaction and stereotyped behaviors and interests. Advice should be elicited from experts in both the field of schizoid personality disorder and autistic/Asperger's disorder to help clarify this distinction for an individual's presentation.

Conceptualization

In individuals with schizoid personality disorder, a set of early experiences in which the themes of peer rejection and bullying are major factors is often present. Alongside this, the individual has often experienced being seen as different from the closer family unit or in some way diminished in comparison with others, and thus has come to view him- or herself as different in a negative sense, others as unkind and unhelpful, and social interaction as difficult and damaging. As a result, a set of rules or assumptions may develop to provide "safety" for such individuals, leading them into a lifestyle of solitude and lack of engagement.

Derek (36) has been unemployed for the last 11 years. He spends much of his time alone in his flat (apartment), listening to the radio or reading books. He goes to church daily, slipping in just after the morning service has started and leaving just before it ends to avoid having to speak to the vicar or members of the congregation. Derek presented to therapy with increasing anxiety and low mood. On initial presentation, Derek avoided eye contact and spoke only minimally to answer questions posed to him by his therapist. He requested that the therapist "get his family to leave him alone and let him be" and reported that their attempts to get him to attend family functions were causing him extreme anxiety. In addition, Derek spoke about an increased sense of the futility of life and his concerns that his oddness meant that nothing could change. It appeared that such beliefs were leading to his increased feelings of low mood. Derek had been unemployed for a number of years and survived on income support and disability allowance.

Derek was one of three brothers born to Jack, a plumber, and his wife, Deirdre, who since their marriage had done the accounts for Jack's plumbing business. The family was outgoing and physical, and Derek's two brothers had followed in their father's footsteps, one working directly for him and the other dealing in hardware for the plumbing trade. In contrast, Derek had been a shy and timid child who had been teased mercilessly at school. Since childhood he had been a solitary person and had been more interested in study than playing football with his father and brothers. Derek formed the following beliefs about himself: "I am different," "I am a loner," "I am an oddity," "I am a misfit," "I'm half a person," "I have an ugly personality," "I'm not normal," "I am worthless," "I am boring and dull," and "I am nothing." He had the following beliefs about the world and others: "People are cruel," "People are unfulfilling," "Others don't like me," and "The world is hostile." He developed conditional assumptions such as "If I try and befriend others, they will notice I am different and ridicule me," "If I speak to others, they will notice how dull I am and will reject and taunt me," "If people don't fit in, they will not be welcome and cannot have friends," and "People should only talk if there is something to say" in order to compensate for these beliefs.

When Derek was young he was called "a square peg in a round hole" and was often told by his father that "he must have been switched in the hospital." Throughout his life, Derek had tried to become involved in sports or the family business, but his efforts were often met with comments as to his ineptitude, and he eventually he gave up. His only regular outing was to his local church, which he attended despite the anxiety it afforded him. On being asked about this, Derek replied that his beliefs about God, heaven, and hell meant that, because he was "half a person" and had an "ugly personality," without his church attendance he would be doomed for a "forever of purgatory." In recent months, due to his parents' retirement and the impending marriage of his younger brother (his older brother is married with two children), his mother had attempted "to pull the family together again." This appears to have exacerbated Derek's anxiety and increased his low mood, based on his beliefs about his difference and the futility of this effort. Figure 7.1 shows the case conceptualization diagram.

Treatment Approach

Axis I Comorbidity

Although Derek clearly presented with low mood and anxiety, the exact diagnosis of the anxiety disorder may be difficult to ascertain. Derek clearly exhibited his anxiety in social situations; however, there appears to be a marked lack of fear of negative evaluation, which would be expected in either social phobia or in avoidant personality disorder. Rather, he exhibited a feeling of being overwhelmed by social contact that he considered excessive. With respect to depression, although this diagnostic group is not particularly prone to strong affective responses, such individuals' moods can be driven down due to their beliefs regarding the futility of life and their existence. Some difficulties which may be encountered in therapy with individuals with schizoid personality disorder are discussed next and illustrated using the aforementioned case example.

EARLY EXPERIENCE
"Square peg in a round hole."
Teased and bullied at school.
"Inept" at family activities.

↓

CORE BELIEFS
"I am different, a loner, an oddity, a misfit, nothing/worthless, boring and dull, half
a person, have an ugly personality, not normal."
"People are cruel, hostile, out to get me, unfulfilling, don't like me, pick on
weakness."
"The world is hostile."

↓

CONDITIONAL ASSUMPTIONS
"If I try and befriend others, they will notice I am different and ridicule me."
"If I speak to others, they will notice how dull I am and will reject and taunt me."
"If people don't fit in, they will not be welcome and cannot have friends."
"If I try and talk to others, there will be nothing to say and no point in this
communication." "People should only talk if there is something to say."
"If people see I am anxious, they will consider me weak and pick on me."
"If I aggravate people, then they will hurt me."

↓

TRIGGER
Attempts by mother to include Derek in family events.

↓

ASSUMPTIONS ACTIVATED

↓

NEGATIVE AUTOMATIC THOUGHTS
"I don't fit in—there is nothing to say."
"Others will taunt me for this."

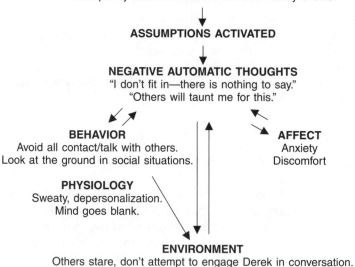

BEHAVIOR
Avoid all contact/talk with others.
Look at the ground in social situations.

AFFECT
Anxiety
Discomfort

PHYSIOLOGY
Sweaty, depersonalization.
Mind goes blank.

ENVIRONMENT
Others stare, don't attempt to engage Derek in conversation.

FIGURE 7.1. Case conceptualization diagram for Derek.

Collaboration Strategy

As therapy is by its very nature an interpersonal event, it is likely that the individual with schizoid personality disorder will have some difficulties in engaging in a collaborative therapeutic relationship. The individuals' beliefs about themselves and their interactions with others are likely to have an impact on the interpersonal therapeutic relationship as they no doubt have on all other interactions in the life of the individual with schizoid tendencies.

On questioning in therapy, it appeared that Derek was ambivalent about engaging in the therapeutic process. Not only did he see the problems as stemming from the fact he has "no personality or character," but he remained extremely fearful that therapy would lead him to discover more flaws in his personality and highlight his sense of inadequacy. Therefore, therapist and client needed to discuss the advantages and disadvantages of attending therapy alongside the advantages and disadvantages of not attending therapy (see Table 7.2). Only when possible advantages appeared to outweigh possible disadvantages was Derek able to engage in the therapeutic process. In therapy, however, this work had to be discussed in five consecutive sessions until Derek felt able and comfortable enough to proceed with therapy.

TABLE 7.2. Examining Advantages and Disadvantages of Therapy

Advantages of attending cognitive therapy	Disadvantages of attending cognitive therapy
• "Curious as to whether therapy may be beneficial." • "Therapy is of an interest to me." • "Therapy may help with my problems." • "Therapy helps me to believe that society cares for me." • "It is nice to talk to a pleasant person." • "Makes the week more interesting."	• "It may lead me to be more introspective, which may add to my difficulties." • "Self-disclosure may be very distressing." • "Self-disclosure may make trouble for myself." • "May lose any remaining illusion about my self-worth." • "If I push myself, things might get worse."
Advantages of not attending cognitive therapy	Disadvantages of not attending cognitive therapy
• "I have no mental vigor (neurological) without therapy I can cope." • "Therapy may be unsettling."	• "I might miss an opportunity to develop myself." • "Life is pretty bad." • "Things will not improve without help."

At the end of the period in which the advantages and disadvantages of therapy were discussed, Derek decided that the disadvantages of not attending cognitive therapy would sway him to attempting to work toward specific goals.

Negotiating a Collaborative Problem List and Goal List. It can also be difficult to negotiate a collaborative problem and goal list with the client. With respect to the individual's problems, it is important that the therapist be able to listen to what clients are saying and ask them to specify what element of their experience is problematic *to them,* as it may differ markedly from what the therapist expects the problematic area to be. Likewise, when developing the problem list, it is important that this information is elicited in a collaborative and Socratic manner from the client. If a therapist begins to speculate regarding an appropriate goal for the difficulties outlined, the therapist is in danger of being completely "off the mark" and client and therapist can become involved in a process with differing goalposts and therefore differing routes and processes.

Derek outlined his problem list as follows: (1) not working, (2) not busy enough, (3) no friends, (4) anxiety, (5) not accomplishing anything, and (6) feeling too low to talk. When attempting to set a goal list for each of the problems, it became apparent in sessions that this was difficult for Derek as "I've always been this way." However, it is extremely important to remember that what may appear as a suitable goal for the therapist may not be suitable for the client. With respect to not having friends, even though the therapist was tempted to suggest that having one or two close friends may be an important and useful goal, Derek wished to aim for the goal that his brothers no longer give him a hard time about having no friends or that he talks weekly to a "friend" made over the Internet.

Therapist Reactions to Client. Working with clients whose sets of beliefs contrast sharply with those of the therapist may raise difficult issues. The expression of the beliefs held by an individual who meets criteria for schizoid personality disorder may differ markedly from that of therapists who have chosen to enter a profession centered on close personal interaction and relationships. This may elicit strong affective responses in the therapist that may need to be understood and worked with in order for therapy to proceed in a collaborative manner.

Derek expressed a number of beliefs pertaining to social relationships. These included "People are cruel," "People are unfulfilling," and "People should only talk if there is something to say." As mentioned previously, it was difficult for the therapist to accept goals that did not incorporate increased social integration and which did not challenge beliefs about other people being cruel, unfulfilling, and unwelcoming and about the futility of directionless communication. In understanding his strong affective reaction to the beliefs and goals of the client, the therapist had to reflect on his own core beliefs and conditional assumptions and how these differed from those of the client. This process in itself created a different perspective on the dissonance, suggesting it could be seen as a rule or belief clash rather than a strong negative affective response to the client. If necessary, further work in supervision or using one's internal supervisor can aid therapists to examine their own beliefs and rules to discover whether they are in fact one way of thinking rather than the "definitive" and only "healthy" rules and beliefs.

Specific Interventions

With respect to the problem list identified in therapy, Derek came up with the following goals for therapy:

1. To help his father out in the business if he was needed
2. To be able to fill his time more
3. For his brothers to respect his lack of friends and to have one person with whom he can discuss difficulties (this did not have to be in person)
4. To be less worried
5. To be able to accomplish tasks which need to be done
6. Feeling better in himself

Anxiety. Derek decided that he would like to work on his anxiety as a first goal of therapy. On exploration of this anxiety, a maintenance formulation was generated (which is the lower part of the conceptualization in Figure 7.1). There appeared to be three main themes to the maintenance of this anxiety. First, he believed that he did not fit in with others. Second, he was concerned that if he did not fit in, others would use this against him. Third, he believed that there is no point to communication with others. This combination of beliefs meant that he would not engage in conversation with others but viewed low conversation as an indication of his oddness. He expected this oddness to be noticed by others, leading them to humiliate or harm him. This sequence was elicited using Socratic dialogue, and the conceptualization was discussed with Derek, who appeared to feel that this was a good summation of his difficulties. The specific beliefs that would need to change in order to enable some reduction in his problematic symptoms were then discussed.

This process began with examining his belief that "If I talk to others, there will be nothing to say and no point in this communication." If this could change, Derek felt that he would be less likely to be the odd one out and thus his fear of reprisal would reduce. However, he felt certain that he did not wish to increase his "small talk" with others. This was followed by an examination of his belief that he was odd and a "square peg in a round hole." However, on questioning Derek remained uncertain about addressing this belief, preferring instead to question his belief that others may attack him as a result of his oddness. Derek felt that countering this belief was likely to be the most effective route to a reduction in his anxiety.

Derek thought it might be useful to examine whether the way he acted as a result of these beliefs affected the likelihood of his being targeted and whether any alterations in the way he acted might reduce the likelihood of this unpleasant occurrence. Therefore, he and his therapist planned the following series of behavioral experiments (following verbal reattribution to challenge this premise) to check out whether others perceived his oddness or his anxiety and would attack him for it.

We discovered that Derek used flat affect and detachment as a safety behavior, believing that if others noticed his anxiety or his "oddness shining through" they would attack him. Therefore, a series of experiments were devised in which Derek would drop his safety behaviors of avoiding all eye contact, gazing at the floor, and hiding all facial expression and see whether he was attacked. This was done following verbal reattribution (considering the evidence and generating alternative explanations) which reduced his belief in attack from 90% to 25%, affording him the possibility of entertaining other possible outcomes and engaging in the experiment.

Reframing Core Beliefs. Despite his certainty earlier in therapy that he did not want to look at his beliefs about oddness, Derek later decided that these may be central to his distress and may need to be addressed. Derek proposed an "I am normal" as an alternative core belief that he would like to hold. Derek was socialized to Padesky's (1993) prejudice metaphor as a way of explaining the mechanism by which information-processing biases could maintain negative self-beliefs despite the availability of evidence to the contrary. This was used as a platform for discussion as to what would be needed for Derek to change his old core belief to the one that he identified would be more helpful for him to hold. Therefore, it was proposed that Derek collect data (as homework) which fitted with "I am normal" using a positive data log, as recommended by Padesky (1994). Questions used to help him elicit such information were: Is there anything that you have done today that seems to suggest that you are normal or that someone else would view as a sign that you are normal? Is there anything that you have done today that, if someone else did it, you would view as a sign that they are normal? The data collected were then used to help Derek rerate his belief in "I am normal" on a weekly basis. Evidence which Derek used to support his new belief included talking with another customer in the line at the supermarket, being able to engage in cognitive therapy, cooking tea for his mother, and saying a friendly hello to a neighbor.

Maintaining Progress

As discussed earlier, Derek was often ambivalent about therapy and considerable time in session was put aside to discuss this issue. During each review session, Derek and his therapist would aim to look at his goal list and evaluate progress with respect to each objective. Joint decisions were then made as to whether the goal had been met. If so, was there another goal that would be useful for this area? If not, was the goal still appropriate and achievable? If so, should they still work toward it, and if not, should they choose a new, more appropriate goal?

Derek's ambivalence about therapy was evident throughout his participation. Even when therapy was in progress and "successful" the negotiation of new therapy goals needed always to be preceded by a review of the advantages and disadvantages of engaging in the therapeutic process. Plans to end therapy were made with Derek once his goals of being less worried and feeling better in himself had been addressed with some success. Therefore, prior to discharge, work revolved around planning to end therapy and to consolidate these new beliefs. Because Derek did not wish for therapy to continue, the work was reviewed to see which of his beliefs had been altered to date and to assess and strengthen his conviction in his new beliefs.

Thus, a blueprint was generated to reinforce helpful work that had been completed, and to provide a conceptual framework for Derek to continue his therapy in the proposed direction, ideally preventing future difficulties. A brief summary of the blueprint follows:

1. A "compassionate" formulation of both the development and maintenance of your difficulties is included here to remind you of how these difficulties developed and, once developed, how they kept going (see Figure 7.1).

2. Following this understanding of your difficulties, we worked on how you used to hide your emotion from others in the belief that if they saw you were afraid, they would attack you. We discussed this in therapy and, finding a lack of evidence to support this, we designed a series of experiments. These experiments appeared to show that you had a belief that hiding your emotions kept you safe. However, the reality was that once you dropped this safety behavior you were not attacked. This

led to a great reduction in your anxiety in some situations. It appears important to remember that this behavior may have kept this anxiety going as it did not allow you to prove that the worst was not going to happen.

3. Again following our conceptualization of your difficulties, we looked at how your beliefs about yourself maintained your anxiety in social situations. These beliefs such as "I am odd" and "I am a square peg in a round hole" contributed to your belief that others would see this and use it against you. We spoke about how such beliefs were able to maintain themselves through changes in the way you process information (like being prejudiced against yourself). We discussed that you would like to believe "I am normal." However, any information which fitted with this was discarded or "squashed to fit" your negative beliefs about yourself. We spoke about how it would be useful to counter this process and set you collecting data in your positive data log. In this book, you collected data on actions that fitted with being normal or that, if others did them, you would see as a sign of their being normal. This prevents such information from being lost. It is helpful to keep reading this and to continue to collect positive data until you feel that this is no longer necessary.

4. At the start of therapy, one of your goals was to find ways of filling your time that may be more satisfying to you. It may be useful, now that some of your concerns about what might happen should you leave the house have been addressed, to consider activities with which to fill your time that may be more satisfying for you.

5. Another goal that you identified was to tackle tasks that needed to be done. We made sense of this avoidance by understanding that your beliefs about being a failure and half a person lead you to predict a negative outcome for tasks. As a result, it made sense not to take on any tasks. However, the problem with this avoidance is that you are not presented with any information to test these predictions. Therefore we spoke about planning a series of tasks that you could attempt in a graded manner, to evaluate the accuracy of your negative predictions.

6. Finally, you identified a goal of wanting to develop an acquaintance over the Internet as a reference to check things out with. You felt confident about how to do this yourself.

SCHIZOTYPAL PERSONALITY DISORDER

There are certain similarities between schizotypal personality disorder and schizoid personality disorder. Both disorders are characterized by avoidance of interpersonal relationships, but people with schizotypal personality also tend to experience psychotic symptoms and have pronounced behavioral peculiarities.

The main feature seen in individuals with schizotypal personality disorder is their acute discomfort with, and reduced capacity for, close relationships, as well as their cognitive or perceptual distortions and eccentricities of behavior. They often have subclinical psychotic symptoms or experiences, such as suspiciousness or believing people are talking about them or mean them some harm. They also lack friendships, feel anxious in social situations, and may behave in ways that others perceive as odd. The DSM-IV-TR (American Psychiatric Association, 2000) diagnostic criteria for schizotypal personality disorder are presented in Table 7.3.

Research and Empirical Data

There has been little research examining the cognitive and behavioral characteristics of people with a diagnosis of schizotypal personality disorder. Much of the research examining the syndrome has focused on neuropsychological and neurodevelopmental processes. There is some evidence to suggest that patient with a diagnosis of schizotyopal personality disorder may have widespread cognitive deficits (Cadenhead, Perry,

---

TABLE 7.3. DSM-IV-TR Diagnostic Criteria for Schizotypal Personality Disorder

A. A pervasive pattern of social and interpersonal deficits marked by acute discomfort with, and reduced capacity for, close relationships as well as by cognitive or perceptual distortions and eccentricities of behavior, beginning by early adulthood and present in a variety of contexts, as indicated by five (or more) of the following:

    (1) ideas of reference (excluding delusions of reference)
    (2) odd beliefs or magical thinking that influences behavior and is inconsistent with subcultural norms (e.g., superstitiousness, belief in clairvoyance, telepathy, or "sixth sense"; in children and adolescents, bizarre fantasies or preoccupations)
    (3) unusual perceptual experiences, including bodily illusions
    (4) odd thinking and speech (e.g., vague, circumstantial, metaphorical, over-elaborate, or stereotyped)
    (7) suspiciousness or paranoid ideation
    (6) inappropriate or constricted affect
    (7) behavior or appearance that is odd, eccentric, or peculiar
    (8) lack of close friends or confidants other than first-degree relatives
    (9) excessive social anxiety that does not diminish with familiarity and tends to be associated with paranoid fears rather than negative judgments about self

B. These should not occur exclusively during the course of Schizophrenia, a Mood Disorder with Psychotic Features, another Psychotic Disorder, or a Pervasive Developmental Disorder, and should not be due to the direct physiological effects of a general medical condition.

Shafer, & Braff, 1999) and attentional impairment (Wilkins & Venables, 1992). There has been some study of developmental factors in the etiology of schizotypal personality. A community-based longitudinal study found that childhood neglect was associated with the development of schizotypal personality disorder (Johnson, Smailes, Cohen, Brown, & Bernstein, 2000). Olin, Raine, Cannon, and Parnas (1997) prospectively collected teacher reports on school behavior as a means of assessing childhood precursors of schizotypal personality disorder. They found that those who later developed the disorder were more passive and unengaged and more hypersensitive to criticism as children. It has also been shown that anxious and avoidant attachment styles are associated with both positive schizotypy, characterized by hallucinatory experiences and unusual beliefs, and negative schizotypy, characterized by withdrawal, apathy, and anhedonia. There is also research demonstrating an association between dissociation and schizotypy.

Arguably the most useful research when examining schizotypy is the work examining psychotic experiences (in both patients and the general population). The individual symptoms of schizotypal personality disorder, such as paranoid ideation, ideas of reference, unusual perceptual experiences, and odd speech or behavior have all been studied in relation to psychosis, and it has long been argued that studying individual symptoms rather than diagnostic syndromes will provide a better understanding of underlying psychological processes (Persons, 1986). For example, there is evidence to suggest that paranoid beliefs are the result of external attribution for negative events (Bentall, Kinderman, & Kaney, 1994) and information-processing biases (Bentall & Kaney, 1989). Similarly, evidence indicates that distress associated with hallucinatory experiences is the result of interpretations made about them (Morrison, 1998). The importance of normalizing such experiences has been demonstrated with psychotic patients (Kingdon & Turkington, 1994), and it is clear that such experiences are highly prevalent in the general population (Peters, Joseph, & Garety, 1999; van Os, Hanssen, Bijl, & Ravelli, 2000). Such a normalizing approach also has the advantage of being less pejorative and stigmatizing than a diagnostic approach, as a label of personality disorder is likely to cause distress.

Differential Diagnosis

Schizotypal Personality Disorder and Delusional Disorder, Schizophrenia and Mood Disorders with Psychotic Features

When such diagnoses are present, in order to give an additional diagnosis of schizotypal personality disorder, the personality disorder must have been present before the onset of psychotic symptoms and must persist when the psychotic symptoms are in remission (DSM-IV-TR). The psychotic experiences of people with schizotypal personality are usually less distressing, cause less functional impairment, and are held with less certainty than those in patients with a diagnosis of schizophrenia.

Schizoid Personality Disorder and Schizotypal Personality Disorder

Although both of these disorders involve a marked lack of social interaction, there are points of distinction. Persons with schizotypal personality disorder usually present with odd beliefs and perceptual experiences, magical thinking, and behavior or appearance that is peculiar or unusually individualistic, whereas those with schizoid personality disorder present as aloof, detached, and unremarkable.

Conceptualization

People who meet criteria for schizotypal personality disorder have often had similar life experiences to those with schizoid traits (e.g., being bullied or rejected). In addition, they may have experienced childhood physical or sexual abuse, which led them to view themselves as different, bad, or abnormal, and may have had other real experiences of persecution. As a result, such people frequently experience unusual beliefs (such as magical thinking, suspiciousness, or ideas of reference) or hallucinations (visual or auditory) and often adopt strategies such as hypervigilance and an unwillingness to trust people in order to compensate for these beliefs.

Joe (25) was referred from a community drugs team (a local, multidisciplinary substance misuse service) for help with his suspiciousness, odd behavior, and unusual experiences. He lived in a community hostel and was working in a bar. He presented with high levels of social anxiety, which made his job problematic as he was expected to interact with the customers. He also had hallucinatory experiences, hearing the voice of his dead mother, although these did not cause him any distress. He was paranoid about other people talking about him and intending him harm and was using alcohol, cannabis, and cocaine to combat these fears. He was having trouble sleeping and was also very concerned about being labeled as having a personality disorder, which meant, the referring drug worker had explained, that he had a defective personality.

Joe was an only child, and his mother died when he was 7 years old. His father had a job that moved him around a lot, so Joe had to change school several times and thus found it difficult to make friends. Joe's dad tried to make up for the loss of Joe's mother by treating him as very special, telling him he was different from other children and that other people should realize his special qualities. Joe took this to mean that his dad wanted him to be noticed by others. His difficulty making friends (both at school and at home in his neighborhood) made Joe a target for bullying. To cope, he spent more time with his dad and on his own when Dad was at work. He developed strategies for entertaining himself that included talking to his dead mother, and he would hear her talk back to him. As a result of these experiences, he developed beliefs about himself as being worthless, vulnerable, and uninteresting (because of isolation from his peers and victimization), as well as being different and special (because of his dad). He viewed others as dangerous and not to be trusted and the world as unfriendly. He developed conditional assumptions such as "If I befriend others, then they will reject me," "If I am very different, then other people will notice me," "If I have unusual experiences, then I can be important," "If I can talk to my mother, then I will not be alone," "If people see how odd I am, then they will be interested," "If I let people see I am upset, then they will hurt me." He compensated for these beliefs using strategies such as adopting eccentric patterns of speech, using vague and metaphorical, or "flowery," language and wore highly unusual clothes that clearly attracted attention, all of which were designed to get him noticed. These were strategies that he adopted from the age of 11 and continued to use in later life. On the other hand, he would avoid social situations, if possible, and would be hypervigilant to social threat at all times, scanning the environment for evidence that others were talking about him or going to harm him. He also believed that he had an innate ability to read other people's body language, so he would pay close attention but often made incorrect inferences. Again, these strategies emerged in early adolescence. He also took illicit drugs and alcohol to remain calm. Sometimes this worked, and at other times it heightened his suspiciousness. Figure 7.2 illustrates the case conceptualization.

Treatment Approach

Collaboration Strategy

Interpersonal aspects of therapy are likely to be difficult for people with schizotypal personality. If they are is socially anxious, therapy is apt to be an activity they wish to avoid. This should be assessed explicitly and compared with reasons to persist in therapy. Similarly, suspiciousness may extend to the therapist, so clinicians should check out whether they are believed to be trustworthy. If not, strategies should be collaboratively developed. For example, suspension of disbelief for a time-limited contract can be useful. Suspicious concerns can be a useful point for the introduction of the concept of an examination of the evidence. A two-column consideration of the evidence for and against the belief "I cannot trust my therapist" can be helpful in reducing suspiciousness, simultaneously helping to socialize the patient to the model.

Ambivalence about the symptoms of schizotypal personality can

EARLY EXPERIENCES
Bullied at school.
Changed school frequently.
Pressure to be noticed.
Death of mother when he was 7.

↓

CORE BELIEFS
"I am different, worthless, uninteresting, and abnormal."
"Other people are cruel, dangerous, and not to be trusted."
"The world is unfriendly."

↓

UNDERLYING ASSUMPTIONS
"If I try and befriend others, then they will reject me or hurt me."
"If I am very different, then other people will notice me."
"If I have unusual experiences, then I can be important."
"If I can talk to my mother, then I will not be alone."
"If people see how odd I am, then they will be interested."
"If I let people see I am upset, then they will hurt me."

↓

COMPENSATORY STRATEGIES
Social avoidance.
Restrict expression of negative emotions.
Dress and speak in an unusual manner.
Allocate attention to hallucinations.

↓

TRIGGERS
Hallucinations of dead mother.
Drug use.
Job in bar.

↓

ASSUMPTIONS ACTIVATED

↓

NEGATIVE AUTOMATIC THOUGHTS
"I ought to be special."
"I have spiritual powers."
"They have a hidden agenda."
"I might be attacked."
"I can pick up other people's intentions."

Behavioral and cognitive responses	**Emotion**	**Physiology**	**Environment**
selective attention to interpersonal threat	anxiety	sleep problems	bar customers
avoidance of social situations	depression	arousal	high frequency of crime
eccentric behavior and dress	anger		
conceal distress			
vague and metaphorical speech			

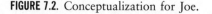

FIGURE 7.2. Conceptualization for Joe.

also be problematic for the process of therapy, particularly for the development of a shared list of problems and goals, as many patients have positive beliefs about these characteristics. For example, Joe valued his unusual perceptual experiences. He also recognized that suspiciousness and paranoia were, at times, functional for him, in that he believed this prevented him from being assaulted. Consideration of the advantages and disadvantages of specific symptoms can be helpful in resolving this ambivalence. For beliefs of paranoia, it is helpful to examine how the beliefs developed, how these beliefs have been useful, whether anything has now changed in the current environment, and whether the beliefs are still useful now. Most important, the cognitive approach explores options for beliefs that would be more useful in current and future circumstances.

Specific Interventions

Negotiating a Collaborative Problem List and Goal List. Joe developed a problem list in collaboration with the therapist. It was prioritized as part of the initial homework task, and, in the following session, considerable time was spent translating these problems into specific, measurable, achievable, realistic, and time-limited goals, which are outlined below:

1. *Social anxiety.* Goal is to reduce anxiety at work from 70% to 35%.
2. *Paranoia.* Goal is to reduce conviction in the belief "Other people are going to attack me" from 75% to 40%, or to reduce associated distress from 95% to 50%.
3. *Paranoia.* Goal is to reduce conviction in the belief "Other people are talking about me" from 80% to 50%, or to reduce associated distress from 80% to 50%.
4. *Drug use.* Goal is to reduce drug use so that it is recreational rather than self-medicating (reduce conviction in the belief "I have to take drugs to cope" from 40% to 0%).
5. *Sleep.* Goal is to stabilize sleep pattern by getting up between 9 A.M. and 11 A.M. and go to bed between midnight and 3 A.M..
6. *Stigma.* Goal is to reduce distress associated with the belief "I have a personality disorder or defective personality" from 50% to 10%.
7. *Friends.* Goal is to develop one social relationship in which he could feel confident about sharing information about himself.

These goals determined the direction of therapy. They were intended to be proximal, going for the smallest meaningful change rather than aiming for elimination of symptoms, although this may happen. They were set in relation to a 10-session contract, with a review planned at the end in which more sessions could be agreed. A total of 30 sessions were delivered throughout the course of therapy. As is often the case with people with schizotypal features, some of these characteristics were not placed on the problem list (e.g., the hallucinatory experiences), as they were not associated with any distress and, in fact, provided comfort.

Anxiety Reduction. Anxiety was selected as the first target for treatment because it was prioritized as the main difficulty, and as there is a large evidence base for cognitive therapy for anxiety disorders (D. Clark, 1999). However, it quickly became apparent with detailed questioning that the social anxiety was not related to concerns about negative evaluation or self-image but rather due to suspiciousness and paranoia. A Dysfunctional Thought Record used for homework confirmed this to be the case. Therefore, social anxiety and paranoia were addressed simultaneously.

Paranoid Belief Change. Because beliefs about being harmed and being talked about appeared interrelated, they were addressed together. Initially, examination of the paranoid beliefs began with a review of their development and a consideration of their advantages and disadvantages. Joe reported that his suspiciousness had come about because of his experiences of being bullied at school and in his neighborhood and that this had kept him safe on numerous occasions, which sounded accurate. He also felt that his beliefs that others were talking about him were useful in providing him with a rationale for avoiding unpleasant social interactions and also meant that he was important, which clearly related to some of his assumptions. However, he acknowledged that these beliefs did cause him some distress and prevented him from achieving his goals of reducing social anxiety and making friends. This was followed by a discussion of what had changed in his life since he developed those strategies, explicitly acknowledging that they were useful at school but questioning their current utility.

On the basis of this, Joe decided that the paranoid beliefs may occasionally be helpful in avoiding real danger, but most of the time he greatly overestimated the danger of interpersonal situations because of his past experiences. This view provided a rationale for collaboratively examining the evidence for and against the beliefs in relation to recent specific situations in which he felt paranoid. A typical example of this kind of situation was a group of people who sat at a table in the bar talking and laughing; Joe would invariably have thoughts such as "They are talking about me" or "They are planning to humiliate me," usually with a level of conviction of about 75%. Joe was encouraged to develop alternative explanations for the situations. He was asked to put himself in the other people's shoes and consider how he has behaved in similar situations and to recognize the distinction between thoughts and facts, or how something can feel real without being real. (See Table 7.4 for an example.) Verbal discussion of such issues helped reduce Joe's belief in the paranoid thoughts to a level where he felt able to take some risks and engage in a series of behavioural experiments.

Behavioral Experiments. There is some evidence to suggest that paranoid beliefs are more likely to be modified by behavior change, within a cognitive framework, than by verbal reattribution methods alone (Chadwick & Lowe, 1990). After Joe had practiced considering the evidence for a couple of weeks, he felt confident enough to change his behavior and test out what happened. Each experiment was planned carefully in session, with a concrete prediction in relation to a specific belief to be tested, and any problems predicted in carrying out the experiments were proactively addressed, including a regular evaluation of whether Joe believed that the therapist was trying to trick him with the aim of humiliating him. On occasions when this appeared to be a factor, a proportion of the session was allocated to examining the events that Joe was interpreting, and alternative explanations were generated and the evidence examined, including a discussion of professional ethics and boundaries. Such mistrust and suspicion can be frustrating for the therapist, and regular supervision is useful in dealing with such feelings.

TABLE 7.4. Review of the Evidence for "They Are Talking about Me and Intending to Humiliate Me"

Evidence for	Evidence against and alternative explanations
• "They are all talking and (at times) look in my direction." • "I have often been humiliated in the past." • "It feels real."	• "I have felt like this many times and have rarely been humiliated recently." • "Most of the occasions were many years ago." • "Just because I think it, does not necessarily mean it is true—I have probably developed a habit of paranoia." • "Even if they are talking about me, they could be saying nice things." • "They might be looking at me because they want to be served."

The experiments included modifying Joe's compensatory strategies, or safety behaviors, such as avoiding social interaction, dressing in a deliberately unusual manner that clearly attracted unwanted attention, and trying not to express negative emotions. Each of these allowed Joe to recognize that his strategies were at times counterproductive. More important, they facilitated the disconfirmation of his fears of being humiliated or attacked. For example, Joe initially believed that if he were to show that he was anxious, everyone in the bar would laugh at him or even assault him. He allowed himself to show his nervousness and deliberately said to customers that he was feeling a bit anxious that night, as had been role-played in the preceding session. Joe found that most people were supportive, and nobody laughed or assaulted him.

Stigma and Other Problems. After Joe had reduced his social anxiety and paranoia, many of the other problems appeared to resolve relatively easily. Joe set himself the task of stabilizing his sleep pattern using a modified activity-scheduling diary. At first, he found this difficult to achieve, as his suspiciousness and social anxiety meant that he had trouble getting to sleep because he would ruminate on the day's interpersonal events. However, once these were less problematic, he was able to change his sleep pattern simply by ensuring a regular bedtime and alarm call. This very concrete change increased his belief that he could change other things in his life. Similarly, once the suspiciousness and social anxiety were diminished, he found his desire to take drugs was correspondingly reduced. He still used alcohol and cannabis at work, and he decided that this was not something he wanted to completely stop. He was also able to share specific pieces of personal information, such as telling several people about having moved around a lot and having been bullied during childhood.

His main remaining concern was the stigma associated with a label of schizotypal personality disorder. Joe addressed this issue by providing information that would help to normalize his experiences. This included information about the continuum of schizotypal personality traits (Rossi & Daneluzzo, 2002), the prevalence of hallucinatory and paranoid experiences in the general population (Kingdon & Turkington, 1994; Peters et al., 1999; van Os et al., 2000), the relationship between cannabis use and schizotypal experiences (Dumas et al., 2002), and the potentially useful nature of certain unusual experiences (McCreery & Claridge, 2002; O'Reilly, Dunbar, & Bentall, 2001). This helped reduce his distress about the label and supported Joe's alternative understanding that he had developed certain ways of thinking and experiencing as a result of his life history rather than having a defective personality. His view of himself as abnormal and his associated distress dramatically reduced as a result of this alternative perspective.

Reframing Core Beliefs

Following the achievement of Joe's goals, the case conceptualization was revisited and new or additional concerns were elicited. The work of examining his suspicious beliefs and the subsequent behavioral experiments had reduced Joe's conviction in suspicious beliefs about others and the world, as well as his view of himself as vulnerable. However, he still viewed himself as being different, worthless, and uninteresting. He was happy with perceiving himself to be different, but decided that he would like to address the beliefs about being worthless and uninteresting. These were examined using schema change techniques, as outlined by Padesky (1994), such as historical tests of the belief, the use of continua in relation to worth and interest and a positive data log for an alternative belief that he decided he would like to replace them ("I am OK").

Possible Variations

Although Joe is typical of a person with a diagnosis of schizotypal personality disorder, many variations can be encountered. Many patients do experience some distress in association with their unusual perceptual experiences. If this is the case, approaches for understanding and intervening with hallucinations can be useful (e.g., Morrison & Renton, 2001). Magical thinking and superstition can be much more prominent than in Joe's case. These preternatural cognitive patterns may respond best to strategies developed for working with obsessional patients, such as experiments designed to test beliefs about thought–action fusion (Freeston, Rheaume, & Ladoucer, 1996) as well as metacognitive beliefs about protection and safety (Wells, 1997).

Maintaining Progress

Therapy finished after 30 sessions. In the third and final review session, Joe decided that he was happy with the progress he had made and did not wish to work on any further goals. Three monthly booster sessions were agreed to keep a check on progress and develop a blueprint for relapse prevention. This incorporated a copy of the formulation, a summary of the strategies that Joe had found helpful, and a list of potential triggers for further difficulties. The latter included possible future life events that could reactivate his assumptions such as actually being assaulted or humiliated, and plans were developed for how to cope with such events. His beliefs about being different were conceptualized as a potential vulnerability for relapse, but he was unwilling to try to change this. Finally, he decided that he should try to maintain at least two social relationships with which he felt comfortable, in order to provide him with social contact and an opportunity to check out his thoughts.

CONCLUSION

It can be seen that both schizoid and schizotypal personality disorders have typical patterns of early experiences involving bullying, rejection, and abuse. These experiences often lead the person to develop beliefs about themselves being different and other people being dangerous and untrustworthy, and sometimes they may decide that interpersonal relationships are simply not worth the effort. People with schizotypal traits also experience paranoia and hallucinatory phenomena and are frequently characterized by unusual or eccentric behavior and appearance. Given these difficulties, developing a good therapeutic relationship is challenging, but regular reviewing of shared goals and consideration of ambivalence about change can assist this. Therapy that targets the characteristic beliefs and strategies, using verbal reattribution and behavioral experiments, can be successful in reducing distress and increasing quality of life for these patients. It is important to remember that the principles of cognitive therapy, such as emphasizing collaboration and guided discovery, facilitate working with this client group and make success more likely.

CHAPTER 8

Antisocial Personality Disorder

Individuals with antisocial personality disorder (ASPD) have both a history of conduct disorder in youth and a pattern of severely irresponsible and socially threatening behavior that persists into adulthood. They may present in a variety of treatment settings, depending on their particular mixture of criminal behavior and clinical psychopathology. They may be inmates in a prison or correctional institution, inpatients in a psychiatric hospital, or outpatients in a clinic or private practice. Whether inmate, inpatient, or outpatient, the motivation for these individuals coming to treatment usually results from an external source (or force) pressuring the individual to "change." Family members, significant others, employers, teachers or, more frequently, the criminal justice system may insist that the person with ASPD seek treatment because of unacceptable behavior or strained interpersonal relations. Often, therapeutic recommendations are really an ultimatum for seeking treatment or else losing a job or being expelled from school. Courts may offer convicted felons a choice—go to therapy or go to jail. The choice is most often to go to therapy. In many cases, probation is contingent upon their attendance in psychotherapy.

Antisocial patients also may come voluntarily to outpatient facilities with various contrived forms of physical problems or psychopathology in order to obtain a prescription for some controlled substance(s). In this latter case, it is most important to separate the identifiable psychological problems and appropriate treatment from the attempted manipulation.

Antisocial personality disorder creates a perplexing and socially relevant problem inasmuch as the disorder is "a pattern of disregard for, and violation of, the rights of others" (American Psychiatric Association, 2000, p. 685). By definition, these individuals create problems for the broader society because this disorder incorporates criminal acts that threaten or injure people and property.

Are individuals with ASPD treatable with psychotherapy? Many authors dismiss them by labeling these individuals as unable to profit from treatment. In exploring the etiology of this perspective, three points emerge. The first stems from the psychoanalytic idea that involvement in psychotherapy requires a superego. The individual with ASPD is therefore untreatable by virtue of his or her lack of empathy and lack of acceptance of community rules and norms (superego) (Kernberg, 1975; Person, 1986). The second source of the untreatability myth stems from the lack of motivation for treatment of most individuals with ASPD. They are brought into therapy against their will with no clear idea of the direction of change and little reason to make changes. A third factor is the prevailing opinion that ASPD as a diagnosis is an amorphous, genetically determined whole rather than a number of related behaviors. The present approach focuses on the composite of related beliefs and behaviors often exhibited by persons with ASPD.

HISTORICAL PERSPECTIVES

The work of Cleckley (1976) and Robins (1966) helped to map out certain personality traits that frequently occur in antisocial individuals. Hare (1985b) has revised a checklist originally developed by Cleckley (1976) for distinguishing these essential traits. Like most trait-based assessments, the psychopathy checklist includes some apt descriptions, but it relies on subjective judgments.

DSM-I (American Psychiatric Association, 1952) included in the diagnosis of sociopathic personality disturbance irresponsible individuals who were always in trouble and those who lived in an abnormal moral environment, as well as those exhibiting sexual deviations, which subsumed "homosexuality, transvestism, pedophilia, fetishism, and sexual sadism (including rape, sexual assault, mutilation)" (p. 39).

DSM-II (American Psychiatric Association, 1968) revised the diagnosis of antisocial personality to include those who "are incapable of significant loyalty to individuals, groups, or social values. They are grossly selfish, callous, irresponsible, impulsive, and unable to feel guilt or learn from experience and punishment. Frustration tolerance is low. They tend to blame others or offer plausible rationalizations for their behavior" (p. 43).

DSM-III (American Psychiatric Association, 1980) added the caveat that there was a chronicity to the behavior that began prior to age 15. This included "lying, stealing, fighting, truancy, and resisting authority" and "unusually early or aggressive sexual behavior, excessive drinking, and the use of illicit drugs" (p. 318). Later, DSM-III-R (American Psychiatric Association, 1987) included physical cruelty, vandalism, and running away from home.

ASPD differs from the other personality disorders in DSM-IV-TR (American Psychiatric Association, 2000). It stands out as the only disorder that it cannot be diagnosed in childhood, whereas all the other diagnostic categories can be used for children and adolescents (p. 687). Further, ASPD requires a history of a precursor diagnosis, conduct disorder.

RESEARCH AND EMPIRICAL DATA

The treatment literature for ASPD has been based primarily on empirical research involving subjects (usually criminals rather than psychiatric patients) defined as psychopaths or sociopaths. The literature on psychopathy has focused on a distinction between "primary" and "secondary" psychopathy (Cleckley, 1976). The primary psychopath is distinguished by an apparent absence of anxiety or guilt about his or her illegal or immoral behavior. Because of his or her ability to do things such as lying purposely for personal gain or physically harming another person without feeling any nervousness, doubt, or remorse, the primary psychopath is regarded as lacking a moral conscience. The secondary psychopath is an individual who might engage in the same exploitive behavior but reports feelings of guilt over having harmed someone else. He or she might fear possible consequences of wrongdoing but continue to behave in antisocial ways, often due to poor impulse control and emotional lability. Inmates classified as primary psychopaths on the basis of significantly lower trait anxiety evince more frequent and severe aggressive behaviors (Fagan & Lira, 1980) and report less somatic arousal in situations in which they perceive malevolence from others (Blackburn & Lee-Evans, 1985) than do secondary psychopathic inmates.

Hare (1986) points out that under many conditions, psychopaths as a group do not differ from normal subjects on autonomic and behavioral responses. For example, psychopaths have been shown to learn from experience when the contingencies are immediate, well-specified, tangible, and personally relevant—such as obtaining or losing access to cigarettes. Thus, according to Hare, laboratory findings regarding the electrodermal underactivity of primary psychopaths may have been overinterpreted, especially given that such responses can be influenced by a wide range of cognitive activities. Alternatively, distinguishing motivational and cognitive features may further clarify response characteristics of psychopaths.

Research in antisocial psychopathology has been built on the assumption that there is a systematically definable disorder distinguishable from criminal behavior alone. However, the degree of importance that criminality is accorded is a controversial issue.

DIFFERENTIAL DIAGNOSIS

DSM-IV-TR (American Psychiatric Association, 2000) criteria for antisocial personality disorder (Table 8.1) are intended to represent an enduring pattern of inner experience and behavior that deviates markedly from the expectations of the individual's culture. The pattern should be manifested in two (or more) of the following areas:

1. *Cognition* (i.e., ways of perceiving and interpreting self, other people, and events). Although we can identify a number of "typical" cognitions of individuals with ASPD, it would be impossible to isolate specific antisocial cognitions. Instead their automatic thoughts reflect common themes of pragmatic strategies for self-advancement. What ap-

---

TABLE 8.1. DSM-IV-TR Criteria for Antisocial Personality Disorder

A. There is a pervasive pattern of disregard for and violation of the rights of others occurring since age 15 years, as indicated by three (or more) of the following:
   (1) failure to conform to social norms with respect to lawful behaviors as indicated by repeatedly performing acts that are ground for arrest
   (2) deceitfulness, as indicated by repeated lying, use of aliases, or conning others for personal profit or pleasure
   (3) impulsivity or failure to plan ahead
   (4) irritability and aggressiveness, as indicated by repeated physical fights or assaults
   (5) reckless disregard for safety of self or others
   (6) consistent irresponsibility, as indicated by repeated failure to sustain consistent work behavior or honor financial obligations
   (7) lack of remorse, as indicated by being indifferent to or rationalizing having hurt, mistreated, or stolen from another.

B. The individual is at least age 18 years.
C. There is evidence of Conduct Disorder . . . with onset before age 15 years.
D. The occurrence of antisocial behavior not exclusively during the course of Schizophrenia or a Manic Episodes.

Note. From American Psychiatric Association (2000, p. 706). Copyright 2000 by the American Psychiatric Association. Reprinted by permission.

pears to be the common denominator for antisocial individuals is that the rules by which they live are significantly and noticeably different from those of the broader community and the goal of their life is to limit or avoid the control of others.

2. *Affectivity* (i.e., the range, intensity, lability, and appropriateness of emotional response). It would be equally impossible to identify a single affective pattern for antisocial individuals. The affective responses of antisocial individuals can run the gamut from the reclusive and disengaged individual whose antisocial actions may be self-focused (e.g., heroin use) to the more aggressive acting-out individual (e.g., physical assault on others). Significant deficits in emotional processing may be one of the characteristic features of the antisocial individual (Habel, Kuehn, Salloum, Devos, & Schneider, 2002),

3. *Interpersonal functioning.* Here again there is no one interpersonal pattern. Some antisocial individuals have poor interpersonal skills and have problems that are rooted in their social skills deficits as they act inappropriately without apparent cause (e.g., taking something without asking). Others have superb interpersonal skills that they use in their manipulation of others (e.g., the "con artist"). Stanley, Bundy, and Beberman (2001) see the need for skill training as potentially useful with the ASPD individual.

4. *Impulse control.* Finally, the range of impulse control runs the range from individuals who evidence excellent impulse control as they patiently wait the chance to get what they want (e.g., embezzlers). Others are opportunists who reach out and grab what they want without thought of consequence (e.g., muggers). Still others show a combination of good impulse control with episodic opportunism.

There are significant gender issues in the diagnostic differentiation between ASPD and borderline personality disorder (BPD). There has been some concern that APD may be underdiagnosed in females because of the aggressive slant of the criteria (American Psychiatric Association, 2000, p. 704). Zlotnick, Rothschild, and Zimmerman (2002) found that men diagnosed as BPD showed more lifetime substance abuse, antisocial behavior, and intermittent explosive disorder than did women. Other related factors are socioeconomic status (DSM-IV-TR; American Psychiatric Association, 2001) and ethnicity (Delphin, 2002).

Avoidance of early contact with the judicial or treatment systems may preclude the ASPD diagnosis because conduct disorder was not established. Further, the report of antisocial or conduct-disordered behavior is often a matter of the patient's report and the clinician's interpretation. Did the individual's behavior amount to early or aggressive sexual experience? Was there *excessive* drug use? Some individuals may meet full criteria for ASPD but lack the validation of their conduct disorder.

Conversely, an individual may want to impress the clinician and regale the interviewer with tales of their adolescent exploits. These exploits may have grown in seriousness and impact over the years and in the need for self-aggrandizement.

A thorough discussion of the patient's life history is necessary for establishing the diagnosis of ASPD. This may include a review of relationships, academic and vocational achievement, military service, and arrest and conviction record, as well as living circumstances, physical health, history of substance use, and self-concept. Attempts also should be made to review additional sources of data, so as not to rely entirely on the patient's viewpoint. Within the spirit of a collaborative investigation, the therapist can invite the patient to bring significant others into a therapy session so that they can provide a different source of information on the patient's functioning. Significant others might include a spouse or other immediate family members, relatives, or friends. With written permission from the patient, the therapist should also obtain a copy of other relevant documents, such as previous treatment records or documents from legal proceedings. From this history, a list of problems can be developed to guide the subsequent work.

CONCEPTUALIZATION

The view of the world of individuals with ASPD is a personal rather than an interpersonal one. In social-cognitive terms, they cannot hold another's point of view at the same time as their own. As such, they cannot take on the role of another. They think in a linear fashion, anticipating the reactions of others only after responding to their own desires. Their actions are not based on choices in a social sense because of these cognitive limitations. Their view of self consists of a system of self-protecting appraisals and attributions. For example, they may be merely "borrowing" funds from their employer, intending to repay the "loan" as soon as their bets pay off. Actions taken in self-interest are appraised more positively than the very same actions in someone else. The antisocial individual views him- or herself as clever, persistent, and constrained by circumstances, but views someone else doing the same thing as a "pathetic thief."

The behavioral dimensions of ASPD can be divided into a number of points on a criminal continuum similar to the divisions used by law enforcement. For example, we might divide the group into several "types" similar to Stone's (2000) "gradations of antisociality" (Table 8.2).

The treatment for each of these "types" would be designed to meet the expressed and subtle variations while factoring in the patient's motivation (interest) and ability (skills) for change.

TABLE 8.2. A Clinical Taxonomy for Antisocial Personality Disorder

Type I. Violates societal rules but destructive action(s) are directed toward self (e.g., alcoholism, drug abuse, prostitution)

Type II. May be highly socialized within subgroup where the identified behavior may be "acceptable" or even overlooked, but comes into conflict with general population episodically. May be volitional or nonvolitional (e.g., fighting, public drunkenness, disorderly conduct).

Type III. Actions are nonviolent and are directed against large institutions (e.g., insurance fraud, income tax evasion, embezzlement, theft from the military or the telephone company or cable company)

Type IV. Nonviolent, volitional actions that are directed against property, without injury to others (e.g., burglary, auto theft, pickpocket)

Type V. Violent, volitional actions against property (e.g., arson, explosives)

Type VI. Nonviolent, volitional actions against people (e.g., conning others, swindler, real estate scams)

Type VII. Non violent, volitional though frightening predatory actions against others (e.g., stalking, verbal threats, physically threatening action[s])

Type VIII. Violent, nonvolitional acts that are accidental or caused by ignorance or naivete (e.g., gun discharge, under the influence of drugs/alcohol)

Type IX. Violent, volitional though not physically damaging actions against others (e.g., kidnapping, carjacking, frottage)

Type X. Violent, though nonlethal dyscontrolled or dysregulated actions (e.g., epileptoid, uncontrolled rage responses)

Type XI. Violent, though nonlethal, volitional physical damage to others (e.g., gangland "enforcer," date rape, pedophilia, sexual abuse)

Type XII. Violent, lethal (or potentially lethal) volitional physical crimes against people (e.g., murder, assault with a weapon, physical assault, spousal abuse).

TREATMENT APPROACH

Treatment intervention for ASPD obviously presents significant challenge. The twin issues of skills and motivation can be equally applied to the patient and the clinician. Is the therapist skilled at working with this population, and is the therapist motivated to enter and maintain the necessary relationship for effective therapy? Treatment effectiveness with such patients is often limited to better management of their disruptive behaviors within an institutional setting or slight alterations in their behavior that can result in their avoiding institutional settings. Not surprisingly, therapists do often view these patients as especially difficult (Merbaum & Butcher, 1982; Rosenbaum, Horowitz, & Wilner, 1986).

Rather than attempting to build a better moral structure through the induction of affect such as anxiety or shame, cognitive therapy of ASPD can be conceptualized as improving moral and social behavior through enhancement of cognitive functioning. Drawing generally from major theories regarding moral development in men and women (Gilligan, 1982; Kohlberg, 1984), and psychosocial development

(Erikson, 1950), we propose that the treatment plan be based on the strategies suggested by R. Kagan (1986) for furthering cognitive growth. This would involve fostering a transition from concrete operations and self-determination toward more formal cognitive operations of abstract thinking and interpersonal consideration. Moral functioning is regarded as a dimension within the broader context of epistemology, or ways of thinking and knowing.

Cognitive therapy is designed to help a patient with ASPD make a transition from thinking in mostly concrete, immediate terms to consider a broader spectrum of interpersonal perspectives, alternative beliefs, and possible actions.

Collaboration Strategy

Symptoms of ASPD can be intense for patients and therapists alike. It is essential that the therapist be able to sail through stormy waters with a firm and stable hand. This requires highly specialized training and supervision. The idea that a patient with ASPD is like all other patients, just more difficult, is a massive under-evaluation.

In formulating a treatment plan, the clinician needs to explicitly inform the patient about his or her diagnosis of ASPD and set clear requirements for his or her involvement in treatment. Otherwise, the antisocial patient is not likely to see any reason or purpose in continuing psychotherapy. Such individuals see their problems as other people's inability to accept them or desire to limit their freedom. It is important in any therapeutic interaction to outline the limits and expected behavior of the therapist and patient; however, this is essential with ASPD patients, due to their generally poor sense of boundaries.

Structuring the treatment should be an explicit process with ASPD patients. It is recommended that therapists clearly outline and adhere to the prearranged length of the session, the policy on session cancellation, the rules about between-session contacts, the homework requirement, and appropriate use of the emergency phone number. More generally, it may be helpful for therapists to highlight for patients the need for commitment to attending therapy even though there may be limited motivation and that there may be times at which they feel like quitting. The treatment contract should include an agreed-on number of sessions and expected behavioral change. The collaborative set involves mutually acceptable goals for therapy that are reasonable, sequential, realistic, meaningful, proximal, and within the patient's repertoire.

Just as the therapist must be aware of and respond calmly and appropriately to the patient's transference behaviors, the therapist must also monitor for his or her own automatic, and often negative, emotional responses to the patient. For example, the therapist may feel manipulated by a patient who repeatedly misses sessions with questionable or even ludicrous excuses. In addition, because of the challenges of forming a strong therapeutic alliance, the collaborative nature of the therapy must constantly be a focus. Therapists must keep in mind that collaboration with many of the patients with ASPD may be 80–20, or 90–10, with the therapist carrying the greater burden. Unfortunately, this imbalance of effort often brings with it a high level of therapist stress and burnout (Freeman, Pretzer, Fleming, & Simon, 1990).

Interviews with "highly committed" therapists indicated that they were able to sustain high levels of work commitment by creating boundaries between professional and nonprofessional life, using leisure activities to provide necessary relief from work, turning work obstacles into challenges and continually seeking feedback from colleagues, among other things (Dlugos & Friedlander, 2001).

As one begins to closely examine both the therapist and the patient responsibilities within the collaboration, rather interesting parallels emerge. Many of the therapeutic issues that are operative for the patient in treatment are active and compelling for the therapist as well. The parallels can help the therapist to maintain an empathic position and maximize the opportunity to use these similarities in helping the patient to best use the therapeutic experience. Both need to understand the long-term, chronic, and pervasive aspects of ASPD, as well as the varied nature and level of impairments experienced by the specific patient.

The therapist treating the patient with ASPD must be trained to work with the problems of anger, dissociation, dishonesty, and relationship difficulty, often within the context of an unstable working alliance. He or she also must have patience, perseverance, and the ability not to take all patient reactions personally. The therapist must continue to maintain hope for the patient, despite the temptation to be drawn, at times, into the patient's own sense of impatience, frustration, and futility.

The therapist must be able to control his or her responses to the patient's often angry, demeaning, or hostile verbalizations or behavior and not become pejorative or inflexible in response. The therapist must also be aware not to be pulled into violations of boundaries be they professional, emotional, physical, or sexual. Those patients who reinforce their view of themselves as "the best therapist" or the "only one who cares" trigger a different vulnerability. This can lead to therapist's bending of the rules, such as working on a Saturday to accommodate the patient's schedule or sharing intimate personal information with the patient. It is particularly important for the therapist working with patients with ASPD to model appropriate behavior and to maintain boundaries and limits, and not to reinforce patients' beliefs that they can live "outside the rules."

Patients with ASPD are apt to respond to the most direct and concrete aspects of the therapist's behavior. Therefore, interaction that conveys undue suspicion, easy suggestibility, or attitudes of superiority, aloofness, or pity is apt to diminish rapport and foster a variety of counterproductive reactions. Inasmuch as the therapist wishes to facilitate psychosocial development characteristic of adolescence, it is important to consider ways in which ASPD patients might develop some "peer-like" identification with the therapist. Characteristics that may help cultivate this rapport include the therapist's being self-assured, relaxed, nonjudgmental, nondefensive, and having a sense of humor. One therapist was positively viewed by her ASPD patient as being "like a sister" to him, primarily because she listened and helped him prioritize his family problems rather than lecturing or admonishing him. Other therapists have accomplished this sort of rapport by spending extra time playing cards with prisoners or patients, or making a point to know the latest jokes being passed around the cellblock, and thus come to be regarded as "one of the guys." There are no simple formulas for accomplishing this rapport, because the right combination will vary according characteristics of the therapist, patient, and setting.

Patients who have been told by their therapists that their disorder can be debilitating and is chronic may understandably feel discouraged about their prospects for improvement. It is therefore crucial for therapists to convey to patients that, although the personality disorder is a chronic condition, it can be highly treatable. In addition, it may be helpful for patients to know that their level of motivation for change will be a contributing factor related to therapeutic success (Freeman & Dolan, 2001; Prochaska & DiClemente, 1983).

Therapists must be careful not to fall into the trap of using pejorative language or statements about their patients if they are to convey optimism regarding change. Though this is often done inadvertently, it can further reinforce patients' perceptions of being powerless and vulnerable, and of their inherent unlovability or untreatability. Patients must be helped to recognize that their chronic disorder needs the same organized treatment as is required by other chronic diseases such as diabetes or asthma.

Due to the range of symptom presentations in patients with personality disorders, and to the strong possibility of co-occurring mental illness, a patient's maximum potential level of psychosocial functioning cannot be predicted based on the personality disorder diagnosis alone. Some ASPD patients may have a long-term, recurring relationship with structured facilities (e.g., in and out of jail), but others may be high functioning, holding jobs and maintaining adaptive marital and family relations with little or no therapeutic support. It is important for the patient to have realistic self-expectations—to understand what his or her strengths, weaknesses, and limits may be—so that treatment gains can be maintained and future problems can be avoided or minimized. Thus, the implications of the ASPD for life functioning, based on the therapist's careful assessment of the individual patient, should be explicitly discussed with the patient.

Specific Interventions

Initiating Problem-Focused Work

As work on the problem list is broached, the therapist is once again likely to encounter the patient's denial of problems. Attempting to coerce the patient into admitting that he or she has problems will probably damage rapport and cause treatment reactance, dropout, or ongoing power struggles. Instead, the therapist can review the criteria for ASPD and compare this with the patient's history. The patient can be apprised that this is a serious disorder affecting judgment and behavior, and that it tends to have very negative long-term consequences for the afflicted individual, such as alienation of friends and family, physical harm from others, or extended incarceration. Treatment options might include an additional 2-week trial for slow starters, referral for alternative services such as family therapy, an intensive inpatient treatment program, a partial hospitalization program, or referral back to a probation officer. When the patient is coming to psychotherapy to avoid going to jail, his or her participation in treatment may need to be reconfirmed at each session. Therapists are encouraged to be mindful of the general rule to continue therapy only if it is reasonably clear that the patient is benefiting, and to be willing to discontinue treatment if this criterion is not met.

Consistent with their style, patients with ASPD may attempt to "control" the sessions, for example, by refusing to talk, expressing suicidal or homicidal ideation, changing the topic at hand, or becoming angry with the therapist, others in their life, or the world in general. Much like substance abusers, patients with ASPD may gain self-reinforcement through the relating of detailed "war stories." The patient may insist on relating the gory details of past incidents when they have engaged in risk-taking behavior or been noncompliant. They may show various forms of "battle scars," such as scars, burn marks, stitches, or open cuts. Throughout therapy, it is important to redirect patients toward building new, successful experiences, as opposed to holding onto the negative, yet comfortable, events in the past.

At the start of treatment, the therapist may need to use some finesse in maintaining the control of the session yet be flexible enough to allow the patients' pressing issues of the day to be addressed. Depending on patients' prior therapy experiences, they may be more or less agreeable to structured sessions. Therapists can systematically shape patients' behaviors into a more structured therapy model over the first several sessions. Patients may regress at later stages in therapy, in which deviation from the structured model should be confronted immediately and discussed as a treatment issue.

It is predictable that the patient will tend to regress to "war stories" during times of particular distress, which should be a cue for the therapist to explore with the patient as a possible control or distraction tactic. It can become a sticky area if not handled directly and carefully. Although possibly frustrating to the patient that he or she is not being encouraged to say and do whatever he or she wishes, the patient must be socialized to the need, purpose, and skills for establishing and maintaining structure within the therapy session. Establishing and maintaining structure allow the patient to be more collaborative, ultimately improving the therapeutic alliance. Further, structured homework assignments and self-monitoring are ways to help clients to establish some structure in their life outside the therapy session.

Case Example. Randy was a 28-year-old male referred by the Federal Probation Office as an alternative to institutionalization in a federal prison. The expectation of his probation officer (PO) was that Randy attend weekly sessions for 1 year. An attendance report was due at the end of every month, and if Randy missed more than two sessions in a month, he risked being sent to prison.

Randy came in for his first session 10 minutes late and stated, "Here I am, I have to check in with you and then I don't have to come back." When informed that the expectation was that he attend weekly sessions, Randy winked and said, "Look, if I don't come in you still get paid. Let's make this simple. I give you a call from time to time and you have a free hour."

When the therapist insisted that therapy was not simply "checking in," Randy became loud and intimidating. "I've done this before. I don't have to come. Forcing me to come to therapy is a violation of my constitutional rights. It's illegal. You can't make me come."

The therapist informed Randy that because he (the therapist) was not a constitutional expert, he would call the PO and have Randy sent to prison until the constitutional issue worked its way through the courts. Randy continued with his loud statements about how the system was simply screwing over people like him, and the therapist was part of that system.

The therapist calmly nodded and accepted Randy's statements, and said, "Why don't we talk for a bit and see where we go."

Randy's response was to ask for clarification. "As a federal prisoner, what I say to you stays confidential, is that right?"

"Yes. That's right."

"So what goes on in these sessions stays between you and me?"

"Yes."

"Good."

At this point Randy took a magazine from his back pocket and started to read it. He did not respond to any questions, prompts, or statements from the therapist.

When the time was over, the therapist stated, "Our time is up for this week. I'll expect you at this time next week. Any session where you come later than 10 minutes after our starting time will be a missed session and I have to report that."

Randy left without a word.

He appeared the next week 10 minutes late. This week he had a newspaper which he silently read throughout the session. The next week the pattern repeated itself. At the end of the session, Randy turned at the door and said, "Next week, doc, bring some work to stay busy."

At the fourth session, the therapist decided to take a schematic approach to treatment. When Randy arrived (10 minutes late) with his magazine, the therapist commented, "It is interesting. Over the last 2 weeks I was thinking about how dumb you are."

At this, Randy looked up from his magazine and asked, "How would you like a punch in the face?"

"I wouldn't," said the therapist.

"What makes you so f___g smart?"

"I didn't say I was smart, I said that you were dumb."

"Yeah, what makes me dumb?"

"Well . . . people pay a great deal of money to talk to me. You can do it for nothing. See all of those books on the shelf? They are all mine. I'm an expert in behavioral change and you are too dumb to use me for your own ends."

The magazine was now on the desk and Randy asked, "How can I use you?"

"Well, is there anyone's behavior that you would like to change?"

"Yes," he said. "My girlfriend. She's a lazy bitch. I would like her to cook dinners and to be more willing for sex."

"I'll need some information." With this the therapist gathered data with the ostensible purpose of helping Randy to "use" the therapist to change his girlfriend.

Randy had lived with Bianca for 3 years. He was verbally abusive but denied any physical violence. As part of the data gathering the therapist asked, "Do you buy her gifts?"

"Like what?"

"Flowers, jewelry . . . you know, presents."

"Yeah, for Christmas and maybe her birthday."

"What do you think would happen if you just brought her a present for no reason other than she might like it?"

"You mean for nothing?"

"No, it would be data for what we're doing. What would she like?"

"She likes flowers."

This was to be Randy's homework. He would see about getting Bianca flowers and evaluate her response.

The next week Randy appeared for the session on time and without a newspaper or magazine. When asked for a homework report, Randy said, "You can't believe it. I got her flowers [he stole them from someone's garden on the way home]. When I came in with the flowers she looked real suspicious. She asked me, 'What's this for?'"

"I said, 'Nothing. I just thought that you would like them.'

"Well, we started kissing and ended up in bed. Then she says to me, 'What would you like for dinner?' "

The therapist asked, "OK, what did you learn from this?"

Randy's response was predictable: "Well, all I have to do to get over on her is to be nice. Does this work on anyone?"

"Who do you want to change next?"

"My PO."

The reader might conclude that the therapist made Randy a better ASPD. Or, we might view the intervention as using the pathology in the service of more effective functioning.

Linking Distorted Thoughts to Maladaptive Behaviors

Within each problem area, it is helpful to identify cognitive distortions that may be linked to problematic behaviors. A patient with ASPD typically holds a number of self-serving beliefs that guide his or her actions. These frequently include, but are not necessarily limited to, the following six beliefs:

1. *Justification.* "Wanting something or wanting to avoid something justifies my actions."
2. *Thinking is believing.* "My thoughts and feelings are completely accurate, simply because they occur to me."
3. *Personal infallibility.* "I always make good choices."
4. *Feelings make facts.* "I know I am right, because I feel right in what I do."
5. *The impotence of others.* "The views of others are irrelevant to my decisions, unless they directly control my immediate consequences."
6. *Low-impact consequences.* "Undesirable consequences will not occur or will not matter to me."

Thus, antisocial patients' automatic thoughts and reactions are frequently distorted by self-serving beliefs that emphasize immediate, personal satisfactions and minimize future consequences. The underlying belief that they are always right makes it unlikely that they will question their actions. Patients may vary in the degree of trust or mistrust they have in others, but they are unlikely to seek guidance or advice on any particular course of action. A person with ASPD who wants something will take it without either understanding the possible consequences or manifesting concern about possible consequences.

For example, the therapist noticed that magazines were disappearing from his waiting room, and he suspected Randy, his ASPD patient. He checked that the magazines were there prior to Randy's session. Afterward they were gone. Asking Randy at the following session about the missing magazines, Randy at first vigorously denied the action. He then switched to the position that he must have inadvertently taken them. But, he reasoned, the magazines were there for the patients, and as a patient he was then justified in taking "his" magazine home to read. Thus, the behaviors of individuals with ASPD tend to elicit negative responses from others without awareness or concern that what he was doing was stealing from someone who was trying to help him.

Because the problems that they manifest are generally chronic and ego-syntonic, the patients themselves are often baffled by the responses of others and unable to see how present circumstances arose. For example, Randy was genuinely astounded that the therapist made such a "big deal" about a "stupid" magazine. Further, even after Randy offered to pay for the magazines, the therapist still saw a need for discussion of the behavior. Typically, the patient with ASPD will see the locus of the difficulties that they encounter in dealing with other people or tasks as external and independent of their behavior, viewing themselves as victims of unfair, prejudiced, or hostile systems.

Building Coping Skills

Even the seemingly simplest of life's endeavors have the potential to generate significant problems. For example, going to work includes dealing with the frustrations of commuting, interacting with people on the job, completing the tasks involved in the job itself, and coping with the demands of authorities. Although managing these challenges involves some degree of stress some of the time for most people, for the individual with ASPD these challenges can be a source of daily frustration and potential humiliation. Many have come from environments with little emotional or behavioral guidance for the tasks of responsible living. Given that many individuals with ASPD have had little support in developing coping skills, they may be operating under the stress of severe skill deficits.

Thus, adaptive problem-solving skills are often a crucial component of treatment for ASPD.

The skills deficits of ASPD patients are often misinterpreted as manipulative behavior. Patients with ASPD can be taught to expand their range of problem-solving skills to include approaches that do not cause harm to themselves and that will be viewed by others as more socially appropriate. Areas of skills development include perspective taking, impulse control, effective communication, emotion regulation, frustration tolerance, assertiveness, consequential thinking, response delay, and cognitive restructuring.

One area in which emotional coping skills almost invariably arise is in the context of persisting without immediate gratification, despite fair effort. Frequent "fire drills" can help the patient be able to withstand "bad days" with a minimum of damage to self, others, or relationships. The patient has to be helped to recognize that they have made it through "bad days" before and that feeling bad is time limited. The key is to appreciate that the deep waves of emotional turmoil are transient, although, in the midst of the feelings, it can certainly seem as though they will never end. The ability to avoid being swallowed up in the moment and to appreciate the transient nature of emotional waves is a very important aspect of tolerating distress. In addition, there are many times when effort does not pay off immediately, but the possible outcome is worth further effort rather than abandonment.

The Systematic Approach to Anger and Impulsivity

The ASPD patient has likely discovered that anger and hostility have an intimidating effect on others. Expressed anger may have the effect of establishing a ring of space between the patient and others that serves a protective function. In other circumstances the anger may be used as a "trial by fire" to see if others care enough to brave the fire and get close. Anger and hostility have become a method for both control of others and for safety and survival. Therapists may wonder whether or not to respond directly or to make pacifying statements that seem traditionally therapeutic. Therapist responses that are avoidant, placating, or rejecting may be reinforcing the very behavior that continues to cause the patient problems in his or her life and work.

Impulsive behavior frequently is a way of meeting the patient's high need for arousal in ways that may not be met in more socially accepted forms. Both anger and impulsive actions have to be mirrored for the patient in a gentle though direct manner. The patient is apt to be working from a "gut" response, and the therapist can offer a more systematic, scientific alternative of testing the advantages and disadvantages of the behavior. Rather than a constant pattern of stimulus–response behaviors, patients can be taught to (1) attend to internal emotional and cognitive cues, (2) evaluate their perception, (3) decide whether it would be of value to respond, (4) identify possible responses, (5) choose a response, and (6) respond.

Self-Monitoring and Functional Motivation

The behavior of an ASPD individual may appear to be both morally bankrupt and lacking in any functional purpose. One can imagine that even Carl Rogers would have been sorely tested to maintain unconditional positive regard having heard of some ASPD conduct. Yet, it is important to separate the person from his or her behavior, and to teach patients to observe their actions and surmise the various functions or rewards associated with a chain of behavior. For example, the patient may express concern for the therapist's "needs" and render an offer to be helpful. Randy, the court-referred patient, commented in the session that he noticed the therapist's old and tired car in the parking lot. He thought that the therapist should have a much better car. The therapist internally agreed. This car was 9 years old, in poor shape and might not pass the next state inspection without a number of expensive repairs. With a new home, the therapist was hard-pressed to get a new car.

Randy then suggested that he could get the therapist any car he wanted, with appropriate papers for registration. All the therapist had to do was "say the word" and it would be "their secret." The therapist, of course, declined and explored the motivation for the offer. He could not help but think on the way home how nice a new car would be. Randy, however, could not benefit therapeutically from such an exchange, as it was merely an effort to attain power and influence via his typical antisocial means.

Patients with ASPD are often nonintrospective and unaware of the different functions served by their patterns of behavior. They must first understand the value of learning to listen to themselves, deal with the discomfort that introspection might bring, and develop the skills to examine what they are thinking and feeling. They must be taught how to be tuned into their internal dialogue, emotional responses, and automatic behaviors. For many patients, these have the theme of survival. This theme might include behaviors of dependence, attachment, seduction, or avoidance. Once patients gain insight into their behaviors, it does not necessarily mean that they will choose to work on replacing them with more adaptive ones. If that were true, therapy would be a far simpler process. The skill of introspection or personal awareness is a sophisticated skill. The introduction and development of that skill can be, in and of itself, a reasonable goal for therapy.

Broadening the Base for Attributions and Appraisals

In the process of helping ASPD patients to test attributions, appraisals, and their associated choices, the overall objective is to expand their range of interests from the strictly personal to include awareness of more interpersonal domains, if possible. We begin with a broad hierarchy that is based on theories of moral and cognitive development. Specific steps are graded according to the individual patient's problematic ways of thinking and acting. At the lowest level on the hierarchy, the patient thinks only in terms of self-interest, basing choices on obtaining rewards or avoiding immediate punishments, without regard for others. This is where the antisocial patient functions most of the time prior to treatment. The dysfunctional beliefs previously described operate as unqualified rules at this level. Antisocial patients at this level do whatever they feel like doing, firmly believe that they always act in their own best interest, and remain impervious to corrective feedback.

At the next major level, a patient recognizes implications of his or her behavior and has some understanding of how it affects others, with an eye toward longer-range self-interest. This is the level toward which the clinician typically attempts to guide the ASPD patient. This is accomplished by helping the patient to grasp the concept of dysfunctional thoughts and behavior and encouraging him or her to test alternative solutions that might modify earlier rules for living. For example, ASPD patients might come to realize that the views of others do have an effect on their getting what they want in the long run, even if such views do not directly control the immediate outcome of a specific situation. Gradually, such patients gain skill in considering something that is "possible" at the same time as something that is immediate or "actual." They are not so firmly convinced that they are always "right," and they are able to take in some new information and alter their behavior accordingly.

The third major level of the hierarchy is more difficult to define, because there is controversy among theorists regarding what constitutes the highest level of moral development. In moral or interpersonal terms, the individual demonstrates either a sense of responsibility or caring for others that includes a respect for the needs and wants of others or a commitment to laws as guiding principles for the good of society. At the second level, the individual shows some concern for specific people under certain conditions in which there is something he or she stands to gain or lose. At the third level, the person shows a greater ability to consider the needs of others or the needs of society in general. He or she may show respect for rules of order or commitment to others because he or she cares about their welfare and considers relationships an important part of his or her life.

A brief example may help to illustrate the general outline of the cognitive hierarchy just described. Consider an antisocial man seeking to fulfill a sexual desire. At the first level, he pursues a partner of his choice without regard for her interests or the consequences of his actions. For example, one young man described his typical relationships as consisting strictly of sexual activity that occurred at his convenience. His current girlfriend repeatedly asked him to accompany her to a public place such as a fast-food restaurant because she wanted him to take her out on a "date." The young man had no intention of responding to any of her interests in expanding their relationship or even her requests for certain sexual techniques. He felt quite comfortable in pursuing his personal sexual purposes, regardless of her feelings.

At the second level, this antisocial young man might be influenced in a limited way by the interests or wishes of others. For example, he might occasionally concede to some of his girlfriend's requests in order to maintain his advantage. "Make her happy once in a while and she will keep giving me what I want" might be his reasoning. At the third level, he might focus more on mutual interests as well as more long-range aspects of his behavior. For instance, he might make an effort to satisfy rather than to frustrate his girlfriend, because that is a better way of treating other people generally, and because it would contribute to a more stable and satisfying relationship for them both.

Making Constructive Choices

Patients whose problems are framed as a set of choices are less apt to feel that they are being manipulated, controlled, or accused of bad behavior. For many problem situations, the patient and therapist can together conduct a systematic review of the "risk–benefit ratio" of different choices. Behavioral changes are most likely to be initiated by antisocial patients when they have selected that change from a range of possible choices because it has distinct, relevant advantages.

For example, Sam, a young man with ASPD, was on the verge of being expelled from dental school. Sam believed that he should do what he felt like doing, such as tell off supervisors or not return from a weekend trip until Wednesday even when he was scheduled to provide clinical services on Monday and Tuesday. He viewed the consequences of these actions as mainly problems for other people and not himself. Sam tended either to dismiss or to become belligerent toward people who tried to convince him that he should feel ashamed of his bad behavior.

As an alternative, the therapist helped Sam to recognize that getting kicked out of dental school was a situation that he wished to avoid. Therapy discussion focused on ways to modify his belief that he could do whatever he felt like doing. Sam worked on reducing behavior that he justified on the basis of immediate feelings. He did this in order to meet his goal of graduating from dental school.

Parts of the "choice review" exercise may be adapted for homework or may be modified to meet the needs of specific patients. The first step is to identify a problem situation and to list all the facts about that situation. Then the patient rates his or her satisfaction with those facts on a scale of 0–100.

Next, as many choices as possible are listed in the second column. The choice column would typically include current maladaptive behavior, as well as presumably more adaptive alternatives. Options in the choice column incorporate the patient's immediate, "automatic" reactions, as well as other possibilities that come out of a discussion between the patient and therapist. In two adjacent columns, the advantages and disadvantages of each choice are listed. At this point, the therapist may be able to point out disadvantages to maladaptive behavior that the patient has overlooked. Advantages of more adaptive choices can also be pointed out. Finally, the patient rates how effective each choice is likely to be, using the 0–100 scale.

An appropriate follow-up for this exercise would include an ongoing review of subsequent behavioral choices made in the problem areas discussed, with a concomitant effectiveness evaluation. Repeated ineffective choices could indicate a need to review the advantages and disadvantages again, or could highlight a need to address some specific skill deficits. Alternatively, the patient may need to review why he or she continues to make ineffective choices. This may be occurring because of some previously undetected dysfunctional belief.

Case Example. Although somewhat complex, the following case example illustrates the benefits of a specific, problem-focused cognitive intervention for ASPD. Over the course of treatment, this patient's cognitions gradually shifted from a predominant focus on her own self-interest and immediate emotional reactions to a greater recognition of the implications of her behavior for other people, and how others' reactions to this behavior in turn affected her.

Susan was a 28-year-old Caucasian female who entered outpatient psychotherapy as part of a complicated family therapy intervention. She had two daughters, 7-year-old Candy, who resided with a custodial father and stepmother (Mr. and Mrs. R), and 4-year-old Carol, who resided with the maternal grandmother.

Susan's history, gathered via interviews with Susan and the Rs, as well as through review of copies of court testimony, revealed a conduct disorder before age 15 and persistent irresponsible and antisocial behavior since age 15. At age 18, she had been convicted of selling controlled substances and served a year in prison. Susan conceived her older daughter, Candy, during a brief relationship with Mr. R, but never told him she was pregnant and did not inform him of his daughter's existence until Candy was almost 3 years old. Susan's impulsive and irresponsible behavior eventually led to the removal of her two daughters from her custody because of her negligence in their care.

At the time of initial therapy contact, Susan was living in a city 150 miles from the Rs. She had been coming to town once a month for a couple of months and visiting with her younger biological child, Carol, overnight in her own mother's house. She also wanted to resume visits with Candy, so she agreed to Mr. and Mrs. R's stipulation of therapy. During the previous several years, Susan had visited Candy very sporadically, once even letting an entire year pass without contact. At the time of treatment, Susan's visitation rights were restricted to being under the direct supervision and discretion of the custodial parents.

Initially, Susan was cordial but also defensive and resentful of the circumstances of therapy. She grudgingly agreed to complete the Minnesota Multiphasic Personality Inventory (MMPI), and produced a valid profile that was characterized by defensiveness and anger, with a spike elevation on scale 4 (Psychopathic Deviance).

After interviewing Candy and Susan separately and observing them playing together, the therapist noted both interpersonal interest and cooperation between them. Susan demonstrated an increased interest in playing a role in her daughter's life by her efforts to expand visitation. The Rs reported that she behaved appropriately when she was with Candy, attending to her, playing with her, and not obviously abusing or neglecting her. Susan claimed that she had been in business school for several months, that she had worked continuously in the same job for more than 6 months, and that she was involved in a romantic relationship of more than 6 months duration—all evidence of increased stability in her life, albeit relatively short term.

Based on this information, the therapist agreed to work with Susan in her reunification efforts with Candy. The therapist informed Susan that her history and psychological test results indicated that she had ASPD. This disorder was explained as a lifestyle disorder of judgments and behaviors that resulted in negative consequences for Susan as well as others, such as Candy. The agreed-on goals of the cognitive therapy were to assist Susan in gaining greater access to visitation with her daughter, as long as there was no decline in Candy's overall adjustment.

Candy responded positively to contacts with Susan but was jealous of her half-sister Carol getting to do more things with their mother and had trouble saying good-bye when their few hours of visitation were up.

Candy had problems of moodiness and noncompliance right after a visit if Carol got to spend that night with her mother, while Candy had to return home to the Rs. By the Rs' report, Candy's behavior also seemed worse in the middle of the month, when she would begin to doubt that her mother was coming back to see her again.

The choice-review intervention with Susan focused on visitation with Candy, as well as other specific concerns that Susan had in handling her two daughters. Figure 8.1 provides an example of Susan's choice-review exercise. In this exercise, Susan listed her immediate, "automatic" reaction to the visitation situation, as well as other possible reactions that she discussed with the therapist. Through the choice-review

Problem	Choice	Advantages	Disadvantages
Visitation. The Rs have a court decree giving them control over my visits with Candy. They only let me visit for 4 hours in their home. S = 10.	Tell the Rs to shove it. E = 40.	Feel better.	May backfire and cause further restrictions.
	Give up and stop visiting altogether. E = 20.	Easy. Least amount of hassle. May be best all around.	Not what I really want. May hurt Candy.
	Just take Candy from school. E = 25.	Get back at the Rs and get time with Candy.	Maybe get arrested. Candy might get scared.
	Enjoy the time we have, and ask for gradual increases. E = 50.	No big confrontation.	Slow progress. Candy wants to stay with me now.
The Rs do not trust me. They think I am an unfit mother. I want to spend time alone with my daughter. S = 0.	Try to convince the Rs that I am not a bad mother. E = 40.	The Rs may believe me and let me have more freedom.	Pain in the ass. I should not have to ask permission to see my own daughter.
	Demand the Rs give me more time with Candy. E = 20.	Show them I have rights too. Feel better.	Won't change their stubborn minds. Might make things harder.
	Stick with the gradual request plan for more freedom with Candy; deal with their negative attitude. E = 70.	May pay off in little ways very soon. Gives chance to build good faith with the Rs.	Pace WAY slow, but I can deal with it.

FIGURE 8.1. Susan's choice review exercise. The "S = __" ratings in the "Problem" column indicate the patient's satisfaction with the facts of the situation, on a scale of 0–100. The "E = __" ratings in the "Choice" column indicate the patient's estimation of the effectiveness of each choice, on a scale of 0–100.

discussion, Susan was able to see that she did have some ability to influence the future of her visitation with Candy. She decided that expressing her resentment of what she believed to be the unfairness of her visitation limits was not as likely to be effective in achieving her goal as was trying to build up a "good-faith" relationship with the Rs. The therapist helped her to determine some steps toward "good faith" through gradual efforts to expand her range of privileges with Candy.

Over the course of approximately 8 months, Susan's privileges with Candy expanded gradually from driving to therapy in a separate car to having lunch alone with Candy after therapy; extending visits from 4 to 8 hours, having half of the 8-hour visit on their own, then most of the visit on their own, and finally having an overnight visit together at Candy's maternal grandmother's house.

Susan made all her own requests for privileges to the Rs, after first practicing her approach with the therapist. Initially, negotiation between Susan and the Rs was conducted in the therapist's presence, in order to facilitate communication. The Rs aired their reservations, to which Susan attempted to respond in a reassuring rather than hostile manner, as she had practiced with the therapist. When Susan did respond with hostility, the Rs backed off and temporarily refused to expand privileges. This was helpful in that Susan could then see how her attitude had interfered with getting what she wanted, with some help from the therapist in mirroring her anger and focusing on the systematic approach. The therapist was careful not to step in and reassure the Rs on Susan's behalf but instead worked with Susan to help her keep her priorities in mind and review the effectiveness of her behavior.

Candy showed improvement in her overall mood and in her cooperation at home and at school. A critical factor family progress was Susan's being responsible enough to continue showing up for visits to the Rs and acting in an appropriate manner when Candy was in her care. Apparently, Susan valued her relationship with her daughter enough to work for it. She was able to function reasonably well in a structured, time-limited parental role. At the same time, that structure had to become flexible enough to allow enjoyable contact with her daughter, rather than emphasizing limitations as punishment for being a poor mother in the past.

Treatment interventions helped Susan to pursue her goal of increased visitation more effectively and helped her to recognize that stepwise efforts were more effective than all-or-nothing demands. Her emotional coping skills were increased through role play and rehearsal of difficult interpersonal situations, emphasizing her skills in tolerating expectations from others without immediate angry reactions. Her ability to use emotional coping skills was greatly influenced by reflecting on the desired functions of her behavior and her increased ability to take an interpersonal perspective.

Susan's thinking and reasoning showed movement up the cognitive hierarchy as she came to recognize that her attitude toward others influenced how she might be treated, and that it was possible for her to be treated differently if she acted differently. She showed some potential for moving toward the third level (general social interest) of the hierarchy by considering several people's wants and needs at once. These considerations, however, were still motivated by a qualified self-interest rather than a commitment to being a good mother because that was important to Candy's adjustment. For instance, she tended to emphasize what she would enjoy doing with Candy rather than what Candy might enjoy doing with her. In another instance near the close of therapy, Susan raised the possibility that she might go to live in Europe with her boyfriend. She was mainly concerned with the possibility that Candy would get angry and reject her, rather than being sensitive to how much Candy might miss her or concerned with how she could fulfill her responsibilities as Candy's mother. However, treatment was terminated when the agreed-on goals of therapy were met. A mutually satisfying visitation schedule was established and maintained for 3 months without incident, and Candy showed significant improvement in her mood and cooperation at home and at school.

MAINTAINING PROGRESS

Both behavioral and cognitive gains are more likely to be maintained if the ASPD patient is able to identify emotionally compelling reasons to implement the strategies learning in treatment. Thus, it is helpful to review with individual patients their potentially high-risk situations in which they may be apt to respond in ways that could be defined as troublesome, and to establish a goal or personal priority that would lead them to review their choices. In addition, the use of environmental supports should be implemented whenever possible, such as participation in sobriety-oriented support groups. However, referral to community support groups should be chosen with care, as ASPD patients may be tempted to take advantage of more emotionally vulnerable individuals.

CONCLUSION

Once intervention takes place, one can never really know how destructive the antisocial patient might have been if no treatment had been provided. Likewise, one cannot predict or promise how many times the anti-social person might decide not to lie, con, cheat, beat, rape, steal, harass, default, or otherwise disrupt social harmony because he or she sees some greater personal advantage in not doing so. However, the case examples described in this chapter illustrate how cognitive therapy can have a pos-itive impact on the life course of an antisocial person. Optimal function-ing might remain an unrealistic goal for treatment, but improvements in prosocial behavior have obvious benefits for the stability of the patient and the well-being of his or her significant others, as well as society at large.

CHAPTER 9

Borderline Personality Disorder

Borderline personality disorder (BPD) can be characterized by the re-markable instability that pervades many if not all aspects of the individuals functioning, including relationships, self-image, affect, and behavior. For example, Natasha, 29 years old, sought help after being unable to work for more than a year. She complained of being too tired to work, lying in bed for most of the day. The problems seemed to have started as the result of a job-related conflict. She had started an affair with her boss but ended it because he did not skip the marriage that he had planned before the affair. She felt strongly disappointed by him and started a relationship with another man. According to Natasha, her boss resented her decision, gave her work below her former level, and criticized her so much in front of other personnel that she became "burned out." The clinician who saw her thought initially of an adjustment disorder with mixed emotional features and a V-code (relational problems). Seeing her for the second time, however, the picture became much more complicated. She described her relationship with her husband as characterized by lots of fights and aggressive threats. She also expressed resentment toward her family and admitted high use of cannabis and alcohol. She repeatedly stated that she found that life had no use and was very distrustful of other people. When asked what should be done in treatment she was rather vague, giving answers such as "I have to feel at home with myself." Although the therapist thought that Natasha probably suffered from high levels of anxiety, sadness, and loneliness, she presented a tough appearance, and it was easy to imagine how this could provoke irritation and anger in other people.

Noting this evidence of further psychopathology, the therapist proceeded with semistructured clinical interviews to establish a thorough diagnosis. In addition to a number of Axis I and Axis II diagnoses, it became clear that Natasha's problems met the criteria of a BPD. It also became clear that Natasha suffered from many unresolved emotional problems related to her youth and her relationships with her parents. The clinician then discussed the possibility that BPD was the main problem and the pros and cons of a treatment directed at her long-standing personality problems. Natasha decided to start with a long-term cognitive therapy focused on her personality problems. She reasoned that something fundamental should be done with the way she felt about herself and about other people, and she wanted to emotionally process the painful experiences she had had with her parents.

BPD is a relatively common disorder (1.1–2.5% of the general adult population), with enormous societal costs, comparable to schizophrenia (Linehan & Heard, 1999; van Asselt, Dirksen, Severens, & Arntz, 2002), high risk of suicide (about 10% die because of suicide; Paris, 1993), and considerable impairment in the individual's life. The proportion of patients with BPD generally rises with the intensity of health care treatment setting, from less than 10% in outpatient facilities to more than 50% in specialized inpatient units (American Psychiatric Association, 1994). Patients with BPD are a burden for relatives, friends, and colleagues, and there is a high risk that they induce psychopathology in their offspring (Weiss et al., 1996). Many individuals with BPD are intelligent and gifted people, but their disorder prevents them from developing themselves, and many have troubles finishing education, do not work at all, or have jobs below their capacities. Relational crises are common, they often injure themselves, and they often engage in substance abuse, usually as a form of self-medication.

Apart from mental health care, they are heavy users of physical health care facilities (Van Asselt et al., 2002). Many patients with BPD seek help because of a crisis related to more chronic problems with posttraumatic stress disorder, depression, social phobia, and relationship disturbance. They should be helped to view their difficulties in the perspective of their personality problems, simultaneously installing hope that these problems can be treated.

Notorious for their angry outbursts and their crises, patients with BPD have a bad reputation in health care, and many therapists are afraid of them. The belief that these people cannot really be helped is widespread. Recent developments however suggest that this view is incorrect. Specialized forms of cognitive therapy are among the most promising treatment options available. Although cognitive therapy for BPD is in no way simple, many therapists discovered that using this framework, treatment of individuals with BPD can be a successful and rewarding experience.

HISTORICAL PERSPECTIVES

The diagnosis "borderline" was introduced in the 1930s to label patients with problems that seemed to fall somewhere in between neurosis and psychosis (Stern, 1938). Object relation theorists have further elaborated on this, and introduced "borderline" as a personality organization related to a hypothesized fixation in the separation–individuation developmental phase of the child. A borderline organization is described as an immature personality, characterized by identity diffusion and the use of primitive defenses such as splitting and projective identification but a largely intact reality testing (Kernberg, 1976, 1996; Kernberg, Selzer, Koenigsberg, Carr, & Appelbaum, 1989). The idea is that object relation representations (including self-representations) are not integrated but split off from each other. They are organized according to their valence, positive (good) versus negative (bad), to prevent the aggressive impulses attached to the bad representations from destroying the positive representations. It should be noted that the concept of borderline organization (or structure) is much wider than BPD and encompasses a range of personality types and symptomatic disorders, including substance abuse/dependence, bipolar disorder, and impulse-control disorders. In the 1970s, Gunderson and Singer (1975) introduced the first operational definition of BPD. The introduction was supported by empirical work so that Gunderson's definition formed the ground for inclusion of BPD in DSM-III. With some adaptations, this definition in its essence is still used in DSM-IV-TR. The more psychotic-like, socially isolated (schizophrenia-like) patients who were formerly diagnosed as "borderline" were from then on diagnosed as schizotypal personality disorder. The essence of the DSM-IV-TR concept of BPD is instability, as expressed in instability of interpersonal relationships, self-image, and affects, and marked impulsivity (see Table 9.1).

RESEARCH AND EMPIRICAL DATA
Psychological Models

Early attempts to test psychological models of BPD have focused on hypotheses derived from object relations theory. By using projective tests such as the Thematic Apperception Test, researchers have attempted to elicit the object relationship representations of patients with BPD and re-

TABLE 9.1. DSM-IV-TR Diagnostic Criteria for Borderline Personality Disorder

A pervasive pattern of instability of interpersonal relationships, self-image, and affects, and marked impulsivity beginning by early adulthood and present in a variety of contexts, as indicated by five (or more) of the following:

(1) frantic efforts to avoid real or imagined abandonment. **Note:** Do not include suicidal or self-mutilating behavior covered in Criterion 5.

(2) a pattern of unstable and intense interpersonal relationships characterized by alternating between extremes of idealization and devaluation

(3) identity disturbance: markedly and persistently unstable self-image or sense of self

(4) impulsivity in at least two areas that are potentially self-damaging (e.g., spending, sex, substance abuse, reckless driving, binge eating). **Note:** Do not include suicidal or self-mutilating behavior covered in Criterion 5.

(5) recurrent suicidal behavior, gestures, or threats, or self-mutilating behavior

(6) affective instability due to a marked reactivity of mood (e.g., intense episodic dysphoria, irritability, or anxiety usually lasting a few hours and only rarely more than a few days)

(7) chronic feelings of emptiness

(8) inappropriate, intense ange or difficulty controlling anger (e.g., frequent displays of temper, constant anger, recurrent physical fights)

(9) transient, stress-related paranoid ideation or severe dissociative symtoms

Note. From American Psychiatric Association (2000, p. 710). Copyright 2000 by the American Psychiatric Association. Reprinted by permission.

lated psychological processes, such as splitting as a defense mechanism. In general, the hypothesis that patients with BPD function on the level of a pre-Oedipal child, as object relation theory states, has not been supported. Patients with BPD appeared to be able to attribute highly developed intentions to figures from projective tests, whereas there was little evidence for splitting. Across studies, however, patients with BPD appeared consistently characterized by attributing malevolent motives to others. According to Westen (1991), malevolence does not characterize the object world of the normal pre-Oedipal child, and the complex attributions produced by subjects with BPD are cognitively far advanced relative to anything a toddler could produce. Similar findings were reported by Baker, Silk, Westin, Nigg, and Lohr (1992) when investigating BPD patients' ratings of their parents.

Various studies have found that patients with BPD are characterized by disorganized attachment representations (Fonagy et al., 1996; Patrick et al., 1994). Such attachment representations appear to be typical for persons with unresolved childhood traumas, especially when parental figures were involved, with direct, frightening behavior by the parent. Disorganized attachment is considered to result from an unresolvable situation for the child when "the parent is at the same time the source of fright as well as the potential haven of safety" (van IJzendoorn, Schuengel, & Bakermans-Kranenburg, 1999, p. 226).

A separate line of research has investigated the developmental history of patients with BPD. Initially, high prevalence of childhood sexual abuse, especially between the ages of 6 and 12, and by caretakers was reported (e.g., Herman, Perry, & van der Kolk, 1989; Ogata et al., 1990; Weaver & Clum, 1993). The association with BPD seemed so strong that it has been proposed to view BPD as a specific posttraumatic disorder (e.g., Herman & van der Kolk, 1987). Severe sexual abuse of the child, especially by caretakers, seemed to explain much of the BPD symptoms and behaviors, including the malevolent views of others and the disorganized attachment patterns. But, some studies also found associations between BPD and childhood physical and emotional abuse.

When traumatic childhood experiences play a role in the pathogenesis of BPD, this might explain why many patients with BPD claim they do not feel pain during self-mutilation. High uncontrollable stress can evoke endogenous opioid release, which reduces the experience of pain (Janssen & Arntz, 2001; Pitman, van der Kolk, Orr, & Greenberg, 1990). Initially extreme stress resulting from sexual, physical or emotional abuse of the child might have led to an unconditioned opioid release. Classical conditioning processes might then lead to a conditioned opioid release in response to stressors such as expectation of a repetition of the abuse. In accordance with this view, studies employing an experimental pain stimulus found support for the existence of stress-induced analgesia in patients with BPD who claimed to feel no pain during self-mutilation (Bohus et al., 2000; Kemperman et al., 1997; McCown, Galina, Johnson, DeSimone, & Poas, 1993; Russ et al., 1992, 1994). The degree to which analgesia in (some) patients with BPD is stress-induced, and is indeed opioid-mediated, is still the subject of discussion.

Although the debate on the role of childhood sexual abuse in the pathogenesis of BPD continues (Fossati, Madeddu, & Maffei, 1999; Trull, 2001; Weaver & Clum, 1993, Zanarini, 1997), there is a general agreement that childhood abuse of some form is highly prevalent among patients with BPD. Almost all patients with BPD seem to have suffered from maltreatment by parents such as physical punishments, emotional abuse, threats, severe psychiatric problems in the parents, or sexual abuse. If the parent was not the perpetrator, he or she failed to protect the child or to help emotionally process the abuse. Instead, patients often report punishing and blaming responses of parents toward them as a child.

A current view is that it is not the trauma itself that caused BPD, but the way the child processed it and attached meaning to it given individual temperament, age, and situational factors (Arntz, 1994; Zanarini, 2000). Some of the traumatic experiences may have taken place at a very early age, notably the kind of punishing, abandoning, rejecting responses of the caretaker that led to disorganized attachment. In cognitive terms, the traumatic experiences may have led to specific childish in-terpretations and oppositional behavior, which may have elicited further negative responses by caretakers, a process that finally led to the forma-tion of pathogenic core schemas and strategies.

Arntz (1994) hypothesized that childhood traumas underlie the for-mation of core schemas, which in their turn, lead to the development of BPD. A structural equation modeling test of this hypothesis, comparing BPD, Cluster C, and nonpsychiatric subjects on childhood traumas and assumptions, demonstrated that patients with BPD could be strongly distinguished from the other groups by a specific set of assumptions. These assumptions mediated (in a statistical sense) the relationship be-tween reports of childhood sexual and emotional abuse, which also strongly discriminated BPD from the two control groups (Arntz, Dietzel, & Dreessen, 1999).

A later, much larger, study provided further support for the hypoth-esis that patients with BPD, in addition to believing in a wide range of assumptions also found in other personality disorders (notably avoidant and paranoid beliefs), are characterized by a specific set of assumptions. The specific themes are loneliness, unlovability, rejection and abandon-ment by others, and viewing the self as bad and to be punished (Arntz, Dreessen, Schouten, & Weertmen, in press). Using a different approach, Butler, Brown, Beck, and Grisham (2002) demonstrated that a set of 14 items of the Personality Belief Questionnaire, originally not formulated as BPD-specific beliefs, discriminated BPD from 6 other personality dis-orders. The BPD-specific beliefs reflected themes of dependency, help-lessness, distrust, extreme attention-seeking behavior, and fears of rejec-tion, abandonment, and losing emotional control. Using an existing instrument, the World Assumption Scale, Giesen-Bloo and Arntz (2003) found evidence for Pretzer's (1990) hypothesis that three themes are dominant in BPD beliefs: "The world is dangerous and malevolent," "I am powerless and vulnerable," and "I am inherently unacceptable." Al-though there is a considerable overlap with the themes found in these three studies, the differences call for further research.

Recently, Young's schema mode model (McGinn & Young, 1996; Young, Klosko, & Weishaar, 2003) has been put to the test. Arntz and coworkers demonstrated that patients with BPD were characterized by higher self-reports of beliefs, emotions, and behaviors related to the four pathogenic BPD modes (detached protector, abandoned/abused child, angry child, and punitive parent mode), and lower ratings on the healthy adult mode scales, compared to Cluster C and nonpsychiatric controls (Arntz, Klokman, & Sieswerda, 2003). Cluster C subjects were charac-terized by significantly higher reports of overcompensation (perfection-ism, etc.) mode items. A stress induction by means of an emotional movie (abuse of a child) led to a specific increase in the detached protector mode in the subjects with BPD, compared to both control groups.

Apart from the content of BPD schemas, early cognitive views have hypothesized that patients with BPD are characterized by hypervigilance (being vulnerable in a dangerous world where nobody can be trusted) and dichotomous thinking (Pretzer, 1990). Three studies tested the hypervigilance hypothesis with the emotional STROOP paradigm. As hypothesized, evidence was found for increased color naming latencies when presented words were threatening (Arntz, Appels, & Sieswerda, 2000; Sieswerda & Arntz, 2001; Waller & Button, in press). The first two studies failed to find stimulus specificity (i.e., all types of threat words elicited the interference), but the last one found that only self-punishing words elicited the bias. One study demonstrated the effect even on a subliminal (i.e., unaware) level (Sieswerda & Arntz, 2001). So far it is unclear to what degree this hypervigilance is specific to BPD or is common to a wider range of personality disorders, as the first study on the subject suggests.

Empirical evidence that dichotomous thinking is highly characteristic for patients with BPD was provided in a study by Veen and Arntz (2000). After viewing specific film fragments with themes such as abuse and abandonment, patients with BPD gave more polarized evaluations of the film personalities than did Cluster C personality disorders and nonpsychiatric subjects. But, after viewing neutral or nonspecific emotional fragments, patients with BPD were as moderate as both control groups. Interestingly, the BPD polarized ratings on a list of character traits were not organized along a good–bad dimension, as would be predicted from object relation theory, which states that patients with BPD tend to view others as either totally good or totally bad (splitting).

When asked to describe the personalities of the specific film clips in an unstructured format, BPD as well as Cluster C patients gave less complex descriptions and used less trait descriptions than did nonpsychiatric controls (Arntz & Veen, 2001). Patients with BPD were the most negativistic, confirming earlier findings with projective tests. Taken together, the findings suggest that patients with BPD are able to function at higher levels (i.e., using more dimensions in their evaluations) in a structured than in an unstructured situation.

Research into affect regulation, which is hypothesized to be disregulated in BPD, has yielded mixed findings. Peripheral psychophysiological indices, facial expressions, and self-report have suggested that responses of patients with BPD to emotional stimuli in experimental settings are comparable to those of nonpsychiatric controls, even at subnormal level (Herpertz et al., 2000; Herpertz, Werth, et al., 2001; Renneberg, Heyn, Gebhard, & Bachmann, in press), but central indices (fMRI, notably amygdala responses) suggested hyperarousability (Herpertz, Dietrich, et al., 2001). This dissociation between periphery and central regions is reminiscent of the contrast between the detached impression patients with BPD often give and their strong inner emotional experiences. Self-report studies in natural contexts have supported the hypothesis that patients with BPD have strong and labile negative affect (Cowdry, Gardner, O'Leary, Leibenluft, & Rubinow, 1991; Stein, 1996).

Psychotherapy Research

Older studies have mainly focused on psychodynamic therapy. In general, high early dropout rates have been reported when more traditional forms of psychodynamic treatment were offered to patients with BPD: 67% within 3 months (Skodol, Buckley, & Charles, 1983); 46% within 6 months, 67% in total (Waldinger & Gunderson, 1984); 43% within 6 months (Gunderson et al., 1989); 64% within 12 months (Yeomans, Selzer, & Clarkin, 1993), and 42% within 6 months (Clarkin et al., 1994). Traditional psychodynamic approaches did not seem to result in a reduction of suicide risk in treated patients. Across four studies, approximately 10% of the patients died during treatment or within 15 years following treatment due to suicide (Paris, 1993). This percentage is comparable to the suicide risk in subjects with BPD in general (8–9%; cf. Adams, Bernat & Luscher, 2001).

Early cognitive-behavioral therapy approaches of BPD mainly focused on problematic behaviors without approaching the disorder as a whole from an integrated formulation. Schema-focused approaches seemed of limited value if treatment was of short duration (Davidson & Tyrer, 1996). But, when more integrated methods of longer duration were introduced, case studies suggested that such approaches were promising (Turner, 1989).

In a landmark study, Linehan, Armstrong, Suarez, Allmon, and Heard (1991) demonstrated that for parasuicidal patients with BPD, 1 year of dialectical behavior therapy (DBT) was superior to treatment as usual (TAU) on three indices: the number of patients who stayed in treatment (83% vs. 50%), median days of hospitalization (17 vs. 51 days), and the number of patients still parasuicidal during the last 3 months of treatment (36% vs. 62%). However, subjective reports of depression, hopelessness, reasons for living, and suicide ideation did not indicate that DBT helped the patients in these respects more than TAU. Similar findings were reported in a Dutch study, comparing DBT with TAU for substance-dependent patients with BPD (van den Bosch, Verheul, Schippers, & van den Brink, 2002). Whereas DBT reduced attrition rate (37% vs. 77% in 1 year), and reduced self-mutilating and self-damaging impulsive acts compared to TAU, no effects were observed on other indices, including substance abuse. Similarly, Linehan et al. (1999) found that DBT was superior to TAU in reducing substance abuse but not on other measures of psychopathology. Thus, DBT might be especially effective in reducing self-damaging BPD behavior but not effective in reducing the emotional suffering of these patients. Although 1 year of DBT leads to improvement of the patient in a number of important respects, which are maintained at follow-up (Linehan, Heard, & Armstrong, 1993), the data indicate that the average patient still suffers from a large number of problems (but, see Koons et al., 2001).

Cognitive-behavioral therapy along the lines of Beck, Freeman, & Associates (1990) has been investigated in at least two uncontrolled trials. Brown, Newman, Charlesworth, and Chrits-Cristoph (2003) found significant decreases on suicide ideation, hopelessness, depression, number of BPD symptoms, and dysfunctional beliefs after 1 year of cognitive-behavioral therapy for suicidal or self-mutilating patients with BPD. Results were maintained at a 6 months follow-up. Effect sizes were moderate (0.22–0.55). Dropout rate was 9.4%. Arntz (1999a) found positive effects of long-lasting cognitive-behavioral therapy in a mixed sample of personality disorders, including 6 patients with BPD. Two patients with BPD dropped out prematurely, but the other four attained good results. In a controlled trial, Berk, Forman, Henriques, Brown, and Beck (2002) and Beck (2002) demonstrated that a short, focused cognitive-behavioral therapy was more successful than a control treatment in reducing suicidal ideation and suicide attempts in highly suicidal patients with BPD.

A cognitive-behavioral therapy approach based on Young's schema-model (McGinn & Young, 1996; Young, Klosko, & Weishaar, 2003) and Arntz's (1994) extension of Beckian cognitive-behavioral therapy is currently being compared to a modern psychodynamic therapy (transference-focused psychotherapy [TFP], developed by Kernberg and coworkers, 1989). Before the study started, therapists treated pilot patients who were not formally randomized across the two conditions. Preliminary findings indicate that 10% of the 20 cognitive-behavioral therapy pilot patients and 47% (3 by suicide) of the 17 TFP pilot patients ended treatment prematurely (Arntz, 1999b). Completers gradually improved in both types of treatments. Results should be interpreted with extreme caution, because patients were not randomly allocated to treatments. Preliminary results of the final multi-center study, which will investigate 3 years of treatment ($N = 88$, now randomized) with most patients being in treatment for less than a year, suggest again that psychodynamic treatment is more strongly related to early termination (at that time 28% (TFP) vs. 7% (cognitive-behavioral therapy); Giesen-Bloo, Arntz, van Dyck, Spinhoven, & van Tilburn, 2001). At 2 years, dropout from TFP was 42%, compared to 13% from cognitive-behavioral therapy (Giesen-

Bloo, Arntz, van Dyck, Spinhoven, & van Tilburn, 2002). Data further
suggest that 1 year of treatment may lead to significant reductions in
BPD manifestations (effect sizes 0.89–1.12) and significant increases in
quality of life, even in domains not directly related to psychiatric symptoms (effect size 0.66), and that these variables continue to improve in
the second year of treatment (cumulative effect sizes for BPD manifestations: 1.00–1.35; for quality of life: 0.67) (Giesen-Bloo et al., 2001,
2002). Complete comparisons of both treatments in these respects are
not yet available.

To summarize, modern versions of cognitive-behavioral therapy
specifically tailored to meeting the problems posed by BPD seem to have
increased the efficacy of psychological treatment of BPD. The proportion of patients who terminate treatment too early has been dramatically
reduced, and effects of treatment seem now broader and deeper than
with earlier approaches that focused on a limited number of problematic
behaviors. Shorter treatments (i.e., of 1 year) are capable of reducing the
most problematic behaviors and improving anger control and social
functioning, but the average patient is far from cured. Longer treatments
appear needed for more extensive remediation.

DIFFERENTIAL DIAGNOSIS

BPD is one of the most common disorders in various inpatient and outpatient settings. Prevalence in the general population is estimated 1.1 to
2.5%, and varies in clinical populations depending on setting, from 10
to 60%. Despite its high prevalence, the disorder is often overlooked.
When a clear, stable, and autonomous Axis I disorder is present and is
the reason for seeking help, this may not be too problematic, because in
such conditions Axis II disorders do not tend to interfere with CBT cognitive-behavioral therapy for Axis I (Dreessen & Arntz, 1998). In many
cases, however, the main problem is the BPD. Underdiagnosis constitutes
a big problem that results in insufficient treatment. In many cases we
saw, it took years of fruitless attempts to treat these patients before it became clear they were in fact suffering from BPD.

The usually high comorbidity associated with BPD makes things
further complicated. Almost all disorders have been found to be associated with BPD: mood disorders, substance abuse/dependence, anxiety
disorders (notably posttraumatic stress disorder), psychotic disorders,
and other personality disorders. Patients with BPD consistently meet criteria of one to five other personality disorders. Because BPD is viewed as
one of the most severe personality disorders, it is recommended to use
BPD as the first personality diagnosis and adapt the treatment to important comorbid personality disorders. Antisocial and narcissistic person-

ality disorders might be an exception, especially when criminal features are present.

With some exceptions, BPD should be the first diagnosis (i.e., focus of treatment) when Axis I disorders are present. Some exceptions are bipolar disorder, severe depression, psychotic disorders (other than transient, stress-related psychosis, which overlaps with criterion 9 of BPD), substance abuse that needs (clinical) detoxification, attention-deficit/hyperactivity disorder, and anorexia nervosa. These disorders should be treated first. These disorders are also problematic, because they partially overlap in criteria with BPD and can make the diagnosis of BPD highly problematic. Bipolar disorder, for instance, can be mistaken for BPD, or the other way round. Finally, some conditions can lead to apparent personality changes that are similar to BPD, such as posttraumatic stress disorder (PTSD) and chronic substance abuse (e.g., cocaine).

Structured assessment of both Axis I and Axis II is perhaps the best safeguard against diagnostic mistakes. Given the high costs (van Asselt et al., 2002; Linehan & Heard, 1999) and suffering of patients with BPD, and the difficult and long treatment, the effort of executing semistructured clinical interviews is minimal.

CONCEPTUALIZATION

There are, roughly speaking, three cognitive-behavioral conceptualizations of BPD: Linehan's dialectical–behavioral view; Beckian formulations, and Young's schema mode model.

Linehan's Dialectical–Behavioral View

According to Linehan's model, patients with BPD are characterized by a dysfunction in emotion regulation that is probably temperamental (Linehan, 1993). This dysfunction causes both a strong reaction to stressful events and a long time until emotions return to baseline. A second assumption is that the environment of the patient with BPD was, and often still is, invalidating. Denying, punishing, or incorrect responses to emotional reactions of the child are hypothesized to contribute to the problems patients with BPD have in regulating, understanding, and tolerating their emotional reactions. Later on, patients with BPD invalidate their own emotional reactions and adapt an oversimplistic and unrealistic view toward emotions. Inadequate emotional reactions, notably the poorly controlled expression of impulses and self-damaging and self-mutilating behavior are the primary target of the treatment. A dialectical stance is taken by the therapist, on the one hand accepting the emotional pain (instead of trying to change this), and on the other hand changing the antecedents of the stress and the way the patient tries to cope with the emotions. Acquiring skills in emotion tolerance and regulation, as well as validating emotional reactions are central to Linehan's DBT. DBT was originally developed to treat self-mutilating patients, before it was clear that most of these patients would be diagnosed as patients with BPD nowadays. Not surprisingly, research has demonstrated that DBT has it strongest effects on self-mutilating and severe self-damaging behavior, including dropping out of treatment.

Beckian Formulations

Early Beckian formulations of BPD stressed the role of assumptions in the disorder. Beck et al. (1990) hypothesized that a large number of assumptions common to other personality disorders are active in BPD. Pretzer (1990) further hypothesized that three key assumptions are central in BPD: "The world is dangerous and malevolent," "I am powerless and vulnerable," and "I am inherently unacceptable." The first assumption in combination with the second is hypothesized to lead to high levels of vigilance and interpersonal distrust. In addition to hypervigilance, two other cognitive characteristics are assumed to be central to BPD: dichotomous thinking and a weak sense of identity (i.e., a poorly articulated self-schema). The three key assumptions and the three cognitive characteristics are assumed to play a central role in the maintenance of the disorder and are consequently major targets for therapy. For instance, the somewhat paradoxical combination of dependent assumptions (the belief of the patient to be weak and incapable, whereas others are strong and capable) and paranoid assumptions (the belief that others cannot be trusted and are malevolent) are thought to fuel the unstable and extreme interpersonal behavior of the patient with BPD, alternating between clinging to other people and pushing others away out of distrust. Dichotomous thinking contributes to the emotional turmoil and extreme decisions of these patients, as lack of ability to evaluate things in grades of gray contributes to the abrupt and extreme shifts patients with BPD make. Consequently, reducing dichotomous thinking is an important ingredient of Pretzer's treatment proposal, which should be addressed early in treatment, as soon as a working relationship is founded.

Layden, Newman, Freeman, and Morse (1993) further elaborated the cognitive model and suggested numerous other biases and processes and related these to early child development and presumed stagnation of development of patients with BPD. Layden et al. also stress the role of nonverbal elements in core schemas of patients with BPD, which they also link to early preverbal development. Consequently, Layden et al. emphasize the use of experiential techniques, notably imagery work, in treatment. Arntz (1994) related Pretzer's observations to findings of high prevalence of childhood abuse in BPD, suggesting that the way the abuse was processed by the child led to the formation of the key assumptions and cognitive characteristics of the patient with BPD. He proposed an integration of Beckian here-and-now cognitive therapy with historical work to process childhood abuse and correct pathogenic conclusions from the abuse. In accordance with Layden et al., the importance of experiential methods in treatment of early childhood memories is stressed (see also Arntz & Weertman, 1999; Smucker, Dancu, Foa, & Niederee, 1995).

Young's Schema Mode Model

The conceptualization of the core pathology of BPD as stemming from a highly frightened, abused child who is left alone in a malevolent world, longing for safety and help but distrustful because of fear of further abuse and abandonment, is highly related to the model developed by Young (McGinn & Young, 1996). To understand the abrupt changes in the behavior of patients with BPD, Young elaborated on an idea, in the 1980s introduced by Aaron Beck in clinical workshops (D. M. Clark, personal communication), that some pathological states of patients with BPD are a sort of regression into intense emotional states experienced as a child. Young conceptualized such states as schema modes, and in addition to child-like regressive states, he also stipulated less regressive schema modes. A schema mode is an organized pattern of thinking, feeling, and behaving based on a set of schemas, relatively independent from other schema modes. Patients with BPD are assumed to sometimes flip suddenly from one mode into the other. As Beck observed, some of these states appear highly childish and may be confusing for both the patient and other people. Young hypothesized that four schema modes are central to BPD: the abandoned child mode (the present author suggests to label it the abused and abandoned child); the angry/impulsive child mode; the punitive parent mode, and the detached protector mode. In addition, there is a healthy adult mode, denoting the healthy side of the patient.

The abused and abandoned child mode denotes the desperate state the patient may be in related to (threatened) abandonment and abuse the patient has experienced as a child. Typical core beliefs are that other people are malevolent, cannot be trusted, and will abandon or punish you, especially when you become intimate with them. Other core beliefs are: "My emotional pain will never stop," "I will always be alone," and "There will be nobody who cares for me." The patient may behave like an upset and desperate child, longing for consolation and nurturance but also fearing it. Many therapists do not like such emotional expressions, because they are afraid of crises and too much dependency from the patient. Usually the patient fears this mode, not only because of the intense emotional pain and the reactivation of trauma related memories and feelings but also because its activation can be followed by an activation of the punitive parent mode. This indicates a severe self-punitive state, during which the patient seems to condemn him- or herself as being bad and evil, deserving punishment. Expressions of negative emotions, opinions and wishes were usually punished by caregivers, attributing these to character, either explicitly ("You are a bad child") or implicitly (e.g., ignoring the child for days). Threats of abandonment ("I'll send you to an orphan home"), verbal or physical aggression, and (threats of) severe punishments by caregivers are supposed to be internalized in this mode. Typical core beliefs are "You are bad (evil) and deserve punishment"; "Your opinions/wishes/emotions are ill founded"; "You have no right to express your opinions/wishes/emotions"; "You are only manipulating." Often the patient not only experiences these punishing thoughts but adds punishing acts to them, such as self-mutilation, damaging the good things in his or her life, and not coming to treatment sessions. Guilt is the prominent feeling. The patient might evoke punishing reactions in others, including the therapist.

One of the other modes the patient (and the therapist!) frequently fears is the angry/impulsive child mode. This denotes a stage of childish rage or self-gratifying impulsiveness that is in the long run damaging for the patient and his or her relationships. Whereas Young states that patients with BPD typically avoid the experience and expression of anger, the tension of suppressed anger may build up and suddenly be expressed in a relatively uncontrolled way. These tantrum-like states are, according to the model, typically followed by an activation of the punitive parent mode. Impulsive, immediate need-gratifying behaviors are also attributed to this mode. Underlying beliefs are: "My basic rights are deprived"; "Other people are evil and mean"; "I have to fight, or just take what I need, to survive."

Although patients with BPD are notorious for their crises and anger, therapists who work for longer periods with these patients have observed that they tend to be detached most of the time. They do not seem to really make contact with other people, or with their own feelings and opinions. According to Young, they are in the detached protector mode, a sort of protective style the child developed to survive in a dangerous world. This mode is hypothesized to serve to protect the patient from attachment (because attachments will be followed by pain, abandonment, punishment, or abuse), emotional experience, self-assertiveness, and development, as each of these signals potential pain and activation of the punitive mode. Core beliefs are that it makes no sense to feel emotions and to connect to other people; that it is even dangerous to do so; that being detached is the only way to survive and to control one's life. Often the patient uses a bulk of strategies to maintain this mode, including cognitive avoidance of feeling and thinking; not talking; avoidance of other people and activities; sleeping, developing, and complaining about somatic discomforts; use of drugs and alcohol; and even (para)suicide. Superficially, the patient may seem rational and healthy, but this is not really healthy because the patient suppresses important issues.

TREATMENT APPROACH

Collaboration Strategy

Before treatment proper starts, the therapist should decide as to what treatment he or she wants to offer. On the one hand, a relatively short treatment directed at reducing the most problematic and dangerous BPD problems can be offered. The objectives of such a treatment are a reduction of impulsiveness and self-mutilating behavior, and perhaps substance abuse, and gaining some control over emotions and insight into the problems, so that the patient is suitable for further psychotherapy. The studies by Linehan et al. (1991) and Brown et al. (2003) demonstrated that these objectives are achievable in a 1-year treatment. But, the studies also demonstrated that longer treatment is necessary to achieve broader and deeper, core schema-level change. We believe that for a real treatment of BPD a longer therapy is necessary, during which usually an intensive personal relationship between therapist and patient develops. One of the reasons for this is that patients with BPD have such a fundamental distrust of other people, especially when they become intimate with them, and their attachment style is so pathological, that it simply takes time to overcome these interpersonal barriers (Gunderson, 1996). Thus, for a real treatment of BPD, time to develop a new secure attachment as a fundamental correction to what went wrong during childhood is necessary. Related to this is the attention that should be given to the treatment of traumatic childhood memories, which also takes time.

The type and objectives of therapy not only affect the duration of treatment but also the type of relationship the therapist tries to develop with the patient. With the first option, the therapist should keep a bit more distance to the patient, because treatment stops soon and discontinuing treatment when secure attachment just develops can be particularly problematic, and even damaging to patients with BPD. Crisis support should always be provided for patients with BPD, but with the first treatment option the therapist does not need to be deeply involved in treatment of crisis. Frequency of sessions can be once or twice a week.

With the second option, on which the remainder of this chapter concentrates, the therapist tries to develop a more personal and caring relationship with the patient. The therapist actively breaks through the detachment of the patient, is actively involved in crises, soothes the patient when sad, and brings in him- or herself as a person. Frequency of sessions can be once or twice a week. This approach almost necessarily provokes difficult feelings in the patient, based on core schemas, which is good because these can be subsequently be addressed in therapy. Thus, this "reparenting" approach is considered an essential ingredient of treatment. To promote secure attachment, we give our patients with BPD a means (e.g., the number of a special phone) by which the patient can reach the therapist in between sessions, when in emotional need. This personal connection in between sessions helps to refute the patient's beliefs that there is nobody who really cares, that expression of negative feelings will be followed by punishment or abandonment, and helps to foster a secure attachment. Talking, and especially listening in an accepting way to patients when in crisis, is especially effective to teach them to tolerate and accept negative feelings and demonstrates to them that with such an approach, negative feelings usually calm down. Giving a means to reach the therapist in between sessions does not imply that the therapist should be always available, or is omnipotent, as that would create too great burden on the therapist. In addition to the option of contacting the therapist, a crisis facility should be available, in case the therapist cannot be reached or the patient is unable to calm down when speaking to the therapist.

Such a therapeutic approach requires from therapists that they feel secure to set limits when the patient goes beyond personal boundaries of the therapist. Frustrating the patient by setting personal limits is essential in a reparenting approach, as it is in real parenting, and can be curative, especially when the patient is able to test negative beliefs about consequences such as "setting a limit means total disapproval of me as a person"; "expression of my anger about the limit will be followed by punishment or abandonment by the therapist." There are two important caveats in communicating personal limits with the patient with BPD. One is that the therapist should only address patient behavior and not make character attributions, as caretakers often did. Further, the therapist should give a personal motivation for the limit and not rationalize solely on the basis of institutional or professional rules. For example, the therapist may limit phone responses to certain times of the day due to other personal commitments. The following is an example of a dialogue concerning the communication of personal limits.

NATASHA: This weekend I'll have my 30th birthday party, and I would like to invite you to be there, so that I can introduce you to my husband and friends.

THERAPIST: That is very nice of you to invite me to your birthday party, but I'm afraid I don't want to do that.

NATASHA: Why not? I so much hoped that you could be with me.

THERAPIST: I like you very much, but I want to spend my leisure time with my family and friends.

NATASHA: (*getting angry*) So you are not considering me as a friend? And you said that I could expect therapy to be a very special place, which would evoke deep feelings, and that you would take a special role and care for me? Like a parent toward a child? And now I'm asking you something personal, something that is very important to me, and you just say no. You lied to me! I must have been a fool to trust you!

THERAPIST: You are right, I don't think of you as a friend, though I like you a lot, and I need my time with my family and friends to recuperate. So this is my personal decision, I like to see and work with you here, but I don't want to come to your party.

NATASHA: Jesus, you don't need to repeat that, you don't need to pour salt into a wound. I know what you said, I heard you. (*getting afraid now*) Oh my God, I shouldn't have asked it. I knew it. I knew that you would refuse and that you would resent me for asking such an impertinent thing. I want to go. I cannot stay here. (*She stands and starts to leave the room.*)

THERAPIST: Don't leave, please stay. I see that my refusal is hurting you very much. I also see that you are now extremely afraid that I will hurt you even more because you dared to ask me. Am I correct? Let's talk it over. It doesn't feel good for me when you leave now. Can we try to do that?

NATASHA: (*sits again and starts to cry*) OK, but I feel so ashamed . . .

This approach requires that the therapist is able to tolerate high levels of negative emotions, especially anger directed to the therapist, and also sadness, and despair. Positive emotions directed to the therapist can be challenging as well, especially lovesickness and other unrealistic expectations of the therapist. Consultation with colleagues who work with similar patients is invaluable when one treats patients with BPD.

The objectives of the therapeutic relationship are clear, but its application is not without hassles. Though patients with BPD long for a caring relationship, they also deeply fear it, and have serious troubles with tolerating the fears and distrust that are evoked by long-lasting personal and intimate relationships. Thus, the therapist should try to balance distance and intimacy and to adapt this to the phase of treatment but also to actively address the fears and distrust that are evoked by treatment. As Pretzer (1990) stated, "trust is most effectively established through explicitly acknowledging and accepting the client's difficulty in trusting the therapist (once this becomes evident), and then being careful to behave in a consistently trustworthy manner" (p. 191). Relating the problem to underlying core schemas (and modes, if the therapist uses a mode model), can also be helpful to get such problems in a new perspective and to install hope that the problems will be overcome by treatment.

As said, one of the biggest problems of treating patients with BPD is their unusually high dropout rate early in therapy. To prevent dropout, the therapist should be active in keeping patients in therapy, by calling patients who do not show up for sessions, asking for (and actively suggesting to break through detachment) the reasons for avoiding therapy, and adapting his or her behavior to what the patient needs. Common reasons for staying away from treatment are related to detaching strategies (not connecting to people, avoiding and pushing away feelings and thoughts about difficulties as ways to survive), fear of being abused or abandoned by the therapist, and self-punishing attitudes (I don't deserve therapy, I should destroy positive things to punish myself). Such underlying beliefs should be clarified and pointed out to the patient in a noncriticizing way that staying away from therapy would mean continuation of pathology and the missing of the chance to correct the underlying beliefs. Recent trials indeed demonstrated that such approaches were highly successful in reducing dropout.

With a time- and objectives-limited treatment, goal setting with the patient can be much easier than with the longer approach. In the latter case, the goals are necessarily global and stated in terms of reduction of the influence of core schemas and dysfunctional strategies and the creation and increase of healthy schemas and strategies. Formulating the latter can be complicated, because many patients with BPD have no idea what healthy views and strategies are. An active and educational stance (again, like in good parenting), not moralistic but explaining why certain views and strategies are more healthy than others, is indicated here. The use of role play and behavioral experiment is also helpful to develop functional schemas and strategies.

As patients with BPD have negative beliefs about experiencing feelings, thinking that their feelings are ill-founded, that they are bad to have such feelings, that they will lose control of urges to act on their feelings, and that other people (including the therapist) will punish or reject them, a primary attitude of the therapist is acceptance and validation of emotions but discouraging of impulsive emotional acts. This is the basis for a healthier schema on emotional regulation. Cognitive therapists who are used to working on Axis I problems should resist their usual habit of immediately looking for biased interpretations that led to dysfunctional emotions: The first issue to be addressed is the pathogenic meaning given to the experience of the emotion.

A last important relationship technique is empathic confrontation, a confrontational message consisting out of three elements: (1) empathic expression that the therapist understands why a dysfunctional strategy is chosen; (2) confrontation with the negative effects of the strategy and the continuation of the disorder if really followed; (3) explicit formulation of a new, functional alternative strategy and asking the patient to follow up that.

> "Although I understand why you are so are upset about what Mark said, because it hurts you deep in your heart, and I understand that you now feel a strong inclination to physically hurt yourself, to demonstrate him what a bastard you think he is, I ask you not to do that, because if you do that, it will further complicate your relationship with Mark. He will get more angry, and you will become more afraid, and this escalation will strengthen your idea that other people are evil, and that there never will be someone for you who you can trust. In other words, by following your old strategy you will continue your problems. Instead, I ask you emphatically to try a new strategy, that is to tell him that what he did was painful for you, and explain to him why it was painful for you, and ask him to stop it. In that way you don't hurt yourself, you remain in control of your behavior. This is a healthy way to deal with the problem. And, if he doesn't stop, we will work on how you can react to that. I know this is difficult and even frightening for you to do, but I insist on it because it will help you to learn more healthy ways to deal with such problems."

Specific Interventions

Hierarchical Approach

In choosing which problem to address, it is wise to use a hierarchical approach. Table 9.2 offers an overview. Issues of life and death should always be given priority. Suicidal impulses and other dangerous behaviors are among them, including behaviors that threaten or endanger the lives

---

TABLE 9.2. Hierarchy of Issues to Be Addressed

1. Life-threatening issues
2. Therapeutic relationship
3. Self-damaging issues
4. Other problems, schema work, and trauma processing

---

of other people, particularly dependent children. Next on the hierarchy are issues that threaten the therapeutic relationship. These include the premature wish of the patient to stop therapy, to move to another city, to not come to therapy, and to start another therapy next to the current one; negative feelings of the patient toward the therapist and of therapist toward the patient; coming too late; using a portable phone during the sessions; etc. The reason that issues that threaten the therapeutic relationship are so high on the hierarchy is that a good therapeutic relationship is a prerequisite for the other issues. Third, although not immediately life-threatening, many self-damaging behaviors are so disruptive that there is no room to address underlying schemas. Self-mutilation, substance and medication abuse, not going to work, impulsive acts and decisions, not having adequate food and housing, and poorly controlled emotional outburst are among the disruptive behaviors. Although it is useful to repeatedly address these behaviors, to ask the patient to stop them, and to work on alternatives and solutions, the therapist should not expect, and certainly not insist on, change early in treatment. The pathology of the patient can be so severe that the therapist has to bear it for a long time, which does not mean that it should not be placed repeatedly on the agenda. Last, but not least, other issues, including schema work and trauma processing should be addressed.

The hierarchy is not only an aid for deciding on agenda issues within a session but also for planning the therapy process as a whole. Therapists should be warned that it can be necessary to readdress issues 1–3 when they are in a phase of therapy in which schema work is done. Addressing childhood traumas can, for instance, bring about life-threatening behavior, which should move into priority position, after which the focus can again be placed upon trauma processing

Handling Crises

Although there should always be a crisis facility, the therapist is the most important person in treating the crisis. As said, most crises are fueled by the patient's negative beliefs about experiencing emotions. The primary strategy to counter these beliefs is to take a calm, accepting, and soothing stance. Empathic listening to the patient, asking for feelings and interpretations, and validating the feelings are important. Often, self-punitive ideas and actions (in Young's model: the punitive parent mode) play a dysfunctional role and it can be important to actively inquire for these thoughts and to counter them (e.g., "That's not true, you are a good person, it is absolutely OK to feel sad and angry when your husband leaves you, and I'm happy that you tell me about your feelings").

Availability during a crisis can be helpful, because an early intervention often prevents worsening, self-mutilation, drug abuse, or other maladaptive actions and reduces need for hospitalization. Early or later in treatment it is possible to come to an agreement with the patient that he or she does not engage in dysfunctional behavior (like self-mutilation) before talking to the therapist. We have learned that in many cases empathic listening and talking to the patient on the phone dampens the crisis in 15 to 20 minutes. During treatment, the patient gradually internalizes this new attitude toward difficult feelings and can apply it to him- or herself, so that immediate help of other persons is less needed. The therapist can help to make this transition by making an audiotape with soothing words spoken by the therapist, and by making flashcards the patient can use to recall soothing thoughts.

One common pitfall occurs when the therapist starts too early to offer practical suggestions on how to handle the problem and the crisis. This generally fuels the punitive beliefs ("so I did it wrong") and counteracts the creation of a healthy attitude toward experiencing emotions. Practical problems should be addressed when emotions are calmed down, and often the patient is then able to handle it for him- or herself. There are, however, circumstances when it is not productive to follow these guidelines. An example is when the patient is so intoxicated (alcohol, benzodiazepines, etc.) that talking to her makes little sense and she cannot control aggressive impulses. More medically oriented help is then indicated. Another example is when the patient engages in self-mutilating behavior while talking to the therapist. The therapist should then set firm limits (e.g., "I want you to stop cutting yourself now, and then we will talk about your feelings, so put away that knife").

Limit Setting

Some behaviors are so unacceptable that they should be limited by the therapist. These include behaviors that cross personal boundaries of the therapist (e.g., stalking, threatening, or insulting the therapist). Unacceptable behaviors also include dangerous actions that threaten the patient's life or the continuation of therapy. Formal limit setting as outlined here should only be done when the therapist feels able to execute the last step, stopping therapy. If not, the therapist should tolerate the behavior, meanwhile continuing to confront the patient with it and working toward a change. In applying this technique, therapists should be firm about the limit, use their personal motives to explain it, and talk about the patient's behavior and not criticize the patient's character. Never assume that the patient should have known that the behavior was unacceptable for the therapist.

"Yesterday you called me when you were in a terrible emotional pain, as I asked you to do. But, I learned that you were drunk and took a lot of benzos. Because you were intoxicated, I didn't think that I could talk to you in any reasonable way. It made no sense. So I want to ask you not to call me when you are already intoxicated. You are welcome to call me before you consider drinking so much and taking pills, so that I can really connect to you. Please call me before, not after you do that."

The patient's behavior may persist, in which case, the therapist firmly repeats his or her limits.

"Two weeks ago I changed the conditions under which you could call me. I asked you not to call me when you are drunk and have used benzos. But, last Wednesday you called me after taking pills and drinking a bottle of wine. I must say that I got a bit irritated when I found out that you were intoxicated. I don't like to talk to drunken people, and I don't want to get a dislike of you because you call me when you are intoxicated. So, let me be clear: call me when you need me because you are in a crisis, but only when you are sober. Don't call me when you are intoxicated. Call me before you start to drink or take pills."

Table 9.3 (based on Young, personal communication) summarizes the steps that should be taken in limit setting. As is clear from Table 9.3, consequences (punishments) are only given after a warning has been given, so that the patient has the chance to change his or her behavior. Furthermore, consequences should initially be light and, if possible, intrinsically related to the undesired behavior (e.g., a patient using too much of the therapist's time gets a shorter session next time). Limit set-

---

TABLE 9.3. Steps to Be Taken in Limit Setting

Explain the rule; use personal motivation.

Repeat the rule; show your feelings a little bit, repeat personal motivation.

As above; add warning and announce consequence.

As above; and execute consequence.

As above; announce stronger consequence.

As above; execute stronger consequence.

Announce a temporary break of therapy so that the patient can think it over.

Execute temporary break of therapy so that the patient can decide whether he or she wants the present therapy with this limit.

Announce the end of treatment.

Stop treatment and refer the patient.

Note. Based on Young (personal communication).

ting can evoke strong anger, which can be dealt with according to the collaboration strategies outlined previously.

Cognitive Techniques

Unraveling Underlying Schemas (Modes). Because patients with BPD have initially poor understanding of their own emotions, thoughts, and behaviors, an important part of treatment is devoted to help the patient understand them. Getting clear what underlying schemas (or modes) play a role helps them to reduce confusion and to gain some control over their behavior. A daily diary of emotions, thoughts, and behaviors is useful in helping the patient to detect underlying schemas and modes. It is particularly useful to link unraveled underlying schemas (or modes) to the patient's history, so that the patient can see how the schema developed and what function it previously served.

As an example, Natasha learned to understand that she adapted a somewhat arrogant, challenging attitude, as if nobody could hurt her, when she felt uncertain and feared harm. This often triggered more hurtful behavior from other people, the last thing she wanted. Natasha and her therapist found out that she had developed this attitude as a child to cope with her mother's threats and physical abuse. Showing her mother how she felt hurt or getting angry inevitably led to even more punishment, and adapting this attitude helped her, in a way, to maintain her self-worth and to punish her mother back. This historical link made clear the protective function of her schema, and that it was adaptive when she was a child. Because it was triggered automatically when she was an adult, and she had been almost unaware of it until therapy, it took her a long time to understand how her own behavior led to more, instead of less, hurt in present situations. After that became clear, she became interested in learning alternative ways to deal with situations that were threatening for her.

Tackling Dichotomous Thinking. Patients with BPD frequently think in dichotomous terms, fueling extreme emotions, polarizing conflicts, and prompting sudden, extreme, impulsive decisions. It is important to help them to become aware of this thinking style, its harmful implications, and to teach them to evaluate situations in more nuanced ways. Structured exercises can be used to develop a more adaptive thinking style. One helpful method is to use a whiteboard to illustrate the difference between black-and-white thinking and nuanced thinking. On the whiteboard, the therapist compares putting an action or a person into one of two compartments (black or white), versus creating a visual analogue scale (VAS) of a horizontal line between two extremes. Thus, different people, actions, or character traits can be placed in the dichotomous system, or they can be places all along a continuum of the VAS. When multidimensional evaluations have to be made, it is wise to draw a separate VAS for each dimension.

Flashcards. What has been achieved in a session is often difficult for patients with BPD to remember when they need it. If a schema has been really triggered, all their thinking and feeling seems to be determined by it, and they have great difficulty taking other perspectives. Flashcards can be particularly useful as an aid to memory, and to fight pathogenic schemas on the spot. Usually, on one side of the card the pathogenic reasoning and the activated schema (mode) are described, so that the patient can understand that his or her emotions are caused by the activation of that schema. On the other side, a healthy view is offered, together with a functional way to cope with the problems. Some patients always take flashcards with them as a sort of safety measure, not only because of the content but also because it makes them feel to be connected to the therapy and the therapist.

Experiential Techniques

Imaginal Rescripting and Historical Role Play. A powerful technique to attain change in painful childhood memories on schema level is imaginal rescripting (Weertman & Arntz, 2001). Detailed procedures are described elsewhere (Arntz & Weertman, 1999; Smucker et al., 1995). In most cases, a present negative feeling is taken as a memory bridge to a childhood memory, which the patient imagines with (if possible) the eyes closed. When the patient clearly imagines the childhood memory and affect is activated, the therapist (or another safe and strong person) should enter the scene and intervene. Patients with BPD are usually, at least in the beginning of treatment, not healthy and powerful enough to intervene themselves, so someone else can serve as the intervener. The intervener stops the abuse, or other painful situation, rescues the child, and asks the child what he or she needs. Special attention should then be given to correction of negative interpretations and soothing of the child, during which imagined physical contact should be offered, as it is the most powerful way to convey comfort and love to a child. If the patient does not accept physical contact, it should not be forced in any way.

In the following example, Natasha imagines a threatening childhood memory with her mother.

NATASHA: I cannot do anything. I'm too afraid.

THERAPIST: Is it OK when I join you? Can you imagine me standing alongside you?

NATASHA: Yes, I can see you beside me.

THERAPIST: Good. I'm talking to little Natasha now . . . what is it what you need? Is there anything I can do?

NATASHA: (*Does not say anything, seems very afraid*)

THERAPIST: OK, listen to what I say to your mother then . . . Madam, you are Natasha's mother, aren't you? I have to tell you that you are doing terrible things to your daughter. Her bike was stolen, there was nothing she could do about that, and she is emotional about that. That is normal, everybody feels emotional when you lose something of importance. But you are humiliating her in front of the rest of the family because she is emotional. And what is even worse, you are accusing her that she caused the theft. You are saying that she has always been a bad lot, always causing problems, and that she is the cause of your misery. But that is not true, Natasha is a good girl. She should get sympathy and consolation from you. Because you are her mother and she is in pain. And if you are not able to give her what she needs, and what every other child needs, that is a problem enough. But in any case you shouldn't accuse her, because you have a problem in handling emotions and being a parent. So, stop accusing her and apologize for having done that!

Natasha, look to Mamma now, what is she doing? What is she saying?

NATASHA: She looks a bit surprised . . . she is not used to be talked to like that . . . she does not know what to say . . . well, she says that I should be taught a lesson because I should have known beforehand that it would go wrong with what I did with the bike . . .

THERAPIST: Listen to me, madam. That's nonsense, Natasha didn't know that beforehand and she feels sad about losing her bike, and if you cannot comfort her, stop talking like this or leave the room . . .

What is she doing now, Natasha?

NATASHA: She stops talking and just sits in her armchair . . .

THERAPIST: How does little Natasha feel now?

NATASHA: I'm afraid that she will punish me when you go away . . .

THERAPIST: Is there anything that I can do to help you? Ask me!

NATASHA: I want you to stay and care for me.

THERAPIST: That is OK, Natasha, I'll stay and take care of you . . . what do you need now?

NATASHA: That you not only take care of me but also of my sister . . .

THERAPIST: Should I send your mother away, or take you and your sister with me?

NATASHA: Take us with you.

THERAPIST: OK, I take the two of you with me: imagine that you take your cuddle toys and everything else you want and that we leave the house together with your sister. We drive to my place. There we enter the house, and you take a seat. Do you want something to drink?

NATASHA: I'm feeling sad now. (*Starts to cry.*)

THERAPIST: That's OK, do you want me to comfort you? Let me take you in my arms . . . can you feel that?

NATASHA: (*Cries even harder.*)

Note that the therapists takes several roles, intervening and protecting the child, correcting dysfunctional ideas about guilt and badness, and comforting the child so that the experience can be emotionally processed. The therapist acts, in other words, as a good parent would have done. The purpose of the rescripting is not to distort or replace the reality of the patient's childhood (which was generally bad) but to correct dysfunctional beliefs, to provide corrective experiences, and to evoke feelings that were avoided or suppressed. Usually imagery with rescripting is highly confrontational, as the patient begins to confront the realization of what he or she has missed and how he or she was abused and is accompanied with a period of mourning. The therapist should help the patient through this period, balancing the focus between here and now and the processing of childhood memories. Role plays of situations from childhood can be used instead of imagery. However, some behaviors are awkward or unethical to practice in a role play (i.e., therapist taking child on his lap), and imagery may provide an easier and safer strategy.

Empty-Chair Techniques. Punitive caregivers, threatening persons in the present, or a punitive schema mode can be symbolically put on an empty chair, and the therapist and/or the patient can safely express feelings and opinions toward them. Often, it is wise that the therapist first models this technique, as patients might be too afraid to express themselves. As Natasha suffered frequently from her punitive schema mode, echoing her mother's verbal aggressiveness, the therapist repeatedly put this mode (i.e., her aggressive mother) on an empty chair, firmly contradicted her, told her to stop, and sent her away. Later in treatment, the therapist helped Natasha to do this herself, and Natasha also started, with success, to do this at home, each time she was burdened by an activation of this mode.

Experiencing Emotions. Patients with BPD should learn to tolerate the experience of strong negative emotions, without acting out behaviors that serve to avoid or escape from the experience. Exposure techniques known from behavior therapy can be helpful, as are writing exercises, such as composing a letter to a former abuser (but not sending it) in which the patient expresses all her feelings. Patients with BPD are especially afraid of experiencing anger, as they fear that they will lose control and get aggressive. As an intermediate stage, the therapist may model verbally expressing anger while banging on a cushion, asking the patient to join. This lowers the fear of anger. Later on, the patient can be asked to try to experience anger without engaging in any behavioral action. The patient than discovers that she can stand high levels of emotions without having to behaviorally express them and without losing control.

Behavioral Techniques

Role Plays. These techniques are useful to teach patients interpersonal skills, such as appropriate assertiveness and expressing feelings toward another person. The therapist usually models assertive expression first, as many patients with BPD are truly confused about how to execute an effective expression of feelings. Even when patients refuse to practice during a session, we have seen that the modeling is helpful to get the patients to start to appropriately express their feelings and opinions outside the session.

Experimenting with New Behavior. A powerful way to reinforce new schemas and strategies is to ask the patient to behave according to them. Thus, even when the patient still feels that this new way of behaving is not integrated in him- or herself, it can be helpful. Later in treatment, Natasha started to show more uncertainty and emotional pain instead of putting on her tough attitude when she was uncertain or hurt inside, and she found out that this was more functional as it led most people to accept her. After she divorced from her aggressive husband, she also tried out new ways of behaving during dating. She found out that other types of men, more caring and less threatening than her former partners, were consequently interested in her.

Pharmacological Interventions

Patients with BPD may experience very high levels of negative emotions while having little tolerance for affect. Consequently, they are often prescribed medication. Studies have indicated that antidepressants may be effective in reducing depressive feelings, and neuroleptics may be helpful in reducing anxiety, anger, impulsive problems, and psychotic symptoms (for reviews, see Dimeff, McDavid, & Linehan, 1999; Soloff, 1994). It should be noted that treatment effects were generally modest, and most medication has been tested only during short periods. In general, pharmacotherapy is considered as a possible adjunct to psychotherapy, not as a treatment of BPD in itself. Moreover, there are specific risks in prescribing medication in this population: paradoxical effects, abuse, dependency, and use for suicide attempts are among them. This is particularly true for benzodiazepines, which might be prescribed when patients are in a state of acute fear. Often, the fear is fueled by aggressive impulses that the patient feels unable to control. Use of benzodiazepines might lead to a reduction of fear of the expression of the impulses and lowered threshold for expression, similar to alcohol (see Cowdry & Gardner, 1988; Gardner & Cowdry, 1985, for empirical evidence). We have often observed the intensification of an emotional crisis, leading to self-mutilation and suicide attempts, after the use of benzodiazepines, especially when used in combination with alcohol. This "paradoxical" effect should be explained to the patient and the patient should be asked to stop the use of benzodiazepines and alcohol. A short use of neuroleptics is often a safe alternative, when anxiety levels seem to become intolerable. Personal contact is often a better alternative. Long-term use of neuroleptics dampens many BPD symptoms but may make it impossible to address important feelings so is generally discouraged.

MAINTAINING PROGRESS

Because termination of treatment might be very frightening for the patient, it should be well prepared and discussed as part of the process of therapy. Feelings and negative beliefs about termination should be clarified. In addition, a list of remaining problems should be made and appropriate treatment strategies chosen. Gradually tapering off the frequency of sessions is recommended, so that the patient can find out how life is without the regular help of the therapist. Booster sessions may be especially helpful, to help the patient maintain functional strategies and to prevent relapse into old schemas. Some therapists recommend an open end, in the sense that the patient can always come back for a few sessions when needed. Paradoxically, this possibility might lead to less relapse and health care use, because it offers a safe base on which the patient can fall back. Because patients with BPD are generally not very healthy in their choice of partners, and treatment usually brings about enormous changes, subsequent relational problems can occur. A referral for marital therapy may be indicated, so that the couple can adapt to the new situation. Many are so unhealthy that the patient decides to leave the relationship. The therapist can help the patient learn to choose healthier partners and prevent a relapse into old patterns by choosing unhealthy partners. Some believe that former patients with BPD are, in the long run, best protected for relapse when in a good relationship with a caring partner.

Similarly, the patient can be encouraged to discover and develop his or her true interests and capacities. This might have implications for choice of study and work, as well as hobbies and friends. Creating a good and healthy context in the broadest sense should be high on the agenda in the final stage of therapy. There is a risk that the patient wants to terminate treatment too early, claiming that there are no longer problems, whereas the therapist knows that important issues were not addressed in treatment. When empathic confrontation with this detached strategy does not work, the best thing the therapist probably can do is offer continuation of treatment if the patient needs it.

CONCLUSION

Although patients with BPD present with remarkable instability in many aspects of their functioning, an intensive and directed cognitive intervention can reduce this instability, modify interpersonal distrust, and alter the underlying core schemas, including the trauma-related schemas so often encountered with this challenging disorder.

ACKNOWLEDGMENTS

Thanks are due to Tim Beck, Christine Padesky, and Jeffrey Young, for what they taught me during their workshops and during discussions I had with them. I also want to express my gratitude to Frank Yeomans for the inspiring discussions we had, although we are from different theoretical orientations. Colleagues as well as clients helped to develop and validate the ideas and methods described in this chapter. Our research on BPD is supported by grant OG 97-001 from the Dutch Fund for Developmental Medicine.

CHAPTER 10

Histrionic Personality Disorder

Histrionic personality disorder (HPD) is characterized by excessive emotionality and attention seeking. Individuals with this disorder are overly concerned with physical attractiveness, often overtly seductive, and most comfortable at the center of attention. Their emotionality seems to be inappropriately exaggerated, labile, and superficial, and they tend to have a global, impressionistic style of speech. These patients are lively and dramatic, with a global, impressionistic style of speech. Their behavior is overly reactive and intense. They are emotionally excitable and crave stimulation, often responding to minor stimuli with irrational, angry outbursts or tantrums. Their interpersonal relationships are impaired and they are perceived by others as shallow, demanding, overly dependent, high strung, and high maintenance.

The interpersonal relationships of histrionic individuals tend to be stormy and ungratifying. Due to their dependence on the attention of other people, individuals with HPD are especially vulnerable to separation anxiety and they may seek treatment when they become intensely upset over the breakup of a relationship. In their study of 32 patients who had been admitted to a psychiatric hospital with the diagnosis of histrionic personality, Slavney and McHugh (1974) found that almost 80% had been admitted due to suicidality, depression, or both. Most of the suicide attempts were not life threatening and most had occurred after anger or disappointment. Anxiety disorders such as panic disorder with and without agoraphobia are also common presenting problems in people with HPD. In fact, studies have shown that HPD is one of the most commonly found personality disorders within panic disorder populations (Diaferia et al., 1993; Sciuto et al., 1991). Other common complications of HPD that may lead to the seeking of treatment include alcoholism and other substance abuse, conversion disorder, somatization disorder, and brief reactive psychosis.

HISTORICAL PERSPECTIVES

The term "histrionic personality disorder" was coined relatively recently. Throughout most of history, this disorder was known as hysterical personality disorder, stemming from the concept of hysteria. Hysteria has a long history, spanning over 4,000 years (summarized by Vieth, 1963). The use of this term has been controversial, and the concept of hysteria has been rejected by feminists as a sexist label that is often used to discount the problems of women whenever they present complaints that are not easily explained or when they make demands that seem excessive. The term "hysteria" has been used to refer to phenomena as diverse as transient loss of control resulting from overwhelming stress, conversion disorder, Briquet's syndrome, a personality disorder, a personality trait, and, perhaps most common, it has been used to describe excitable female patients who are difficult to treat. In their review of this phenomenon, Temoshok and Heller (1983) state that " 'hysteria' as a diagnostic label is as impressionistic, labile, diffuse, unstable, and superficially appealing as the various phenomena with which it has been associated" (p. 204). In an attempt to reduce the confusion (and possible sexist connotations) regarding the use of the term "hysteria," the American Psychiatric Association (1980) did not include the term "hysteria" anywhere in DSM-III. Instead, separate categories of somatization disorder, conversion disorder, hypochondriasis, dissociative disorders, and histrionic personality disorder have been designated.

The concept of hysteria began with the Egyptian idea that if the uterus were unmoored, it would wander throughout the body, lodging in one place and producing hysterical symptoms there. Treatment consisted of luring the uterus back to its normal position by fumigating or anointing the vagina with sweet-smelling or precious substances, or by chasing the womb away from its new location by inhalation or application of foul-smelling, noxious substances at the distressed site. Hippocratic prescriptions often included marriage and childbirth, which physicians have recommended to their hysterical patients ever since.

Although psychoanalytic theory had its origins in Freud's explication of hysterical symptoms, his primary interest focused on conversion hysteria, not on hysterical personality traits. Early psychodynamic descriptions emphasized unresolved Oedipal conflicts as the primary determinant of this disorder, with repression seen as the most characteristic defense (Abraham, 1949; Fenichel, 1945; W. Reich, 1972). Based on the belief that the discharge of repressed sexual emotions would result in a cure, early analytic treatment of hysteria consisted of using suggestion and hypnosis to facilitate abreaction. Later, Freud modified his method to include the use of free association and the interpretation of resistance and transference in order to develop insight and abreaction. Although the treatment of hysteria has been characterized as the foundation of the psychoanalytic method, few empirical, controlled studies of this treatment approach have been published.

Marmor (1953) challenged classic psychoanalytic thinking by raising the question whether the fixation involved in hysterical personality is primarily oral rather than phallic in nature, suggesting a more pervasive and primitive disturbance. Several psychoanalytic thinkers have reached a compromise between these two views by suggesting differentiations within the spectrum of hysterical personality (Baumbacher & Amini, 1980–1981; Easser & Lesser, 1965; Kernberg, 1975; Zetzel, 1968).

RESEARCH AND EMPIRICAL DATA

An epidemiological study of HPD found that it had a prevalence of 2.1% in the general population, could be diagnosed reliably, and was a valid construct (Nestadt et al., 1990). Despite the clinical impression that most individuals with HPD are female, this study found that males and females were equally affected.

In factor-analytic studies, Lazare, Klerman, and Armor (1966, 1970) found that four of seven traits classically associated with hysterical personality clustered together as expected. The traits of emotionality, exhibitionism, egocentricity, and sexual provocativeness were strongly clustered together, while the traits of suggestibility and fear of sexuality did not cluster together. Dependency fell into an intermediate position.

As early as DSM-I (American Psychiatric Association, 1952), a discrimination was made between what were considered neurotic aspects of hysteria (conversion reaction) and the personality aspects (then called emotionally unstable personality). In DSM-II (American Psychiatric Association, 1968), the distinction was made between the hysterical neuroses (including conversion reaction and dissociative reaction) and hysterical personality.

There has been some research on the specific trait of emotional lability. In a series of studies, Slavney and his colleagues demonstrated that variability of mood was positively correlated with self-ratings on hysterical traits in normal men and women, and that patients diagnosed as hysterical personality disorder had greater variability of mood than did control patients (Rabins & Slavney, 1979; Slavney, Breitner, & Rabins, 1977; Slavney & Rich, 1980). Standage, Bilsbury, Jain, and Smith (1984) found that women with the diagnosis of HPD showed an impaired ability to perceive and evaluate their own behavior as it is perceived and evaluated by others in the same culture.

The relationships between HPD, antisocial personality disorder, and somatization disorder have been studied by Lilienfeld, VanValkenburg, Larntz, and Akiskal (1986). They found the three disorders to overlap considerably within individuals, with the strongest relationship being between antisocial and histrionic personality. In addition, they reported that histrionic personality appeared to moderate the relationship between antisocial personality disorder and somatization disorder, because it was only in individuals without histrionic personality that the relationship between antisocial personality and somatization disorder was significant. This led the authors to suggest the possibility that histrionic individuals develop antisocial personality if they are male and somatization disorder if female. Some authors have hypothesized that psychopathic personality features manifest themselves into different sex-typed personality disorders, such as HPD and antisocial personality disorder. Data regarding this hypothesis have been inconsistent and are summarized in Cale and Lilienfeld (2002).

HPD is the only personality disorder explicitly linked to a person's physical appearance. An interesting study by Robert Bornstein (1999) found that women with HPD were rated higher in physical attractiveness than women with other personality disorders or women with no personality disorder diagnoses. However, a similar link between attractiveness and HPD was not found in males.

Although patients with any personality disorder showed more functional impairment on the Global Assessment of Functioning Scale (Nakao et al., 1992) than did patients without personality disorders, HPD was one of the personality disorders with the least functional impairment. In a study of the family environments of nonclinical samples of subjects with histrionic personality (Baker, Capron, & Azorlosa, 1996), histrionics were characterized by a family of origin that was high in control and intellectual–cultural orientation and low in cohesion. This would fit to some extent with Millon's (1996) theories about the families of histrionics. The low cohesion score may reflect Millon's hypothesis that the parents in these families are self-absorbed.

Little has been written about the treatment of hysteria from a behavioral point of view, and most of the limited behavioral research has been confined to the treatment of conversion and somatization disorders (summarized by Bird, 1979). Even less has been presented about behavioral treatment specifically for HPD. Fairly positive results were reported in two uncontrolled studies using at least partly behavioral treatments of hysteria (Kass, Silvers, & Abrams, 1972; Woolson & Swanson, 1972). Although it has often been shown that clients with personality disorders have poorer outcomes in standardized treatments, this has sometimes been shown to be the opposite with HPD. Both Turner (1987) and Chambless, Renneberg, Goldstein, and Gracely (1992) found that in structured cognitive-behavioral treatments for anxiety disorders, those subjects with HPD showed a better response than others on measures of panic frequency. It is hypothesized that the focus on relabeling affect may have been particularly useful for the histrionic clients.

DIFFERENTIAL DIAGNOSIS

As the name indicates, the strongest indication of HPD is an overly dramatic, or histrionic, presentation of self. Asking house officers and faculty members to rank-order the diagnostic importance of trait items describing hysterical personality, Slavney (1978) found that self-dramatization, attention seeking, emotional instability, and seductiveness were ranked as most diagnostically important and most confidently recognized. Vanity, immaturity, and conversion symptoms were seen as relatively unimportant and less certainly recognized.

Clinical Example

Cathy was a 26-year-old woman who worked as a salesclerk in a trendy clothing store and who sought therapy for panic disorder with agoraphobia. She was dressed flamboyantly, with an elaborate and dramatic hairdo. Her appearance was especially striking as she was quite short (under 5 feet tall) and at least 75 pounds overweight. She wore sunglasses indoors throughout the evaluation and constantly fiddled with them, taking them on and off nervously and waving them to emphasize a point. She cried loudly and dramatically at various points in the interview, going through large numbers of Kleenex. She continually asked for reassurance ("Will I be OK? Can I get over this?"). She talked nonstop throughout the evaluation. When gently interrupted by the evaluator, she was apologetic, laughing and saying, "I know I talk too much"; yet she continued to do so throughout the session.

Pfohl (1991) discusses some of the criteria for the diagnosis of HPD that were subsequently changed in DSM-IV-TR (American Psychiatric Association, 2000). The two criteria "constantly seeks or demands reassurance, approval, or praise" and "is self-centered, actions being directed toward obtaining immediate gratification; has no tolerance for the frustration of delayed gratification" were removed and no longer appear in DSM-IV-TR. They were eliminated as criteria not because these features are not prevalent in HPD but because they are so frequently present in other personality disorders that they did not distinguish it from other personality disorders. DSM-IV-TR has an additional criterion which was not present in DSM-III-R. The criterion of "considers relationships to be more intimate than they actually are" was based on concepts in the historic literature and helped to maintain the same number of criteria as were present in DSM-III-R.

The patient with HPD has been conceptualized as a caricature of what is defined as femininity in our culture—vain, shallow, self-dramatizing, immature, overdependent, and selfish. When asked to rate the concepts "woman," "man," histrionic personality," "antisocial personality," and "compulsive personality" using a semantic differential technique, psychiatric residents and psychiatrists showed a stronger connection between the connotative meanings of the concepts "woman" and "histrionic personality" than was found between the concepts of "man" and either "antisocial personality" or "compulsive personality" (Slavney, 1984).

Clinically, HPD is most frequently diagnosed in women, and when it is diagnosed in men it has been associated with homosexuality. This gender differential, however, may be more a product of our societal expectations than a true difference in occurrence. It has been suggested that HPD is more appropriately seen as a caricature of sex roles in general, including extreme masculinity as well as extreme femininity (Kolb, 1968; MacKinnon & Michaels, 1971; Malmquist, 1971). The extreme of femininity is fairly commonly diagnosed as histrionic, yet a caricature of masculinity (an overly "macho" male who is dramatic, sensation seeking, shallow, vain, and egocentric) is rarely diagnosed as HPD even though he would meet the DSM-IV-TR criteria (see Table 10.1). Also, such a man would not be likely to seek treatment and therefore would not receive a diagnosis.

Emotions of the histrionic individual are expressed intensely, yet seem exaggerated or unconvincing, as if the patient is dramatically playing a role. In the assessment of HPD, the clinician can use his or her own reactions as a useful indicator of when to consider this disorder. If a patient is expressing extreme distress, yet the clinician has the sense of watching a performance rather than having a feeling of empathy for the individual, it may be helpful to explore further for possible HPD. These patients appear quite warm, charming, and even seductive, yet depth or genuineness seems to be missing.

In a group therapy session, one of the therapists commented on the fact that Cathy always brought a large glass of water. Cathy responded by saying, "The water is nothing, look what else I have to carry with me!" She then dramatically grabbed her large handbag and pulled out a

TABLE 10.1. DSM-IV-TR Diagnostic Criteria for Histrionic Personality Disorder

A pervasive pattern of excessive emotionality and attention seeking, beginning by early adulthood and present in a variety of contexts, as indicated by five (or more) of the following:
(1) is uncomfortable in situations in which he or she is not the center of attention
(2) interaction with others is often characterized by inappropriate sexually seductive or provocative behavior
(3) displays rapidly shifting and shallow expression of emotions
(4) constantly uses physical appearance to draw attention to self
(5) has a style of speech that is excessively impressionistic and lacking in detail
(6) shows self-dramatization, theatricality, and exaggerated expression of emotion
(7) is suggestible, i.e., easily influenced by others or circumstances
(8) considers relationships to be more intimate than they actually are

Note. From American Psychiatric Association (2000, p. 714). Copyright 2000 by the American Psychiatric Association. Reprinted by permission.

Bible, salt, washcloth, paper bag, and a medicine bottle, explaining how she would use each of these items in case of a panic attack. Although she was describing how anxious she was, and how she could not stand to go out without all of these items, she seemed proud of her display of equipment and seemed to enjoy the "show and tell."

These patients often present their symptoms, thoughts, and actions as if they were external entities involuntarily imposed upon them. They tend to use dramatic nonverbal gestures and make all-inclusive statements such as "These things just always seem to be happening to me!" Their speech may be strong and dramatic, including a great deal of hyperbole. They tend to use phrases that seem quite powerful and striking at the time, yet later, the clinician realizes that he or she does not really have any idea what the patient meant. They use theatrical intonation with dramatic nonverbal gestures and facial expressions. They often dress in ways that are likely to attract attention, wearing striking and provocative styles in bright colors, and overusing cosmetics and hair dyes.

Although dramatic portrayals of the self can serve as useful cues to the presence of a HPD, a dramatic style or unusual clothing alone are not sufficient data on which to base the diagnosis. For the term "histrionic personality disorder" to do more than just substitute for "hysteric" with all its biases, clinicians must be careful to use the full DSM-IV-TR diagnostic criteria and not to classify patients as histrionic merely on the basis of indications of dramatic flair (e.g., red dress indicates histrionic patient). However, these characteristics can indicate a need to probe more carefully for further diagnostic information.

Data from interpersonal relationships are integral to HPD assessment. Details should be obtained as to how relationships started, what happened, and how they ended. Indications to watch for include a romantic view of relationships that is soon shattered, relationships that start out as idyllic and end up as disasters, and stormy relationships with dramatic endings. Another area to ask about is the way that these individuals handle anger, fights, and disagreements. The clinician should ask for specific examples and look for any signs of dramatic outbursts, temper tantrums, and the manipulative use of anger.

Cathy had a history of stormy relationships with men. When she was a young teenager, she had a boyfriend who was jealous and followed her without her knowledge. Even though this relationship finally ended with a knife fight, Cathy still saw him on and off at the time she began treatment. In her early 20s, when her boyfriend suddenly stopped calling her, she found another boyfriend who she "married just for spite." When asked what was good about the marriage, she said that they were compatible in that "we both like clothes." She reported that the relationship was great before marriage but that soon after the marriage "he began to control me." However, this report was contradicted by later descriptions of how she had begged him not to marry her on the night before the wedding, with him threatening to kill her if she did not go through with the wedding. It was only when questioned carefully as to what she meant by being controlled by him that she specifically disclosed his alcoholism, compulsive gambling, physical abuse of her, and infidelity. They were divorced a few months later.

Many people would not readily acknowledge possessing the negative traits of HPD, but relevant material can be elicited by asking patients how other people tend to view them. One way to phrase this is to discuss previous relationships that did not work out well, asking what complaints the other person made about them. With any patient, details should be gathered about suicidal ideation, threats, and attempts to determine whether there is currently a risk of a suicide attempt. With a patient who is potentially histrionic, this information is also useful to help determine whether there is a dramatic or manipulative quality to the threats or attempts. It can also be useful to ask for details of the types of activities the patient most enjoys, to see if he or she seems to especially enjoy being the center of attention or shows a craving for activity and excitement.

Hypomanic periods can be found in patients with HPD as well as in patients with the Axis I syndromes of cyclothymic disorder or bipolar disorder. Millon (1996) describes an urgency, restlessness, and intensity about the hypomanic phase of cyclothymia that is not typical of the histrionic patient. Although the behavior of the histrionic patient can occasionally be inappropriate, the histrionic generally has learned reasonable levels of social skills and can experience some hypomania without serious interference with routine social and occupational functioning, whereas the hypomanic periods are much more disruptive for the cyclothymic patient.

There may be overlap between histrionic and other personality disorders, and multiple dimensions may coexist. Both histrionics and narcissists desire to be the center of attention. However, histrionics are more willing to act subservient to maintain attention, but narcissists will sacrifice attention to maintain their superiority. Both borderlines and histrionics show labile and dramatic emotions; however, borderlines are much more likely to exhibit self-destructive behaviors and extreme discomfort with strong affect.

CONCEPTUALIZATION

Shapiro (1965) wrote of the hysteric's general mode of cognition as global, diffuse, and impressionistic regardless of content. Among cognitive and behavioral theorists, Beck (1976) presented a cognitive conceptualization of hysteria but examines hysteria in the sense of conversion hysteria rather than HPD. Millon (1996) presented what he refers to as a biosocial learning theory view of HPD, seeing this disorder within an active-dependent personality pattern. Figure 10.1 graphically outlines a cognitive-behavioral conceptualization of HPD combining some of the ideas of Millon and Shapiro with Beck's cognitive theory.

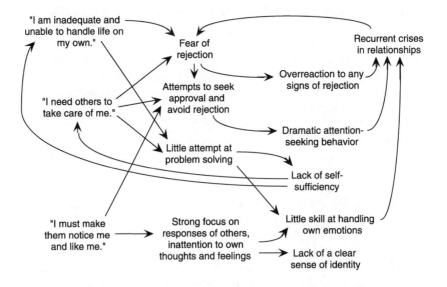

FIGURE 10.1. Cognitive model of histrionic personality disorder.

One of the underlying assumptions of the individual with an HPD is "I am inadequate and unable to handle life on my own." Individuals with other disorders may hold a similar assumption; however, the way the person copes with this assumption is what distinguishes among the disorders. For example, depressives with this basic belief might dwell on the negative aspects of themselves, feeling worthless and hopeless. Individuals with a dependent personality disorder may choose to emphasize their helplessness and passively hope that someone will take care of them. However, histrionic persons tend to take a more pragmatic approach, without leaving anything to chance. They conclude that because they are incapable of caring for themselves, they will need to find ways to get others to take care of them. Then they actively set about seeking attention and approval in order to find ways to ensure that their needs are sufficiently met by others.

Given that other people hold the key to survival in the world, histrionic patients tend to also hold the basic belief that it is necessary to be loved by everyone for everything one does. This leads to a very strong fear of rejection. Even entertaining the notion that rejection is possible is extremely threatening to these individuals, because this reminds the patient of his or her tenuous position in the world. Any indication of rejection at all is devastating, even when the person doing the rejecting was not actually that important to the patient. Feeling inadequate yet desperate for approval as their only salvation, people with HPD cannot relax and leave the acquisition of approval to chance. Instead, they feel constant pressure to seek this attention in the ways they have learned are effective, often by fulfilling an extreme of their sex-role stereotype. Female histrionics (as well as some of the males) seem to have been rewarded from an early age for cuteness, physical attractiveness, and charm rather than for competence or for any endeavor requiring systematic thought and planning. The more "macho" male histrionics have learned to play an extreme masculine role, being rewarded for virility, toughness, and power rather than interpersonal competence or problem-solving ability. Understandably, then, both male and female histrionics learn to focus attention on the playing of roles and "performing" for others.

Cathy's parents were divorced when she was still an infant, after which her father moved to New York City and went into show business. As a child, she saw him once a year and clearly felt that she had to compete with all his exciting show business friends and "all the women" he had around. She reported that he had always wanted her to be "the perfect little girl," and she had been constantly worried that she would disappoint him.

In the discussion of one case of HPD, Turkat and Maisto (1985) formulated her problems as "an excessive need for attention and a failure to use the appropriate social skills in order to achieve attention from others" (p. 530). Thus, although winning approval from others may be the primary goal, these individuals have not learned effective ways to achieve it. Instead of learning to carefully observe and analyze the reactions of other people and systematically plan ways to please or impress them, the histrionic person has been more frequently rewarded for the global enactment of certain roles; thus it is only in the enactment of these roles that he or she learns to excel. The striving to please others would not necessarily be dysfunctional in and of itself. Histrionic people, however, get so involved in this strategy that they take it far beyond what is actually effective. Carried away with dramatics and attracting attention, they lose sight of their actual goal and come to seek stimulation and drama for its own sake.

People with a HPD view themselves as sociable, friendly, and agreeable, and, in fact, they are often perceived as very charming at the beginning of a relationship. However, as the relationship continues, the charm seems to wear thin and they gradually are seen as overly demanding and in need of constant reassurance. Given that being direct involves the risk of rejection, they often use more indirect approaches such as manipulation to try to gain attention but will resort to threats, coercion, temper tantrums, and suicide threats if more subtle methods seem to be failing.

Histrionic people are so concerned about eliciting external approval that they learn to value external events over their own internal experience. With so little focus on their own internal life, they are left without any clear sense of identity apart from other people and see themselves primarily in relation to others. In fact, their own internal experience can feel quite foreign and uncomfortable to them and at times they actively avoid self-knowledge, not knowing how to deal with it. Having some vague sense of the superficial nature of their feelings may also encourage them to shy away from true intimacy with another person for fear of being "found out." Because they have paid little attention to their own internal resources, they have no idea how to respond when depth is required in a relationship. Thus, their relationships tend to be very shallow, superficial, and based on role playing.

The HPD cognition is global and lacking in detail, leading to an impressionistic sense of self rather than one based on specific characteristics and accomplishments. If one does not view one's own actions and feelings in a sufficiently detailed fashion, it is difficult to maintain a realistic impression of oneself. In addition, given that cognitive theory argues that thoughts exert a strong influence on emotions, it follows that global, exaggerated thoughts would lead to global, exaggerated emotions. These global emotions can be very intense and labile so that the histrionic patient gets carried away by affect even though it does not feel totally connected to him or her. Without the availability of complex, cognitive integration, these undifferentiated emotions can be very difficult to control, leaving the person subject to explosive outbursts.

The histrionic patient's characteristic thought style leads to several of the cognitive distortions outlined by J. Beck (1995), especially dichotomous thinking. The histrionic patient reacts strongly and suddenly, jumping to extreme conclusions whether positive or negative. Thus, one person is seen immediately as wonderful while someone else is totally awful. Because such patients feel their emotions so strongly and lack sharp attention to detail and logic, they are also prone to the distortion of overgeneralization. If they are rejected once, they dramatically conclude that they always have been rejected and always will be. Unlike the depressive, however, histrionic patients can be equally extreme in their positive conclusions about people and relationships and can easily switch between the two extremes. They are also subject to the distortion of emotional reasoning—taking their emotions as evidence for the truth. Thus, histrionic individuals tend to assume that if they feel inadequate, they must be inadequate; if they feel stupid, they must be stupid.

TREATMENT APPROACH

Obviously, in the course of working on specific problem situations, the full range of cognitive-behavioral techniques (outlined in J. Beck, 1995) can be useful. Depending on the goals of the patient, it may be helpful to use a variety of specific techniques including pinpointing and challenging automatic thoughts, setting up behavioral experiments to test thoughts, activity scheduling, and training in relaxation, problem solving, and assertion. The foregoing conceptualization of HPD would suggest a treatment strategy that integrates work on changing the patient's interpersonal behavior and thought style in addition to making the changes typically needed to achieve the patient's immediate goals. Finally, the underlying assumptions, "I am inadequate and unable to handle life on my own" and "It is necessary to be loved (by everyone, all the time)" will need to be challenged in order to make changes that will persist long after the treatment has ended.

Collaboration Strategy

Conflicting thought styles between the histrionic patient and the cognitively oriented therapist can make treatment quite difficult and frustrating at first. However, if this conflict in styles can be gradually resolved, the cognitive changes facilitated by therapy can mediate the patient's emotional difficulties. The primary challenge in doing cognitive therapy with the histrionic patient is for the therapist to maintain steady, consistent effort and to be sufficiently flexible to enable patients to gradually accept an approach that is initially so unnatural to them. The systematic, problem-focused approach of cognitive therapy exposes the histrionic patient to an entirely new way of perceiving and processing experience. Thus, the process of learning cognitive therapy is more than just a means to an end; the skills acquired by participating actively in cognitive therapy may constitute the most significant part of the treatment.

At least initially in therapy, the patient is likely to view the therapist as the all-powerful rescuer who will make everything better. This may feel good, but it can seriously interfere with the effectiveness of treatment. The more active a role the patient is required to play in the treatment, the less this image can be maintained. Thus, the consistent use of collaboration and guided discovery is especially important given the tendency of the histrionic patient to play a dependent role in relationships. Whenever the patient begs the therapist for help, the therapist needs to be careful not to be seduced into the (sometimes tempting) role of savior but, rather, to use questioning to help the patient arrive at his or her own solutions to the problems.

The unwary therapist can easily be maneuvered into taking on the role of "rescuer," taking on too much of the blame if the patient does not work toward change and giving in to too many demands. This may lead to the therapist feeling manipulated, angered, and deceived by the histrionic patient. A therapist who strongly wants to be helpful to others may inadvertently reinforce the patient's feelings of helplessness and end up embroiled in a reenactment of the patient's usual type of relationship. When the therapist finds him- or herself having strong emotional reactions to the histrionic patient and being less than consistent in reinforcing assertive and competent responses, it may be time for the therapist to monitor his or her own cognitions and feelings (see Chapter 5, this volume).

Cathy's therapist had mixed feelings about her. On the one hand, he found her to be quite likable and could see how it could be fun to know her as a friend. As a therapy patient, however, he felt frustrated with her. For example, when he would try to probe for thoughts and feelings before or during a recent panic attack, all he could get were repeats of the superficial thought "I'm going to faint" over and over again. He experienced a sense of futility and wanted to just throw up his hands and give up. He had thoughts such as "Why bother with this? Nothing sinks in. It won't make any difference. Nothing is going to change anyway." At times like these, he needed to challenge some of his thoughts by thinking, "I can't be certain of the effect of what we're doing. She is getting better, so things are in fact progressing. This is just a challenge. I simply need to continue to help her process events, because the idea is so foreign to her."

It is important to reinforce patients with HPD for competence and attention to specifics within the therapy sessions. Learning that attention to details and assertion can pay off in the sessions is the first step toward teaching these individuals that being assertive and doing active problem solving can pay off more than manipulation and emotional upheaval in the world outside the therapy sessions. Thus, it is important for the therapist to avoid falling into the patterns of so many of the patient's previous relationships. This can be quite a challenge even to the experienced therapist, because the style of the histrionic patient can be very appealing and attractive and dramatic renditions of experience can be quite absorbing, entertaining, and amusing. It is crucial for the therapist to avoid getting too wrapped up in the drama of the patient's presentation and to be aware of attempts at manipulation within the therapy, so that clear limits can be set by the therapist without rewarding these attempts.

Cathy tried for months to get special fee arrangements of various kinds, at times trying to go "over the head" of the therapist and contacting administrators throughout the hospital to make special "deals" without the therapist's knowledge. Fortunately, all such attempts were promptly brought to the attention of the therapist so that he could clearly and repeatedly enforce the same fee arrangements for Cathy as for the other patients. When she viewed refusals to comply with her requests as rejection, her feelings were discussed, but no exceptions to the fee arrangements were made. She tested the limits by insisting that she would need to schedule appointments only every other week because she could not afford treatment and was surprised and angry when the therapist agreed to this instead of making exceptions so that she could come weekly. After coming to therapy biweekly for a few weeks and seeing no hopes of special considerations, she returned to weekly therapy. Later in the treatment, when her income actually did change and she assertively raised the issue with her therapist, her assertion was rewarded and an appropriate fee adjustment was made.

Specific Interventions

The individual with HPD needs to learn how to focus attention on one issue at a time. The setting of a session agenda is an excellent place to begin teaching the patient to focus attention on specifics. The natural tendency of the histrionic patient is to spend most of the session dramatically relating all the exciting and traumatic events that occurred throughout the week. Rather than fighting this tendency, it may be important to schedule a part of each session for that purpose. Thus, one agenda item could be to review how things went during the week (with a clear time limit) so the therapist can be supportive and the patient can feel understood; then the rest of the session can be spent on working toward other goals.

One of the biggest problems in the treatment of individuals with HPD is that they usually do not stay in treatment long enough to make significant changes. As with other activities and relationships, they tend to lose interest and move on to something more exciting. One key to keeping histrionic patients in treatment is to set goals that are genuinely meaningful and perceived as important to them, and that present the possibility of deriving some short-term benefit as well as longer-term gain. They have a tendency to set broad, vague goals which fit their image of what is expected from a therapy patient but that do not seem particularly genuine. It is crucial, however, that goals be specific and concrete, and that they are genuinely important to the patients (and not just an image of what they think they "should" want). The therapist can help them to operationalize goals by asking questions such as "How would you be able to tell if you had achieved your goal?," "What exactly would look and feel different, in what ways?," and "Why exactly would you want to accomplish that?" It may be useful to have patients fantasize in the session about how it would feel to have changed their lives, in order to help them begin to fit their ideas together into a tentative model of who they would like to become. Once the goals have been set, they can be enlisted as an aid to help teach the patient to focus attention during the session. When these patients wander off the subject or go into minute detail about some extraneous topic, the therapist can gently but persistently ask how it is related to the goal that they had agreed to discuss.

Cathy originally came into treatment with the very practical goals of going back to work, being able to drive alone, and staying alone in her own apartment. However, Cathy was much more able to get excited about treatment when the goals were expanded to include being able to go into situations that were more immediately rewarding to her. Working on goals such as going to shopping malls ("especially to buy shoes!"), going to rock concerts, eating out at restaurants, and going to church (a charismatic congregation) kept her interest longer than her more pragmatic goals. One of the most powerful motivators for Cathy came when she had the opportunity to fly on an exotic vacation. This was such a compelling goal that she made rapid progress in the short period before the trip.

After the initial stages of treatment, the actual interventions will depend to some extent on the patient's particular presenting problem and goals. However, it is important to address each of the various elements of the cognitive conceptualization of HPD (Figure 10.1) in order to make a lasting change in the overall syndrome.

Because the histrionic patient's problems are exacerbated by a global, impressionistic thought style (which includes failure to focus on specifics), teaching the patient to monitor and pinpoint specific thoughts is an important part of treatment regardless of the presenting problem. In teaching these patients to monitor thoughts using the Dysfunctional Thought Record (DTR), it is likely that a great deal of time will have to be spent specifying events, thoughts, and feelings in the first three columns. Although many other types of patients may be able to go home and monitor thoughts accurately after a simple explanation and demonstration in the session, it is an unrealistic expectation for histrionic patients. It is much more likely that histrionic patients will forget the purpose of monitoring automatic thoughts and will instead bring in a lengthy narrative of exactly what happened to them throughout the week. The therapist needs to reward them for all attempts to do the homework; however, the DTR will probably need to be explained several times before the patients fully understand that the goal is not just to communicate with the therapist. They will need to be reminded that the primary purpose of the DTR is to learn the skill of identifying and challenging thoughts in order to change emotions in the moment. Some histrionic patients strongly feel the need to communicate all their thoughts and feelings to the therapist and, if so, it can be suggested that they write unstructured prose in addition to the thought sheets (but not as a substitute). DTRs can be especially useful in helping patients to distinguish reality from extreme fantasies and to make more accurate attributions regarding cause and effect.

Cathy would attribute any slight change in her physical condition to a terrible disease and immediately conclude that she had cancer or AIDS and was about to die. It made no difference to her whether she became dizzy and had trouble breathing because the room was hot and crowded or because she was having a panic attack. Whatever the actual cause of her dizziness, she immediately concluded that she was going to faint or die. Teaching her to stop and explore the possible alternative causes for her physical symptoms helped her to make more appropriate causal attributions and interrupt her cycle of panic.

Written homework assignments will likely be viewed as boring and dull, so extra time may be needed to challenge these thoughts with the potential benefits. Rather than fighting patients' sense of drama, their vivid imagination can be used in the tasks of therapy. For example, patients can be encouraged to be dramatic when writing rational responses, making the rational responses more compelling and powerful than the automatic thoughts. Cognitions often take the form of vivid imagery rather than verbal thoughts; thus vivid imagery modification can also be encouraged. Dramatic types of verbal challenges to automatic thoughts, such as externalization of voices, where the therapist role-plays the patient's automatic thoughts and the patient role-plays more adaptive responses, can be particularly convincing to histrionic patients.

Cathy's therapist found that she paid more attention when he used her own, dramatic words when setting up homework assignments. They therefore ended up with unusual-sounding assignments, such as "meeting with The Creep," instead of using more mundane terminology such as "meeting with my boss." Cathy found externalization of voices to be a dramatic, and therefore, powerful method of rational responding to thoughts. After having done a dramatic externalization of voices in a session, she was more able to go home and challenge her automatic thoughts on her own in writing.

Setting up dramatic behavioral experiments can be another powerful method of challenging automatic thoughts. For example, every time Cathy felt dizzy, she had thoughts such as "I'm going to faint and make a total fool of myself." To challenge these thoughts, it was important to set up exposure to the interoceptive cue of dizziness, which could be done in a dramatic way in group therapy.

THERAPIST: Cathy, it seems like the main symptom that frightens you is the dizziness.

CATHY: Yeah, I hate it. It's awful, isn't it?

THERAPIST: Well, I know that it feels that way to you. But I can't help but wonder if you've convinced yourself that it's awful when it may simply be unpleasant. Can you tell us what makes feeling dizzy seem awful?

CATHY: It's just terrible. You know, I'll pass out and I'll embarrass myself.

THERAPIST: So you believe that if you become dizzy you will pass out. And if you do pass out, what is it that you find frightening about that?

CATHY: I just have a picture of myself getting up and passing out again and again, forever.

THERAPIST: You picture that happening continuously? For how long?

CATHY: Just forever, like I'll never snap out of it. (*Laughs.*)

THERAPIST: You're laughing as you say that. Are you doubting your prediction?

CATHY: Well, I know it sounds a little silly, but that's the way it feels to me at the time.

THERAPIST: So you are making a prediction based on your feelings at the time. And how many times have you felt dizzy?

CATHY: Oh, thousands of times. You know I'm always talking about it.

THERAPIST: Then, how many of the thousands of times that you felt dizzy, and assumed that you would faint, did you actually faint?

CATHY: None. But that's only because I fight the dizziness. I'm sure it I didn't fight it I'd faint.

THERAPIST: That's exactly what we need to test out. As I see it, the problem here is not the dizziness per se, but rather the fear that you've come to associate with the dizziness. The more accepting you become of the dizziness and the less you catastrophize it, the less your life will feel ruled by the agoraphobia. So the job we have is of working on your becoming more comfortable with the dizziness. Does that make sense?

CATHY: Yeah, I guess it make sense. But I don't see how to do that. We talk about it but it seems just as scary to me.

THERAPIST: That's right, and that's because you need real evidence that nothing catastrophic will happen if you become dizzy. The evidence we have at this point is too weak. You also need to intentionally expose yourself to the dizziness rather than just let it hit you whenever. Are you willing to try an experiment that will be useful to you?

CATHY: Not if you're going to tell me to do something ridiculous.

THERAPIST: Do you agree with everything I've said so far?

CATHY: I guess.

THERAPIST: Then, while what I'm going to ask you to do may seem a little awkward, it will fit with what you've already said makes sense. I'd like for you to go to the center of the group and twirl until you get very dizzy.

CATHY: I don't want to do that.

THERAPIST: Here, I'll demonstrate. (*Gets up and twirls a number of times.*) There, like that. I was able to get dizzy quickly. I used to do that all the time when I was a kid. Didn't you?

CATHY: Yeah. Except now it's different. Then it was fun and now it scares me.

THERAPIST: If you are unwilling to twirl until you become very dizzy, would you be willing to do it a more limited number of times?

CATHY: I'll go around twice. No more.

THERAPIST: Great!

CATHY: (*Reluctantly gets up and very tentatively rotates two times.*) I hate that feeling!

THERAPIST: All the more reason to do it. As you directly face the feeling, rather than try to avoid it, I expect that you will eventually become more accepting of it. What did you discover today?

CATHY: I didn't faint. But that's probably only because I know I'm in a hospital and help is right around the corner. (*Laughs.*)

THERAPIST: That's why I'm going to ask that you practice twirling daily, first at home, so you can face the dizziness in your natural environment. Then in the next group, we'll see if you can twirl a bit longer.

CATHY: You mean I have to do this again?

THERAPIST: I think it's the quickest way to work on your problems. Your hesitancy gives an even stronger indication that we're right on track. But we can work on this at a pace that you can tolerate.

CATHY: It seems crazy, but I guess it make sense.

Another advantage of learning to pinpoint automatic thoughts is that the process can be used to reduce impulsivity. By learning to stop before reacting long enough to record thoughts, the patient has already taken a major step toward self-control.

One cognitive technique that is valuable in improving the coping skills of the individual with HPD is the listing of advantages and disadvantages of options. This technique is best introduced early in the treatment, as soon as the patient resists efforts to focus on the agreed-on topic. If the therapist simply insists that the patient focus attention on goals, a power struggle may ensue with the patient deciding that the therapist is "mean" and "doesn't understand." On the other hand, if the therapist consistently points out that it is the patient's choice how to spend the therapy time but that the advantage of focusing on the goal is that there will be some chance of achieving the desired goals, the patient is left to make his or her own decision. Whatever is chosen then feels more like it came from the patient than from the therapist. Helping the patient to make conscious choices within the therapy session by examining the "pros and cons" of various courses of action is a useful antecedent to learning to make such choices and do active problem solving in daily life.

Although Cathy had listed "being able to stay alone in my own apartment" as one of her primary goals, she never seemed to follow through on homework assignments involving spending even short periods in her apartment (e.g., 5 minutes). Rather than trying to push her into increased compliance, her therapist raised the issue of whether Cathy really wanted to work on this as a goal. Writing a list of the advantages and disadvantages of staying at her mother's house versus staying at her own apartment helped her to make her own decision that she did indeed want to pursue this goal (see Table 10.2). After coming to this de-

TABLE 10.2. Cathy's Analysis of the Pros and Cons of Staying Alone in Her Apartment

Advantages	Disadvantages
Staying at Mother's House	
"A lot of things are done for me (meals, cleaning)."	"My grandmother likes it warm and I like it cooler, so it is uncomfortable for me."
"There is someone here for companionship."	I don't have the independence."
"We've been doing a lot of craft projects together."	"I have my own place."
"I'm not as frightened when I'm here than I am alone."	"My mom can nag alot at times (re losing weight, smoking)."
"My mom is fun to be with most of the time."	"I feel like a failure not being in my own apartment."
	"No stereo."
	"Mom's VCR is acting up, so I can't tape while I'm away."
Staying at My Own Apartment	
"I love the way the apartment looks and feels."	"I don't feel comfortable in my apartment now."
"All my clothes and things are there."	"The rent is high and I'm not using it now."
"I have call waiting."	
"I can have my TV or stereo up as loud as I want."	"I think of how I was before the agoraphobia and I feel bad that I don't enjoy it like that now."
"I can keep my apartment cool."	
"I feel independent."	
"My VCR is working so I can tape while I'm away.	

cision on her own, she began to work more consistently on homework assignments toward this goal.

In addition to these cognitive strategies, these patients can also benefit from specific problem-solving skills. Given that they rarely consider consequences before action, it is helpful to introduce "means–ends thinking" (Spivack & Shure, 1974). This problem-solving procedure involves teaching the patient to generate a variety of suggested solutions (means) to a problem and then to accurately evaluate the probable consequences (ends) of the various options.

Treatment of the individual with HPD is rarely complete without attention to problematic interpersonal relationships. These individuals dominate relationships in indirect ways which seem to carry less risk of rejection. The methods that they most generally use to manipulate relationships include inducing emotional crises, provoking jealousy, using their charm and seductiveness, withholding sex, nagging, scolding, and complaining. Although these behaviors may work well enough to be maintained, long-term costs are often not apparent to patients due to their focus on the short-term gains. Challenging immediate thoughts may not be sufficient, however, because histrionic individuals so often use emotional outbursts as a way to manipulate situations. Thus, if a patient has a tantrum because her husband came home late from work, her immediate thoughts may include, "How can he do this to me? He doesn't love me any more! I'll die if he leaves me!" As a result of her tantrum, however, she may well receive violent protestations of his undying love for her, which satisfy her desire for reassurance. If she only challenges her automatic thoughts, she might not be addressing one of the most important aspects of the situation. Thus, in addition to directly challenging her thoughts when she gets emotionally upset, she also needs to learn to ask herself, "What do I really want now?" and explore alternative options for achieving this.

When patients have learned to pinpoint what they want out of a situation (which, with histrionic patients, is often reassurance and attention), problem-solving skills can be applied. Thus, rather than automatically having a temper tantrum, they are confronted with a choice between having a temper tantrum and trying other alternatives. Rather than asking them to make permanent changes in their behavior (such as giving up temper tantrums completely), the therapist can suggest that they set up brief behavioral experiments to test out which methods are the most effective with the least long-term cost. Brief experiments are typically much less threatening than the idea of making lasting behavior changes and may help prompt new behaviors.

Having spent so much time focusing on how to get attention and affection from others, histrionic patients typically have very little sense of their own needs, wants, or identity. Thus, therapy effort needs to focus on helping them pay attention to what they want and begin to develop a sense of identity. From there, it is helpful to consider the advantages of assertiveness, including the notion of one's personal rights for having needs met. Before patients can learn to more clearly and effectively communicate their wishes to others, they must first have a clear communication with their self.

In one group therapy session, the group leader encouraged Cathy to take on a difficult homework assignment. She agreed to the assignment but then skipped the next group session and sat pouting in the session after that. When another group member confronted her on her behavior, she became very anxious and had a full panic attack. At first, she was unable to identify what she was thinking and feeling and just reported vague feelings of not liking being in group anymore. Eventually she was able to identify her thoughts and assertively tell the group leader that she felt he was pushing her too hard and had set too difficult a homework assignment. She was strongly rewarded for her assertion by the other group members as well as by the group leaders and concluded that it had been worth enduring the anxiety.

The concept of "identity" or a "sense of self" is likely to be a source of many dysfunctional thoughts for the histrionic patient. These patients tend to see identity as a big, magical thing that other people somehow have but which they are lacking. The idea of exploring their sense of self seems totally overwhelming, and they tend to see identity as something one either already has or does not. Once the patient has started using some of the cognitive techniques discussed previously, he or she is already paying some attention to his or her emotions, wants, and preferences, but he or she may not see these as important parts of an identity. It can be helpful to describe the development of a sense of self as simply the sum total of many, varied things one knows about oneself and begin listing some of these in the therapy session, starting with mundane, concrete items such as favorite colors, types of food, and so on. The elaboration of this list can be an ongoing homework assignment throughout the rest of the therapy, and every time the patient makes any type of statement about him- or herself during the sessions (such as "I really hate it when people keep me waiting"), the therapist can point it out and have it added to the list.

It is important to eventually challenge the belief that loss of a relationship is disastrous. Even if the patient's relationships seem fine, it will be difficult to take assertive risks if the patient still believes that he or she could not survive if the relationship ended. Fantasizing about the reality of what would happen if the relationship should end and recalling life before the relationship began are two ways to begin helping the patient to "decatastrophize" the idea of rejection. Another useful method is to design behavioral experiments that deliberately set up small "rejections" (e.g., with strangers) so the patient can actually practice being rejected without being devastated.

Ultimately, the patient with HPD needs to challenge his or her most basic assumption: the belief that "I am inadequate and have to rely on others to survive." Many of the procedures discussed earlier (including assertion, problem solving, and behavioral experiments) are designed to increase the patient's ability to cope, thereby increasing self-efficacy and helping the patient to feel some sense of competence. Given the difficulty these patients have in drawing logical conclusions, however, it is important to systematically point out to them how each task they accomplish challenges the idea that they cannot be competent. It can also be useful to set up small, specific behavioral experiments designed with the explicit goal of testing the idea of their adequate independence.

MAINTAINING PROGRESS

Histrionic people can be lively, energetic, and fun to be with and they stand to lose a lot if they give up their emotionality completely. They may fear becoming drab, dull, and boring to others. It is therefore important to clarify throughout the treatment that the goal is not to eliminate emotions (which is impossible), but to use them more constructively. In fact, the therapist can encourage the adaptive use of their vivid imaginations and sense of drama throughout treatment, by helping them use dramatic and convincing means for challenging automatic thoughts. Other constructive avenues for sensation seeking can be encouraged, including involvement in theater and drama, participating in exciting activities and competitive sports, and occasional escape into dramatic literature, movies, and television. For Cathy, her newfound Christianity provided a more constructive avenue for some of her sensation seeking, and she was able to get very absorbed in the drama of her baptism and the laying on of hands that was part of her church.

For patients who feel reluctant to give up the emotional trauma in their lives and insist that they have no choice but to get terribly depressed and upset, it can be useful to help them gain at least some control by learning to "schedule a trauma." Patients can pick a specific time each day (or week) during which they will give in to their strong feelings (of depression, anger, temper tantrum, etc.) but rather than being overwhelmed whenever such feelings occur, they learn to postpone the feelings to a convenient time and keep them within an agreed-on time frame. This can have a paradoxical effect. When patients learn that they can indeed "schedule depression" and stick to the time limits without letting it interfere with their lives, they may not feel the need to schedule such time on a regular basis. It always remains as an option for them, however, so that long after therapy has been terminated, if they convince themselves that they simply have to "get it out of their system," they have learned a less destructive way to accomplish this.

Because the histrionic patient is so heavily invested in receiving approval and attention from others, a structured cognitive group therapy can be a particularly effective mode of treatment. Kass et al. (1972) demonstrated that group members could be enlisted to assist in the reinforcing of assertion and the extinction of dysfunctional, overly emotional responses. As in the cognitive therapy of most personality disorders, treatment overall tends to be longer in duration than with Axis I diagnoses.

Cathy's treatment began with individual therapy. As she mastered the basic concepts of cognitive therapy, she was moved into a cognitive therapy group as one step toward completion of treatment. Being the most histrionic member in the group, she quickly took on the role of "social director" and set the tone for dramatic reinforcement of progress on exposure hierarchies. With Cathy's encouragement, group members applauded and, at times, gave each other standing ovations for accomplishing particularly difficult items. The group provided an ideal arena for her to work on assertiveness and her need to entertain and please the group. For example, in one session, Cathy made a joke that did not get the response she had expected. In the following session, the group decided that they wanted to spend some time discussing assertiveness. Cathy responded, "Well, since we are talking about assertiveness, I want to share how I felt last session." She was able to pinpoint thoughts such as, "I said something funny, so now they'll kick me out," "I did something wrong," and "People want me to be different than I am." In discussing this, she was able to clarify for herself that she was especially concerned about how the male group leader would react. This discussion, and the challenging of these thoughts, led to her working for the next several sessions on the goal of deciding what she wanted and what was best for her, separate from other people, including men in authority.

For patients who are currently involved in significant relationships, couple therapy can also be especially useful. In couple treatment, both spouses can be helped to recognize the patterns in the relationship and the ways in which they each facilitate the maintenance of those patterns.

Cathy was seen for a total of 101 sessions over the course of 3 years. When she began therapy, she was unable to work due to her agoraphobia and had a Beck Depression Inventory score of 24. After six sessions, she was back at work and her Beck Depression Inventory score has dropped to 11 (within the normal range). Although she showed rapid symptomatic improvement in the early stages of therapy, it took a much longer period to make lasting changes in not only her agoraphobia and depression but also her HPD. Two years after she completed therapy, Cathy reported that she had not had any recurrence of agoraphobia or serious depression, despite having to go through several major crises including the breakup of a relationship, euthanizing her dog (and beloved companion), and the serious illness of her mother. When dealing with these major stresses, she reported that she continually told herself, "If I can get over the phobia, I can deal with anything." She had ended a problematic relationship and was engaged to be married to a man that she reported was stable, mature, and treated her well. She reported that for the first time in her life, she had a good solid relationship with great sex.

CONCLUSION

Although 101 sessions over a period of 3 years is hardly short-term therapy, it should be noted that Cathy was treated for agoraphobia and recurrent depression in addition to HPD. Although changes in the Axis I symptoms can be achieved in a much shorter period, the author's experience has been that changing the characteristics of the HPD itself often requires 1 to 3 years. Clearly, uncontrolled case reports are limited in their usefulness. Empirical research is needed to substantiate the effectiveness of this treatment with this population, to clarify the necessary components of the treatment, and eventually to determine which types of patients are most appropriate for which variations of the treatment.

CHAPTER 11

Narcissistic Personality Disorder

Narcissistic personality disorder (NPD) is an extensive pattern of distorted regard for self and others. Although it is normal and healthy to take a positive attitude toward oneself, narcissistic persons exhibit an inflated view of self as special and superior. Rather than strong self-confidence, however, narcissism reflects aggrandizing self-preoccupation. The narcissist is very active and competitive in seeking status, as outward signs of status are used as the measure of personal worth. When others fail to validate the special status of the narcissistic person, he or she is apt to view this as intolerable mistreatment and become angry, defensive, and depressed. The failure to be superior or regarded as special activates underlying beliefs of inferiority, unimportance, or powerlessness and the compensatory strategies of self-protection and self-defense.

Narcissistic individuals take pride in their social standing yet show some startling lacunae in adhering to norms and expectations of social reciprocity. Self-centered and inattentive to the feelings of others, the narcissist can turn a friendly exchange into an irritating display of self-preoccupation. A deceptively warm demeanor may be marred by arrogant outbursts, heartless remarks, or insensitive actions. Attention to the needs and feelings of others is lacking, whether in simple matters such as recognizing the contributions of others or in respecting more complex and deeply meaningful emotions. They may begrudge the successes of others and jealously judge or discredit those they view as encroaching competitors. The narcissist can also be masterful in twisting confrontations toward attributing blame and fault to other people.

When faced with limits or criticism, narcissists are apt to turn nasty and defensive. Others may find them to be demanding, insensitive, and unreliable—particularly as a source of emotional support, difficult to influence, and irritating because of their arrogant behavior. Narcissistic individuals may be able to maintain a coterie of admirers who are caught in a vortex of obligation, but intimacy is often lacking and long-term relationships are strained. Significant others see beyond the well-tended external image and may find their personal experiences with the narcissist to stand in stark contrast with public impressions. Narcissistic persons may have a history of rejecting others, sometimes abruptly, because they do not want to associate with people who make them "look bad," or fail to advance their status.

Challenges from the external environment that pose a threat to self-esteem are typically the precipitants for individuals with NPD to enter treatment. Precipitating events may include relationship disturbance, trouble at work, loss, or limitations that threatens their self-image. They do not see their problems in ordinary terms, however, and may expect to fascinate the therapist by being a uniquely complex patient. Sometimes unmet grandiose expectations accumulate over time, triggering despondence over a passing window of opportunity or unrealized entitlements. Depressed NPD patients often seem to be seeking quick restoration of their power and status and may tend to focus complaints on circumstances and people who disappoint or mistreat them. A sense of grandiosity may be evident in the bitter resentment of modest successes or inability to maintain a "special" status enjoyed at a previous point in life.

The narcissist may also enter treatment at the behest of frustrated significant others, or as a result of being in trouble because of exploitive or aggressive behavior or abuse of power. Conflicts presented by the narcissistic individual typically reflect discrepancies between attitudes of grandiosity and entitlement and realistic limits.

For example, 27-year-old "Misty," a medical technician who had a minor career in beauty pageant competitions, came to treatment at her grandmother's urging after a series of problems in her work and personal life caused a depressed mood. She complained bitterly about the boyfriend who recently broke off their relationship, citing her "selfishness" and "spoiled brat" behavior, which she viewed as an outrageous perspective "after all I've done to promote his career." She expressed hopes of suing him for damages. This was the first relationship breakup she had ever experienced that was not initiated by her; she had dated a great deal and had always been the one to "move on to someone better." At work, she had been told that she "had issues" and should seek counseling. This advisory came after she got into a shouting match with the chief surgeon because he corrected her behavior in front of another technician. Finally, she was in danger of losing her driver's license due to a history of moving violations, including a recent collision with a police vehicle that was parked in an interstate access lane while attending to another accident. Misty was caught in the traffic backup caused by the prior accident but decided that she "was not about to sit and wait with all those other sheep." She was speeding down the access lane when she rammed into the parked police car. Misty's problems are a composite example of issues encountered with several different NPD patients, and her hypothetical case illustrates the cognitive therapy applications to follow.

HISTORICAL PERSPECTIVES

The term "narcissism" has its origins in a classical Greek myth about Narcissus, a young man who fell in love with the image of himself he saw reflected in water. He was so taken with his self-image that his fate was to become rooted to the spot and transformed into the narcissus flower. The first reference to this myth in the psychological literature appeared in a case report by Havelock Ellis (1898), describing the masturbatory or "autoerotic" practices of a young man.

Freud (1905/1953) subsequently incorporated the term "narcissistic" into his early theoretical essays on psychosexual development, and eventually he conceptualized narcissism as a phase of normal development following an autoerotic phase, eventually maturing into object love. Major conflicts in the development of object love were thought to cause a fixation at the narcissistic stage (Freud, 1914/1957).

The work of object relations theorists elaborate narcissism as a character deficit that stems from inadequate parenting during early development (S. Johnson, 1987; Kernberg, 1975; Kohut, 1971). In the phase of development during 15–24 months, called "rapprochement" because of the alternation between exploring moves into the environment and returning to the safekeeping of a caregiver, the child sometimes receives inadequate support in these alternating efforts because caregivers are inconsistent, unavailable, or place self-centered demands on the child. The vulnerable child then suffers injury to his or her emerging self, which is called "narcissistic injury." To compensate, the child develops a grandiose, false self that will satisfy the needs of the caregivers. Rage and entitlement are split off from the conscious mind, which focuses on striving to attain perpetual adoration through the false self. In this conceptualization of narcissism, there is emotional pain evident as a nagging sense of worthlessness, inadequacy, and lack of meaning or pleasure in achievements meant to sustain the fragile esteem based on the false self (S. Johnson, 1987).

An interpersonal perspective, developed by Alfred Adler (1991/

1929), an early associate of Freud, holds that one of the major motive forces in personality development is the striving to overcome feelings of inferiority arising out of comparisons to others. He termed this process "compensation." Thus, an individual who perceives him- or herself as deficient relative to others might work exceedingly hard to achieve in that very area. The narcissistic personality, according to this model, would be the result of compensatory actions of an individual who perceived him- or herself as unimportant and inferior compared to others.

A social learning theory of narcissism advanced by Millon (1985) dispenses with the caregiver injury or compensation hypotheses and focuses primarily on parental overvaluation. According to Millon, when parents overinflate the child's sense of self-worth and entitlement, the internalized self-image is enhanced beyond what external reality can validate. The overinflated self image generates rage when disappointment occurs, and intermittent reinforcement maintains the self-image distortions. Inferred intrapsychic structures are limited to the person's inflated self-image.

The schema-focused cognitive approach to personality disorders detailed by Young (1990) lists several early maladaptive schemas (EMS) which are unconditional, self-perpetuating beliefs learned from interaction patterns beginning in early childhood. NPD appears to overlap with the EMS of impaired limits and unrelenting standards. Impaired limits schemas refer to self-centered and exploitive behavior, and unrelenting standards reflect a constant striving to achieve superiority.

The narcissistic theme of self-involvement has evolved from an explanation for masturbation to a disorder of arrested personality development to a personality impaired by maladaptive beliefs or an inflated self-image. The psychodynamic literature on narcissism provides extensive phenomenology but lacks empirical support for many assumptions. The cognitive approach may be more closely tied to emerging data on narcissism and offers treatment strategies that are more accessible to both patients and clinicians.

RESEARCH AND EMPIRICAL DATA

There is some empirical evidence to contradict the prevailing notion that narcissism is somehow linked to "underlying" low self-esteem (Baumeister, 2001). Narcissists characteristically regard themselves as superior to others and typically have moderate to high self-esteem on self-report measures. Narcissism and high self-esteem have been linked to aggression and violence in laboratory studies and some selected clinical populations. However, more investigation of both clinical and non-

clinical populations is needed to clarify these relationships, as narcissistic individuals often present clinically with self-esteem impairments, and
they are typically highly reactive to self-esteem threats.

According to self-verification theory, self-esteem is the motivating
force behind feedback seeking (Swann, 1990). Across a broad range of
contexts, individuals with an inflated self-image tend to create and maintain a positive illusory bias where they solicit confirming positive feedback, avoid self concept change, place uncomfortable demands on others, and deal with dissonance via hostility and aggression, a behavioral
composite quite unlike those with low self-esteem (Baumeister, Smart, &
Boden, 1996). A positive illusory bias in self-image has been linked to
aggressive behavior, interpersonal deficits, undesirable traits, and peer
rejection among adults (Colvin, Block, & Funder, 1995) and hospitalized youth (Perez, Pettit, David, Kistner, & Joiner, 2001). Bullies have
been shown to overrate themselves on academic and interpersonal skills
and to endorse unrealistically high self-esteem (Gresham, MacMillan,
Bocian, Ward, & Forness, 1998). Similarly, studies of inner-city gang
members typically find notably high rather than low self-esteem among
these violent youths (Baumeister, 2001).

The link between narcissism and hostile aggression has been noted
in a variety of laboratory studies (Kernis, Grannemann, & Barclay,
1989; Rhodewalt & Morf, 1995). Narcissism is positively correlated
with dominance and hostility (Raskin, Novacek, & Hogan, 1991), as
well as grandiosity, exhibitionism, and disregard for others (Wink,
1991). The readiness of narcissists to behave aggressively toward others
appears to be mediated by specific ego threats such as a bad evaluation
(Baumeister, Bushman, & Campbell, 2000; Bushman & Baumeister,
1998). In a population incarcerated for violent offenses, high levels of
narcissism and narcissistic personality disorder were identified as risk
markers for violence against family members, particularly when combined with a history of abuse within the family of origin (Dutton &
Hart, 1992). In another study of violent criminals, the range of moderate
to high self-esteem was comparable to the typical male college student.
On the other hand, the mean narcissism score of the violent offenders
was higher than for any other published sample (Baumeister, 2001).
However, Baumeister notes that "narcissists are no more aggressive than
anyone else, as long as no one insults or criticizes them" (p. 101).

Bushman and Baumeister (1998) apply a psychodynamic, motivational theory to discriminate between high self-esteem per se and narcissism, separating emotion from cognition. They note that "high self-
esteem means thinking well of oneself, whereas narcissism involves
passionately wanting to think well of oneself" (p. 228). They consider
narcissism to be a subcategory of high self-esteem where the self-image is

inflated and stable, albeit reactive to external ego threats. The specific role of cognition is not elaborated in their formulation.

Although self-esteem and narcissism are correlated, the two traits are not the same. Individuals with high self-esteem are not necessarily narcissistic but rather confident of their personal worth. Their esteem is apt to be based on realistic self-appraisals of demonstrated talents, achievements, and relationships viewed in a context of social norms and opportunities. Corrective feedback does not trigger a dramatic loss of self-esteem. For the patient with NPD, self-esteem is established by outward success, and any experience that challenges this success becomes a threat to self-esteem. He or she remains firmly rooted in the importance of a flawless or powerful image, much the same as Narcissus remained rooted to the spot while admiring his reflection. Without a flawless image, core beliefs of inferiority become activated.

DIFFERENTIAL DIAGNOSIS

NPD occurs in 2–16% of the clinical population (DSM-IV-TR; American Psychiatric Association, 2000; see Table 11.1). Other co-occurring disorders include mood disorders, especially with hypomania; anorexia nervosa; substance-related disorders, especially related to cocaine; and other personality disorders, notably histrionic, borderline, antisocial, and paranoid personality disorders. As developmental changes affect self-image and sense of potency in life, the person with NPD may be quite vulnerable to adjustment disorders. Narcissism may be underestimated as a co-occurring disorder because it is difficult to pinpoint in the context of other symptoms, or gender expectations. Thorough clinical evaluation should rule out any psychotic process indicating a delusional disorder, particularly erotomanic or grandiose type.

It is important to note that the traits of narcissism can also characterize highly successful individuals (American Psychiatric Association, 2000, p. 717). The defining feature that may distinguish narcissistic psychopathology within the cognitive formulation is the belief that without superior success and distinction, one is unimportant and worthless.

Evidence of functional impairment may be found in the individual's current and past work performance, interpersonal relationships, unethical behavior or exploitation of others (e.g., deceit, sexual harassment), legal difficulties, and financial problems resulting from grandiosity and entitlement, as well as the affective impairments associated with Axis I disorders. Subjective distress may be focused on resentment, disappointment with the inadequacies of others, or perceived unfairness of external situations or consequences, where insight about the entitlement is minimal or absent.

TABLE 11.1. DSM-IV-TR Diagnostic Criteria for Narcissistic Personality Disorder

A pervasive pattern of grandiosity (in fantasy or behavior), need for admiration, and lack of empathy, beginning by early adulthood and present in a variety of contexts, as indicated by five (or more) of the following:
(1) has a grandiose sense of self-importance (e.g., exaggerates achievements and talents, expects to be recognized as superior without commensurate achievements)
(2) is preoccupied with fantasies of unlimited success, power, brilliance, beauty, or ideal love
(3) believes that he or she is "special" and unique and can only be understood by, or should associate with, other special or high-status people (or institutions)
(4) requires excessive admiration
(5) has a sense of entitlement, i.e., unreasonable expectations of especially favorable treatment or automatic compliance with his or her expectations
(6) is interpersonally exploitative, i.e., takes advantage of others to achieve his or her own ends
(7) lacks empathy: is unwilling to recognize or identify with the feelings and needs of others
(8) is often envious of others or believes that others are envious of him or her
(9) shows arrogant, haughty behaviors or attitudes

Note. From American Psychiatric Association (2000, p. 717). Copyright 2000 by the American Psychiatric Association. Reprinted by permission.

CONCEPTUALIZATION

A schema of oneself as needing to be special and superior to escape inferiority may develop via a number of possible pathways. Narcissistic tendencies are apt to be inherited (Livesley, Jang, Schroeder, & Jackson, 1993) and shaped by parents who overcompensate for feelings of inferiority or unimportance. Instead of learning to accept and master normal and transient feelings of inferiority, these experiences are cast as threats to be defeated, primarily by acquiring external symbols or validation. In some cases, there may be negative circumstances that the individual is powerless to address, triggering even more profound feelings of inferiority or unimportance. Attempts to defeat feelings of inferiority at all costs and maintain positive self-esteem become magnified into overdeveloped strategies of self-aggrandizement. Other people are thought to be powerful, and their recognition and validation are crucial to the narcissistic person's sense of worth. At the same time, it is part of the narcissistic compensatory strategy to be alert to flaws in others, and to associate only with those who reflect their most positive, superior image. Broader experiences also reinforce the overdevelopment of self-aggrandizement. The actual presence of some culturally valued talent, attribute, or special position elicits social responses that reinforce the superior/special schema. Affiliations with social groups or institutions that espouse beliefs of exclusiveness and superiority while condemning outsiders can further extend this schema. Insulation from negative feedback and inter-mittent reinforcement of self-display and exploitive behavior support the compensatory beliefs of self-superiority. Fantasy provides cognitive re-hearsal of grandiosity and self-preoccupation, further maintaining the overdeveloped strategies.

Although their active strategies have the potential to be quite adap-tive in pursuit of success, narcissistic patients seem to cross the line to maladaptive in compulsively pursuing self-interests, rigidly overreacting to self-image threats, exploiting positions of power, and failing to de-velop or use adaptive skills, particularly sharing and group identifica-tion. Looking bad, feeling bad, losing a special status, or confronting limits are all perceived threats to self-image. We term this threat to self-image a "narcissistic insult." When faced with the stress of narcissistic insult, the NPD patient will become angry and self-protective and may act with surprising disregard for others.

A downward spiral may occur when self-centered behavior pro-vokes controversy, disapproval, perhaps disgust among others. The pa-tient experiences this as a narcissistic insult and will predictably become angry, defensive, and demanding of special treatment. The patient also may become depressed or anxious and harbor critical, punitive thoughts toward self and others, because his or her sense of value or importance depends on unremitting success and external admiration. Further, the NPD patient has a poor tolerance for discomfort and negative affect. Complaints, demands, and temper tantrums make such a patient feel powerful, and often work effectively in restoring a sense of superiority.

Misty, the medical technician with work problems, relationship loss, and poor driving record, grew up believing that being a "pretty girl" meant that she was entitled to be "spoiled" by others, and that she was superior to less attractive people. Her mother and grandmother de-voted considerable resources to Misty's beauty pageant competitions, and they took great pride in her successes. Misty's father died tragically in an automobile crash when she was very young. Her mother remar-ried, to a man who promised to "spoil" both she and Misty, to make up for the unfortunate circumstances of their loss. This primarily meant providing material things, with an associated expectation that Misty and her mother would idealize him and be evidence of his success in life. The couple then had two sons, allowing Misty to remain the "special girl" in the family. However, her brothers were regarded as the "smart ones," and they often teased Misty about being an "airhead." In fact, she was an average student. Her mother was absorbed in running their large home and participating in social commitments, and she focused her rela-tionships with all her children around their competitive endeavors. Her family also belonged to a religious congregation that endorsed ethno-centric beliefs about being morally superior and exclusively saved from hell and entitled to heaven on the basis of their particular worship. A cognitive conceptualization presented in Table 11.2 summarizes the relationship of Misty's early experiences, maladaptive beliefs, and strategies and how these patterns influence her current problems.

Core Beliefs of Narcissism

The core belief of narcissistic personality disorder is one of inferiority or unimportance. This belief is only activated under certain circumstances and thus may be observed mainly in response to conditions of self-esteem threat. Otherwise, the manifest belief is a compensatory attitude of superiority; "I am a rare and special person," or "I am superior to others." Another compensatory belief holds that "Other people should

TABLE 11.2. Cognitive Case Conceptualization: Misty

Childhood data

Parents inattentive but generous with material things; pay most attention to children's competitive endeavors.
Felt inferior in intellect compared to her brothers.
Exceptional good looks make her special and important.

Core beliefs

"I'm inferior; to compensate, I have to be special."

Assumptions

"Being pretty means I am special and superior."
"I deserve special treatment."
"I need people to admire me."

Coping strategies

Demanding and exploitive in seeking attention and gratification. Complains or attacks others when challenged or frustrated.

	Situation		
	Criticism at work	Stuck in traffic	Loses in beauty competition
Automatic thought	"How dare he speak to me like that."	"I shouldn't have to deal with this."	"I deserved to win."
Meaning of AT	"I can't stand to look bad."	"I am above petty problems."	"They think I am inferior."
Emotion	Angry	Impatient	Angry, Anxious
Behavior	Stomps off; vents to coworkers.	Honks horn; tailgates; speeds.	Files complaint on judge; goes on shopping spree.

recognize how special I am." In therapy, the narcissistic patient seeks admiration for special qualities but resists exploring feelings of inferiority, preferring to see the source of problems as external.

In therapy, Misty talked at length about her beauty pageant experiences and dating prowess, but she was reluctant to address her financial, interpersonal, or legal problems. Her speeding and reckless driving citations were attributed to unfair circumstances. "There are just too many people out there who don't know how to drive, and won't get out of my way," she griped.

Conditional Assumptions

Evidence of Superiority

The narcissistic person assumes that certain circumstances or tangible assets provide evidence and validation of superiority, special status, and importance. Thus, this patient believes that "I must succeed in order to prove my superiority." Such proof might include community influence, income level, physical attractiveness, material trappings such as the "right" car or living in the "right" neighborhood, personal awards, or associations that are exclusive or coveted by others. Not everyone, however, regards these things as markings of a generalized personal superiority. It is a narcissistic assumption to believe that achievements, position, possessions, or public recognition indicate personal value, or lack thereof. Conversely, the narcissist also assumes that "If I'm not successful, then it means I'm not worthwhile." Thus, self-esteem may plummet if these outward signs are lost, compromised, or unattainable.

Relationships Are Tools

Other people are viewed as objects or tools in the quest for distinction, and the narcissistic patient expends a great deal of mental energy comparing him- or herself and judging the worth of others. If others have the potential to advance the narcissist in some way, they will be idealized and pursued. If others are perceived as ordinary or inferior, they will be dismissed, or perhaps exploited for some gain, then discarded. As one narcissistic patient stated, "Very few people are worth my time. The rest bore me." The value of others rests in how they can serve or admire the narcissistic person. If they fail to treat the narcissist as special, this may be viewed as an indication of others regarding them as inferior, triggering defensive reactions. Narcissistic patients also experience anxiety if they believe someone else is commanding special attention from a person they hold important, and this may create a relationship crisis. Friendships can crack or family relationships become strained and fail simply because other people have legitimate competing interests. For example, a narcissistic man responded to the loss of attention from his partner when their child was born by initiating an affair with someone who provided unremitting admiration.

Misty rated the worth of people on a hierarchy, with looks, celebrity, and competitive victory being the prevailing criteria for superiority. She only wanted to associate with people who were "in style," or "winners." She was heavily invested in competing for opportunities to validate her good looks as better than others. She felt quite humiliated by being rejected by a man and perceived this as a terrible loss of status.

Power and Entitlement

Narcissistic individuals also use power and entitlement as evidence of superiority. The narcissist believes that "If I am powerful enough, I can be totally confident and free of doubt." As a means of demonstrating their power, narcissists may alter boundaries, make unilateral decisions, control others, and determine exceptions to rules that apply to other, ordinary people. The loss of power is apt to be a crisis for this patient, something that will provoke significant hostility, resistance, and possible depression.

Narcissistic individuals can be quite judgmental, opinionated, and forceful in communication, because they believe that superior people have superior judgment. Cognitive processes, however, are characterized by categorical, black-and-white reasoning, striking confirmatory biases, arbitrary inferences, and generalizations to others. The opinions or judgments of others are easily dismissed, no matter what the person's expertise. On the other hand, when the narcissist does seek input, it is typically important that their consultant have some claim to superiority. Interestingly, other "superior" people arbitrarily know what is right, even if the matter at hand is far afield from their expertise (e.g., a social celebrity can give financial advice—without any financial credentials). Out of their vehement certainty of judgment, boundary violations of all sorts may occur, as narcissists are quite comfortable taking control and dictating orders ("I know what's right for them") but quite uncomfortable accepting influence from others. Narcissists are puzzled or downright angry when others do not obsequiously follow their direction. To be challenged or proved wrong can literally undo their sense of personal esteem and worth.

Misty was quite irritated that her coworkers did not back her up in her work dispute with the chief surgeon. "I know how things should be done around there, and that surgeon doesn't know what he is talking about," was her take on the situation.

Another conditional assumption of power is the belief of exemption from normal rules and laws, even the laws of science and nature. Risk is viewed as remote, minimal, or easily managed. The patient may dismiss or actively distort evidence indicating risk, even when overwhelming, because of the firm belief in being the "exception." "I'm special; I can get away with it," where the "it" may be smoking, drinking, reckless driving, spending, overeating, substance abuse, emotional abuse, even sexual abuse or physical harm. The fallacy of this exception will not be casually accepted. "This can't be happening to me," is the refrain when exception fails. When faced with an unremitting loss, perhaps as in a life-threatening illness, the patient with NPD may persist in believing that he or she will not have to cope but will be excepted from the emotional stresses experienced by other, "lesser" individuals. Other normal expectations such as compromising in a marriage may be resisted or resented, based on the belief that "it should be easy for me, and I should not have to make that effort."

The narcissistic patient also assumes as a condition of power that "other people should satisfy my needs," and that "no one's needs should interfere with my own." Thus, he or she is apt to approach any number of situations feeling automatically entitled to personal gratification. From simple examples such as hogging the best seat, biggest steak, or choice bedroom; dominating entire conversations with personal concerns; commanding excessive portions of a family budget; or relentlessly demanding an outrageous inheritance claim, the assertion of his or her needs seems to lack the constraint of consideration for others. If others fail to satisfy the narcissist's "needs," including the need to look good, or be free from inconvenience, then others "deserve to be punished."

Misty believed that if she dated someone, she was entitled to be "spoiled" by that person with gifts, jewelry, cash, trips, and such. She was quite proud of her power to "play the male ego" by telling her dates about previous gifts and additional things on her wish list, provoking the current male interest to "spoil" her with bigger and better items, regardless of her interest in the person. If the man declined to become involved in this extortion, she would retaliate by spreading ridiculing lies about his sexual performance.

Image Preservation

Narcissistic individuals believe that "image is everything," because it is the armor of their self-worth. Checking and maintaining their image is a paramount concern, and they perceive themselves always on display. Typical automatic thoughts exaggerate the likelihood of being noticed in a positive sense, and make comparisons with other high-status individuals or celebrities. One narcissistic patient stated quite confidently that "God admires me." Failure to look good or be admired is cause for extreme disturbance, as this can trigger angry, self-doubting ruminations and fears associated with negative core beliefs.

The belief about the importance of appearances will frequently, although not always, extend to those whom the patient views as an extension of him- or herself (e.g., spouse, child): thus the assumption, "My child (spouse) has to make me look good." Perplexing double binds may arise out of this view for significant others. If they fail to perform in an admirable way (according to the narcissist), they may be ridiculed, punished, or tormented. If they succeed in admirable performance and challenge or surpass the narcissist, they may be ridiculed, punished, or tormented.

Amanda and Lewis arrived at their marital therapy session in a private limousine, courtesy of Amanda's parents, who always wanted the best for her. Marital tension was focused on Amanda's growing dissatisfaction with Lewis, and his "unwillingness" to please her. It seems that at 42, his hair was thinning and receding, and he was getting a bit flabby in the middle, although as a sports professional, he remained physically well toned. Slim Amanda proudly pointed out that at size 1, she was the same size as she had been at age 16. Lewis's unwillingness to please her involved his reluctance to undergo hair implants which, she reasoned, would ensure that he retained some hair as the natural process of thinning progressed. "I just can't be married to a flabby, bald guy," she complained. "It would make me look bad."

Assumption of Meritorious Contribution

Narcissistic individuals tend to create a market of personal opportunity by exaggerating the needs and weaknesses of others, and embellishing their own virtues and merits. "They need me," and "I'm doing them a service," may rationalize actions that are primarily self-gratifying or exploitive. Seeing oneself as a generous, noble benefactor or mentor allows minimization or denial of possible risks or harm to others. Although there may be a kernel of reality to the efforts made, the narcissist greatly exaggerates the benefits accruing to others, and misconstrues reactions of others as overly favorable. Even when punishing others out of intolerance or entitlement, the narcissist sees this as "a lesson they need, for their own good."

Misty lived rent-free in her grandmother's house, and also asked her grandmother for a "maintenance allowance" to help cover the costs of her expensive cosmetic procedures and regular salon services, as well as designer clothing and accessories. Although the grandmother worked part-time as a retail sales clerk to provide this allowance and coped with advancing arthritis, Misty believed that her grandmother "needed" to give her money to feel useful and happy.

Assumptions about Affect

Persons with NPD appear to overestimate the negative implications of emotions such as sadness, guilt, and uncertainty by viewing these affects as personal weaknesses that threaten their positive self-image. On the other hand, the possible risks associated with unbridled anger or self-admiration are minimized or denied altogether. The patient with NPD often has a low tolerance for frustration and expects not only to have wishes easily gratified but also to remain in a steady state of positive reinforcement. When this does not occur, the individual experiences what we have previously termed "narcissistic insult." Conditional assumptions may include the notions, "If I want something, it is extremely important that I get it," and "I should feel happy and comfortable at all times," and "If I'm not happy, no one can be happy," and "I need to feel special to be happy." The narcissistic patient may be ridiculing or intolerant of vulnerability as a "weakness." He or she may be quite reluctant to discuss problems or concerns because this is tarnish on their personal image and would allow others to see their "weaknesses." Expressed concerns of significant others will only be tolerated, not welcomed, because the narcissist fears being viewed as inferior. In therapy, the NPD patient may be reluctant to discuss "weaknesses" but at the same time expects the therapist to somehow restore his or her feelings of well-being.

Active Compensatory Strategies

Narcissistic individuals are quite active in their attempts to reinforce self-aggrandizing beliefs and avoid experiences of discomfort or vulnerability. They have big dreams and seek fame, ideal romantic love, or power. Desired power may be objective, as in wealth or positions of control, or interpersonal, as in having significant authority and influence over others. The goal of these endeavors is to gain admiration, demonstrate superiority, and become invulnerable to pain or loss of esteem. There are at least three types of strategies that express this action orientation. Within any of these strategies, there is the potential for the behavior to become abusive and even violent toward self or others if the patient is criticized or challenged.

Self-Reinforcing Strategies

Narcissistic individuals seek reinforcement of their power and importance by solicitation of flattering feedback and behaving in an arrogant, condescending manner toward persons in subordinate positions. These strategies seem to say, "See how important and influential I am!"

Self-Expanding Strategies

Narcissistic individuals take seriously the accumulation of symbolic measures of status, perfection, and power. Some gravitate toward material possessions and are emotionally invested in the status of things. Their motto might be "the best is good enough for me." For others, self-expanding strategies are focused primarily on achievement or recognition, and they may even appear to care little about appearance or material things.

The narcissistic individual may pursue risky self-expanding endeavors such as high-stakes business deals, extreme sports, trophy dating and marriage, multiple cosmetic surgeries, world travel, nonstop entertainment, whatever demonstrates a distinctive lifestyle. These ventures can resemble manic or hypomanic activity but are more purposeful and sustained, lacking the disorganization of manic mood states. When there is the possibility of looking good in the eyes of others, achieving a higher status, or winning an important competition for power, the narcissist will have very few, if any causes to stop the action or consider the consequences.

Self-Protecting Strategies

Most pernicious of the narcissistic strategies are those where the aim is to ward off threats to the distorted self-image. Threats are idiosyncratic and may be perceived in many forms. However, predictable threats involve personal feedback or evaluative comments, which, if not precisely flattering, will be received as criticism. Disagreement with their opinion, failure to display appropriate "respect" or admiration, or challenging their beliefs are all possible self-esteem threats. Because "image is everything," the situations most likely to threaten the narcissist are those that make them "look bad" in front of an audience (or in the eyes of someone important). Casual, trivial remarks made in the presence of friends might be cause for a subsequent "blow up" due to the narcissistic insult. Others are apt to find the narcissistic person defensive, unreceptive, or unresponsive to constructive feedback, even when delivered in the most tactful and caring way.

Narcissism is a risk factor for situational defensiveness to cross the line toward interpersonally destructive, even violent actions. The narcissistic individual may be socially destructive toward others by engendering gossip, shunning, or publicly devaluing challengers. Making threats of implied violence to scare the challenger ("You'll be sorry. You don't know who you're dealing with!"), or engaging in overt acts of physical violence to punish are, unfortunately, a distinct, albeit rare possibility.

"Chief" was arrested for the serial murder of six family members, and subsequently diagnosed with NPD. Chief's violent episode followed a series of hardships and stresses. He separated from his wife but retained custody of their several small children. A layoff from his laborer job caused financial loss and repossession of his furniture, leaving his home without beds or chairs. Chief's estranged wife had reportedly telephoned on several occasions to taunt him with stories of her new boyfriend's sexual prowess and material possessions, including a new gun. Chief became increasingly angry and preoccupied with thoughts that the boyfriend "had a bigger gun than mine," and that his children would abandon him for the material offerings of their mother and her boyfriend. To reassert his power, he planned to murder his wife and her boyfriend. On the day he set out to do this, however, he also "took care of" his four children by shooting each of them, so the wife and boyfriend could not have them. He found his wife at her mother's home and shot both victims to death. He then stalked the boyfriend for 6 hours, finally wounding but not killing him. Extensive psychological evaluation supported the notion that the murders were all committed to ward off insults to Chief's self-esteem, to punish those who threatened him, and to protect his entitlements.

TREATMENT APPROACH

Narcissistic patients can be expected to enter treatment in a stage of change that Freeman and Dolan (2001) describe as "anti-contemplation." In this stage between precontemplation and contemplation, the patient's stance is opposed to change. In essence, to say, "I'm fine the way I am, I do not need to be here or to change. What's more, you can't make me change!" Even when in distress, narcissistic patients are ambivalent about treatment and reluctant to engage in self-evaluation because it threatens to activate the core negative belief of inferiority. The self-protecting strategy of this disorder is to externalize sources of distress. Something needs to be different, but it is not they who need to change. When the well-intentioned therapist attempts to recommend actions to initiate change, in the manner more typical with Axis I disorders, unproductive power struggles and defensive resistance may be the result.

Collaborative Strategy

The defensive characteristics and active strategies of this disorder can easily provoke therapist annoyance, defensiveness, anxiety, or errors in judgment. Both criticism and flattery are interpersonal strategies used by the narcissist. Even in the first meeting, patients with NPD may criticize the therapist's office décor or location, challenge the therapist's worth, act arrogant toward staff, or expect special treatment. Such inappropriate behavior can make it hard to empathize and establish an emotional bond with this person. Alternatively, the narcissistic patient may attempt to bedazzle the therapist and use flattery to draw the therapist into his or her personal entourage of "exceptional" people. It is important to spot aggrandizing and idealizing comments as potential psychopathology. Such comments are notable for deviation from the kinds of positive reactions that may be typically encountered across a range of patients. For example, patients may frequently comment on the pleasant view from the therapist's office windows. The narcissistic patient, however, covets the view for his or her own office and evaluates the windows as a measure of status.

Remaining attuned to these strategies and one's own expectations for and response to reinforcement is crucial. The most important therapist strategy may be to work consistently from a conceptualization of narcissistic beliefs and strategies and adjust one's expectations for patient responses. Therapists may become discouraged if they expect a smooth process of applying cognitive techniques. Narcissistic patients have significant problems that interfere with collaboration, including a lack of insight and external focus of change. They may need to be guided repeatedly through contemplation of problems before they will accept any influence from the therapist. They may view therapy as a threat and need assistance in viewing therapy as a self-enhancing process. They are likely to feel entitled to special treatment and will trivialize concrete and standard recommendations. They expect to feel better without effort or risk and may resent the expectations for their input. More important, the maladaptive aspects of the personality may not be addressed if the therapist is too quick to give up on the cognitive approach or attributes these difficulties only to his or her own technical skills.

With narcissistic patients, it is important to provide praise or support for the patient's strengths and successive approximations and vary the structure as needed. Favorable reflections and comments are necessary to meet the patient's relationship expectations and keep the patient involved in treatment, but it must be done strategically to reinforce desired behaviors.

Sometimes emotional reactions to narcissistic patients go beyond the normal parameters in either a positive or negative direction and significantly challenge the therapist's usual coping skills. The therapist may experience revulsion or disgust in response to a patient's illegal, immoral, or abusive actions. Alternatively, the therapist may be charmed or seduced by the flattery and endorsement of this apparently discerning and powerful individual. Either kind of reaction suggests some possible threat to the integrity of the treatment and indicates a need to conceptualize possible therapeutic responses. It is particularly helpful for the therapist to use the cognitive therapy tools, such as a Dysfunctional Thought Record, to work out alternatives and coping strategies for any uniquely strong emotional reactions to the patient. As always, it is wise to be mindful of ethical, legal, and clinical guidelines for handling threats or dangerous behavior, or potential boundary violations, and to seek consultation as needed.

Specific Interventions

Key target areas with the narcissistic personality include (1) improving mastery and goal-attainment skills and examine the meaning of success; (2) increasing awareness of boundaries and the perspectives of others; and (3) exploring beliefs about self-worth and emotions and developing constructive alternatives. A variety of cognitive tools can be useful in guiding NPD patients in a process of gathering data and testing hypotheses about problem situations in these target areas. Pie charts of contributing factors can be a useful method for thinking in broader, or more complex terms, as well as clarifying priorities. Role plays, particularly with the inclusion of role reversals, can be effective in fostering empathy and understanding of boundaries and external perspectives. Magnified emotional reactions to situations of criticism or frustration of entitlements may attenuate with the use of scaling procedures and the review of options and alternatives. Goal setting and persistence in graded tasks can be a useful way to address problems of excessive reliance on fantasy gratification. Various guided discovery questions can be used to explore self-aggrandizing beliefs and assumptions and to develop more affiliated alternatives. Cognitive hypnotherapy may also be a useful tool for modifying narcissistic thinking, particularly at the structural or schema level (see Dowd, 2000). As Dowd (2000) notes, it is important that both therapist and patient are adequately prepared to use this specialized intervention.

Problem List, Agenda, and Motivation for Treatment

Because patients with NPD fear exposure of their feelings of inferiority, a concrete problem list based on specific difficulties presented by the patient must be established as quickly as possible. Ambivalence about being in therapy can be addressed by reviewing the pros and cons of using therapy as a way to deal with the problems on the list. This structure empowers the patient to choose to view therapy as a positive, self-enhancing option. Sometimes it is helpful to suggest that people from all walks of life use therapy, including highly successful and famous people, and that, typically, patients view therapy as a positive experience overall.

Although specific issues might provoke some discomfort, patients enjoy the therapist's help and guidance and positively anticipate coming for sessions. Further, they will work together with the therapist to assess progress and the usefulness of the therapy.

As rapport develops in the process of working on specific functional problems, a structured tool such as the Personality Belief Questionnaire (PBQ) can be useful to assess specific narcissistic beliefs and their intensity. This assessment can then further guide the case conceptualization as it is shared between patient and therapist, and possible modifications of core beliefs can be explored. When the problem list includes felonious criminal behavior, additional treatment strategies will be needed (however, it is beyond the scope of this chapter to extensively address problems of criminal proportions—e.g., violent assault).

It is typically useful (1) to address any immediate crisis or destructive behavior, (2) to focus on any symptoms of Axis I disorders, and (3) to modify the underlying beliefs through experiments and guided discovery. Instead of broad goals of personality restructuring (e.g., "I need to make Misty become a humble, altruistic individual"), a more limited focus on promoting adaptive strategies ("Help Misty stop exploiting her grandmother and others, attain some realistic career goals, cope more effectively with narcissistic insults, and construct more adaptive beliefs about self-esteem") is needed.

As previously mentioned, Misty came to therapy because a confluence of suggestions, including her grandmother's, convinced her to give it a try. She admitted that she did not see how she had any need to change but still agreed to an initial 12 sessions of therapy, with an option to continue if she felt it was useful, to focus on her relationship disappointments, her frustration with her career goals, and her driving/legal problems. She leaned more favorably toward the idea of therapy after learning that a famous leading actress she admired had revealed in a magazine interview that she relied on marital therapy to "help her stay normal." With that in mind, she also liked the idea that she could, in fact, choose to look forward to the sessions as an opportunity for self-enhancement, not as a threat of weakness or embarrassment.

Misty did not have a preference for which problem to address first, but she did have a tendency to use sessions to tell self-aggrandizing stories. Her therapist provided brief, but frequent orientation to the cognitive model when this occurred.

THERAPIST: Misty, I notice that you show wonderful initiative in getting our sessions started, and I imagine that quality serves you well in many situations.

MISTY: Thank you!

THERAPIST: It's helpful to take note of what makes us feel good, and to learn from our successes. However, let's be sure we allot enough time to work on at least one problem from our list. Which one should that be today?

MISTY: Well, I want to be sure and tell you about my great experience on Saturday.

THERAPIST: OK, I would like to hear about it. If that doesn't automatically take us into one of our problem topics, I'll help us shift gears in about 10 minutes so we can work more on the career stuff. How does that sound to you?

MISTY: Fine. Now back to Saturday . . .

Goal Attainment and the Meaning of Success

High goal attainment is central to the NPD sense of worth and identity. However, the incremental efforts and frustration inherent in most mastery experiences are highly likely to trigger negative core beliefs. Actual mastery and achievement are often thwarted by attitudes of entitlement, excessive reliance on fantasy, inflexible grandiose expectations, and insufficient effort. Even when there is a measure of achievement, even notable achievement in some cases, the derived meaning of that success continues to be problematic because it is the measure of individual worth. Both cognitive and behavioral strategies can be used for more effective goal attainment and for examining beliefs about the meaning of success.

In exploring her career aspirations, Misty reported that she had frequent fantasies of winning major beauty titles, becoming an actress, and eventually winning awards for her work in films. She would watch the televised Oscar awards and think, "That should be me up there." However, a good part of her frustration seemed to come from doing little more than wishful dreaming to advance an acting career. As she was fantasizing her ideal future (and doing little about it), she was paying scant attention to other personal goals.

To help Misty clarify her priorities, her therapist asked her to help develop a pie chart of potentially desirable life accomplishments (dreams). Besides her aspirations to be a famous actress, she also acknowledged hopes for relationships and family connections that would be both happy and enduring. In allocating relative portions of 100% of her current priorities, she established that acting was about 40%, dating was 30%, friends and family were 20%, and earning a living was 10% (with some therapist prompting). Misty and her therapist then mapped out possible steps that she could take to realize her priorities rather than just waiting for her dreams to come true. Graded tasks that Misty chose to advance the reality of her acting dream were to audition for "extra" roles in films and videos, enrolling in an acting workshop, and working part time at a local venue where major productions were staged.

An important part of this exercise was discussing Misty's reactions as she took small steps and catching negative reactions such as minimizing or ridiculing these efforts. Dysfunctional Thought Records were useful in tracking these reactions during the course of her daily activities. As she was able to explore reasons for negative reactions, she pinpointed some key beliefs about superiority and worth connected to success (e.g., "I need to have a starring role. If I don't, then I'm worthless.") This allowed further testing of the underlying belief, by setting up an experiment to see whether persistence and flexibility in her goals (bit part rather than starring role) did result in any worthwhile gains.

When failed expectations or dreams are the presenting problem, it may be that ruminative comparisons, minimization of the necessity of effort, and contempt or dismissal of partial results stem from similar rigid expectations for superlative achievement. Further, the NPD patient may be minimizing or denying some exploitive or aggressive actions that have impaired their advancement.

Scott, an investment broker terminated from his third firm, complained that "this shouldn't be happening to me." He ruminated constantly about the success he "deserved," and angrily compared himself to former classmates now in business, noting that "their successes just grind at me." He expected to be earning "at least" a $1 million salary, and he did not see that the complaints about his sexual harassment of employees should have anything to do with his lost positions. Scott accepted the idea that it probably was not in his best interest to constantly measure his potential against the past successes of others. More grudgingly, he explored the viability of expecting a $1 million contract with a "prestige" firm despite repeated (and well-substantiated) claims of sexual harassment and other unprofessional conduct. Most difficult but crucial was exploration of the meaning of his expected success and modifying the beliefs about the worthlessness of alternative goals.

When envy and anger over frustrated entitlements are problematic, another helpful strategy is to agree on the advantage to the patient while also directing attention to an assessment of the costs and benefits of current behavior and a problem-solving discussion of alternatives. For example, Misty believed that other people should get out of her way on the road, so that she could achieve her goal of getting to her destination in a hurry. The therapist agreed that, yes, it would be nice if people could just get out her way, so she could travel unimpeded. However, given that the chances are low that they will, what are the options for coping with this frustrating situation? The costs of trying to run them over had Misty on the verge of losing her license, not to mention paying hundreds of hard-earned dollars in various fines, insurance increases, and auto repairs. Misty agreed to try a few self-restraining changes, including giving up tailgating slow drivers and practicing self-calming thoughts when traffic was too heavy for speeding. Additional strategies for dealing with entitlement anger have been effectively demonstrated by DiGiuseppe (2001).

If the therapeutic rapport is sufficiently well established, the therapist may choose to explore the reasoning behind beliefs of entitlement, gently challenging support for this position and exploring the meaning associated with surrendering the entitlement. What is realistically lost with a given concession? What might be gained by choosing to let something go? For example, Misty was encouraged to consider what she might gain by not demanding that her dates "spoil" her with gifts. Scott was asked to compare what he was losing by sitting, day after day, in the coffee shop, ruminating about what he deserved, as opposed to what he could gain by applying for some jobs in "second- or third-tier" firms, and adhering to the employee relations guidelines.

Interpersonal Boundaries and Perspectives of Others

A central task with the patient with NPD is improvement of interpersonal skills, although this patient would likely view the idea of social skill training as a narcissistic insult. More than basic social skills, it is the intimacy skills of listening, empathizing, caring, and accepting influence from the feelings of others that are lacking in NPD. Instead, the narcissist tends to judge, manipulate, or dominate in dealings with others. Keeping the focus on boundaries and perspectives may offer a way to approach these issues with minimal reactance. Specific boundaries to be reviewed may include physical, sexual, social, and emotional boundaries of others, as well as the boundaries for attention to self and others. The strategy of attending to the perspective of others can be modeled and shaped by the therapist's solicitation of feedback during sessions. Further, judgments and comparisons can be labeled as emotional boundary violations, with nonevaluative description and acceptance as the more empathic or respectful alternative.

After several inquiries about the health and well-being of her grandmother, Misty agreed to discuss their relationship in terms of what boundaries were being kept and how much she understood her grandmother's perspective. Although she tended to be dismissive, she agreed that her grandmother was an important person in her life. By using role-reversal imagery and empathic confrontation, the therapist guided Misty toward greater empathy for grandmother's needs and limits.

THERAPIST: So, your grandmother is irritable in the evenings sometimes, especially when you don't come home for dinner. Let's try to get an image of what she might be thinking. Can you imagine being your grandmother, and telling Misty what's making you so cranky?

MISTY: I'm tired from work, and stiff from my arthritis. It's hard to get around, and making dinner is almost impossible. I just want to go to bed.

THERAPIST: Is it possible that your grandmother is stressed by going to work at her age, and having you rely on her for so many things?

MISTY: Oh, she enjoys spoiling me and making me happy.

THERAPIST: I'm sure that she loves you and she does enjoy making you happy. But is it possible that the stress of working when she is exhausted, in pain, and needs money for herself might be physically or emotionally harmful to her?

MISTY: I don't know; I guess it's possible.

THERAPIST: Would you be willing to gather some evidence to check this hypothesis, perhaps by asking her more about her feelings?

MISTY: I suppose so.

THERAPIST: OK, let's talk about how you might actually do that.

Narcissistic patients, like those in manic states, are particularly prone to overestimate the positive responses of others and to inflate the positive impact of their sometimes highly questionable actions. Those patients who may be at risk to hurt others need intensive and repeated focus on distortions of risk, harm, and exception and development of an understanding of the potential impact of their actions.

Maladaptive Beliefs about Self and Emotion

Rigidity of judgment and maladaptive beliefs about self and emotion are a third cluster of issues to address in therapy for NPD.

First, the distorted self-confidence of narcissism may significantly affect this patient's ability to engage in critical thinking about his or her beliefs. Accepting influence and changing position to accommodate information from external sources may be viewed as a weakness or loss of power that is dangerous to his or her self-image. For instance, the patient with NPD may believe, "Once I make a decision, I should stick with it at all costs." Further, "If I change my mind, I'll appear weak and inferior." Still further, "Accepting influence is letting the other win, and conceding defeat is humiliating." In the narcissist's mental image, "Confident, successful people never back down or change their position." Exploring the alternatives to these beliefs is an important step in the process of working with the range of narcissistic beliefs. One option is to define the reasons and circumstances for implementing the alternative beliefs. For example, even confident people change their position when certain things are at stake, or within certain contexts such as a close personal relationship.

The NPD belief that one should feel comfortable, happy, and confident at all times is another important potential issue. There may be implicit or explicit demands that the therapist (among others), should take action to restore the patient's continuously positive state. However, this automatic reaction may very well be an avoidance strategy to minimize negative schema activation. Some patients with NPD believe that if they feel bad, that means they are powerless and inadequate, and that confident, superior people never grapple with disappointment, fear, sadness, anxiety, or other negative emotions. Related to this are beliefs about the necessity of defending one's positive self-image, as in "I have to defend myself if I'm challenged," or "I can't allow anyone to criticize me."

The first step toward accepting emotional experiences may be simply to provide empathic support and validation. Second, it may be useful to point out how the expectation for uninterrupted positive affect is directly self-defeating because it creates a context in which any negative feeling becomes a threat to self-esteem. In addition, the therapist can draw attention to the patient's contemptuous or rejecting attitudes toward certain emotions, noting the evaluative nature of these automatic thoughts, as in "I'm stupid and weak for feeling hurt," or "It's intolerable if I don't feel happy all of the time." These evaluative statements can be further explored in terms of advantages and disadvantages of holding the belief, as well as advantages and disadvantages of an alternative position, for example, believing that a range of emotions as normal and human, and even part of the vitality and challenge of living. In an appeal to their self-interest, patients with NPD can be invited to test the effects of accepting emotions to see what happens, and whether or not they are able to become more confident by valuing rather than devaluing this important dimension of their personality.

Misty acknowledged feeling embarrassed, angry, and defensive when her behavior was corrected at work. However, because she "couldn't stand" feeling this discomfort, she lashed out at what she perceived to be the source, her supervising surgeon, much to her detriment as her work evaluation and subsequent pay was affected. She also identified the operative belief that "I have to defend myself to prove I'm right." When asked specifically what she "couldn't stand," she identified "looking bad in front of coworkers," and "not having my contributions recognized." Then her therapist asked whether her discomfort was alleviated by lashing out, and she admitted that still felt angry and embarrassed. Further, lashing out did little to actually get her contributions recognized, she agreed. The therapist then invited her to consider whether or not there was anything to be gained from allowing the feelings of discomfort to happen if she was corrected. Misty agreed that this could be an opportunity for self-acceptance and understanding of the demands she placed upon herself to be in command of every situation. The discomfort came more from her personal interpretation of what it meant to be corrected, and from the associated arousal. This opened to door to considering the possibility that the surgeon was actually trying to help her by giving her feedback that, if taken, would enhance her contributions and opportunities for recognition.

Testing Maladaptive Beliefs and Strengthening Functional Beliefs

Based on her responses to the PBQ, Misty's therapist brought up her strong belief in the importance of being admired and feeling special and explored with her the many ways that this belief affected her behavior and her life. One way that she acted on this belief was participating in beauty pageants. To test the idea that admiration and competitive victory made her life happy and worthwhile, Misty was asked to review what the experience of competition was actually like, how long the pleasure of winning lasted, and how adversely the experience of losing affected her overall life. Meaningful schema change began to occur when she acknowledged that competition was actually quite stressful and expensive. Winning made her happy only briefly, and that was because it allowed her to think of herself as a special person. Further, she did not philosophically accept the idea that human worth could be established on the basis of titles or victory in beauty contests.

Further change in this belief was achieved by exploring the childhood origins and messages she had received from her family about how important it was to have status, how her appearance was the special quality that established her worth, and how her value and importance in her family seemed tied to her contribution to the family image rather than her personal presence or relationships with family members.

Misty and her therapist explored the idea of what it would feel like and mean not have status or be special but rather just average or ordinary, and Misty realized that this provoked anxiety and underlying fears of inferiority and worthlessness. By activating this core belief, Misty was better able to understand that she thought she needed to be special because she felt inferior and unimportant without notable distinction. Her therapist suggested that her intense emotional reactions to challenges were signposts that this core belief was being activated. Triggering of this core belief was characterized as a good opportunity to challenge it, and to introduce productive new alternative beliefs. Different beliefs were offered to her for experimentation, as possible alternative sources of self-esteem that had been underdeveloped in her life so far. Because Misty had had little exposure to these ideas, her therapist suggested a menu of options to help her consider the possibilities, drawing from the beliefs (see Table 11.3).

TABLE 11.3. Possible Beliefs for Building Self-Esteem through Sharing and Belonging

"One can be human, like everyone else, and still be special."

"Self-esteem can come from participating and belonging."

"It's good to do some things just to have fun, build relationships, or contribute to others, without regard for recognition."

"I can be ordinary and be happy."

"There are rewards in being a team member."

"Relationships are experiences, not status symbols."

"Other people can be resources, not just competitors."

"Feedback can be valid and useful, even if it's uncomfortable."

"Everyone is special in some way."

"Superiority and inferiority among people are value judgments and thus always subject to change."

"I don't need constant admiration and special status to exist and be happy."

"I can enjoy being like others, rather than always having to be better."

"Status is the measure of my worth only if I believe that to be true."

Misty agreed to test the idea "I don't always have to feel special to be happy." In each session after this, her therapist inquired about evidence that supported this new belief. For example, Misty found that she had a good time out at lunch with her coworkers when she made a point to not seek admiration from them but to focus on their lives instead. Events that challenged the new belief were discussed and reframed. For example, she saw her former boyfriend out on a date with a rising recording artist and became quite upset over the idea that this meant she was worthless, as he had found someone more special. In reframing this incident, she realized that her old beliefs had been automatically triggered. When she systematically considered both advantages and disadvantages of not being involved with him, she agreed that in most ways she was happier without this relationship. Further, the status of his current interest had no reflection on her personal value or importance.

Misty was also intrigued by the idea that one could build self-esteem by doing things for just for fun, to build relationship connections, or to contribute to others without self-advancement as the primary objective. She was not sure how this could be true, but she agreed to try some homework in the interest of having possible new sources of self-esteem. She came up with some creative personal ideas, including driving her grandmother to visit relatives in the area at least one Sunday per month and joining a book discussion group. As she became involved in these experiences, her therapist asked her to rate how much she valued the exchange with others, and how well she could tolerate participating in something "ordinary." Misty noted a fairly high level of enjoyment, something that she did not expect because she did not initially think of these as things worth doing. She was also surprised to think that others might think well of her for these simple things that anyone could do.

MAINTAINING PROGRESS

It is helpful to maintain contact with the narcissistic patient on a consulting basis over time, even if sessions do not occur with great frequency. Such ongoing or follow-up contact can support persistence with functional efforts and adaptive beliefs and note any regression toward self-aggrandizing strategies. Possible challenges or transitions can be anticipated, and it may be helpful to make an individualized summary of useful tools discussed in therapy.

Misty completed 40 sessions of treatment over 1½ years. During the last several sessions, she and her therapist made a list of the changes in her problems over the course of therapy. These included taking concrete steps to realize goals and not to live in dreams concerning her acting, being able to find common ground with the people at work, showing empathy and care for her grandmother by not taking her money and paying attention to her physical health, not taking advantage of the "male ego," and managing her expectations for driving conditions. She gave a 90% endorsement for the belief that she could be happy without necessarily being special or admired, and she felt good about her efforts to be useful to others. She had received an improved evaluation at work, and had retained her driver's license without further citation. She terminated with a favorable attitude toward therapy, agreeing to return if she experienced further mood or interpersonal impairments.

CONCLUSION

The cognitive conceptualization of narcissism holds that distorted core beliefs about personal inferiority lead to self-preoccupation and conditional assumptions about superiority, image, power, merit, and emotion. Narcissistic insults are experienced when circumstances create dissonance with these beliefs and self-esteem is threatened. Active, self-aggrandizing strategies reinforce the compensatory beliefs but impair relationships and functional adjustment. Alternative skills to improve adjustment, relationships, goal attainment, and reinterpret maladaptive beliefs about self and emotion are proposed as a means of developing more resilient and less reactive self-confidence.

CHAPTER 12

Dependent Personality Disorder

Feelings of dependency and attachment are said to be universal, and perhaps defining, mammalian behaviors (Frances, 1988). It clearly is adaptive for individuals to rely upon others to some extent, but excessive amounts of dependency can be quite problematic, and the extreme of dependency has been defined in DSM-IV-TR (American Psychiatric Association, 2000) as dependent personality disorder (DPD). According to DSM-IV-TR, the essential feature of DPD is "a pervasive and excessive need to be taken care of that leads to submissive and clinging behavior and fears of separation, beginning by early adulthood and present in a variety of contexts" (see American Psychiatric Association, 2000, p. 725; Table 12.1). Unwilling to make everyday decisions unless they have an excessive amount of advice and reassurance, dependent individuals typically concur with what other people suggest. They have difficulty initiating projects or doing things on their own, feeling so uncomfortable when alone that they go to great lengths to be with other people. They feel devastated and helpless in response to disapproval or relationship distance and tend to be preoccupied with fears of being abandoned. They tend to subordinate themselves to others and will go to great lengths to get other people to like them. Rejection is so threatening that they will agree with others even if they believe the other person is wrong. These individuals lack self-confidence, tending to discount any of their own abilities and strengths.

Treatment of DPD presents an interesting dilemma to the therapist. Initially in therapy, these patients can seem deceptively simple to treat.

TABLE 12.1. DSM-IV-TR Criteria for Dependent Personality Disorder

A pervasive and excessive need to be taken care of that leads to submissive and clinging behavior and fears of separation, beginning by early adulthood and present in a variety of contexts, as indicated by five (or more) of the following:

(1) has difficulty making everyday decisions without an excessive amount of advice and reassurance from others
(2) needs others to assume responsibility for most major areas of his or her life
(3) has difficulty expressing disagreement with others because of fear of loss of support or approval. Note: Do not include realistic fears of retribution.
(4) has difficulty initiating projects or doing things on his or her own (because of a lack of self-confidence in judgment or abilities rather than a lack of motivation or energy).
(5) goes to excessive lengths to obtain nurturance and support from others, to the point of volunteering to do things that are unpleasant
(6) feels uncomfortable or helpless when alone because of exaggerated fears of being unable to care for himself or herself
(7) urgently seeks another relationship as a source of care and support when a close relationship ends
(8) is unrealistically preoccupied with fears of being left to take care of himself or herself

Note. From American Psychiatric Association (2000, p. 725). Copyright 2000 by the American Psychiatric Association. Reprinted by permission.

They are so attentive and appreciative of the therapist's efforts that they provide a welcome relief in contrast to the many other patients who do not seem to listen to or respect what the therapist has to say. They are easy to engage and are so cooperative at the beginning that they create the expectation of rapid therapy progress. However, this can add to the therapist's frustration in the later stages of treatment, when the patient seems to passively cling, resisting the therapist's efforts to encourage greater autonomy. D. Hill (1970) summarizes some of the frustration of working with these patients. "Invariably each patient has a setback when she realizes that therapy is not a passive experience" (p. 39).

Depression and anxiety are common presenting problems with DPD. Because dependent individuals count on other people for their survival, they are especially prone to separation anxiety and worry over being abandoned and left to fend for themselves. Panic attacks may occur as they anticipate and dread new responsibilities that they do not believe they can handle. Phobias tend to elicit care and protection from others as well as enabling avoidance of responsibilities, providing secondary gains that are fully consonant with their basic dependent orientation (Millon, 1996). Other common presenting problems in individuals with DPD include somatic complaints, ranging from conversion symptoms to hypochondriasis and somatization disorder. Alcoholism and other substance abuse are also common presenting problems.

HISTORICAL PERSPECTIVES

Early descriptions of dependent individuals were often pejorative. In the writings of 19th-century psychiatrists, the passivity, ineffectuality, and excessive docility characteristic of these patients were seen as failures in moral development, and terms such as "shiftless," "weak-willed," and "degenerate" were used. Although frequently observed, the overly dependent personality type was not given its own diagnosis in most early classification systems.

A very different view was taken by early psychoanalytic theorists. Both Freud and Abraham described their "oral–receptive" character as due to either overindulgence or deprivation in the oral or sucking stage of development. Abraham (1924/1927) stated that "some people are dominated by the belief that there will always be some kind person—a representative of the mother, of course—to care for them and to give them everything they need. This optimistic belief condemns them to inactivity . . . they make no kind of effort, and in some cases they even disdain to undertake a bread-winning occupation" (pp. 399–400).

The forerunner to the diagnostic categorization of passive–aggressive and dependent personality types was the World War II category of "immaturity reactions," defined as a "neurotic type reaction to routine military stress, manifested by helplessness or inadequate responses, passiveness, obstructionism or aggressive outbursts" (Anderson, 1966, p. 756). Dependent personality was mentioned only briefly in DSM-I (American Psychiatric Association, 1952) as the passive–dependent subtype of the passive–aggressive disorder, characterized by inappropriate clinging in the face of environmental frustration. The dependent personality was totally overlooked in DSM-II (American Psychiatric Association, 1968), with the closest category being the inadequate personality disorder, characterized by "ineffectual responses to emotional, social, intellectual and physical demands. While the patient seems neither physically nor mentally deficient, he does manifest inadaptability, ineptness, poor judgment, social instability and lack of physical and emotional stamina" (p. 44).

Using the classic polarities of active–passive, pleasure–pain and self–other as a basis, Millon (1969) derived a classification system producing eight basic personality types. The passive–dependent pattern (originally known as the Millon submissive personality) involves seeking pleasure and avoiding pain by looking passively to other people to provide reinforcement. This classification was expanded in several drafts by Millon into dependent personality disorder as it first appeared in DSM-III (American Psychiatric Association, 1980).

The contemporary psychodynamic conceptualization of DPD states that either overindulgence or deprivation can lead to fixation in a psychosexual stage, with excessive and maladaptive dependency result-ing from fixation in the oral-sucking stage of development. In his study of maternal overprotection, Levy (1966) saw this overindulgence as leading to overdependent traits such as demandingness, lack of initiative, and the insistence that others do for them what they felt unable to do for themselves. In some cases, overdependence is seen as representing a re-gressive expression of unsatisfied phallic longings, with the individual hoping that through a dependent attachment she will get the penis she believes is necessary for self-esteem (Esman, 1986). Esman (1986) stresses the prominence of latent and unconscious aggression and hostil-ity toward the dependent individual's primary figures, with cloying sweetness and submissiveness seen as a reaction formation against the expression of hostile feelings that could threaten the existence of what is viewed as a vital relationship.

West and Sheldon (1988) view DPD as a clear example of a disorder of the attachment system, which has been most thoroughly discussed by Bowlby (1969, 1977). The attachment pattern most characteristic of DPD is the "anxiously attached" pattern, which Bowlby views as devel-oping from experiences leading the individual to doubt the attachment figure's availability and responsiveness. When these individuals do estab-lish relationships, they become excessively dependent on attachment fig-ures and live in constant anxiety over losing this attachment figure. Fur-ther work on attachment and dependency by Pilkonis (1988) supports the association between anxious attachment and excessive dependency.

RESEARCH AND EMPIRICAL DATA

Major depression and adjustment disorder were the Axis I diagnoses found to be most frequently associated with DPD by Koenigsberg, Kaplan, Gilmore, and Cooper (1985). Using personality questionnaire criteria, Reich and Noyes (1987) found that 54% of their depressed sub-jects qualified for a diagnosis of DPD. Because they rely excessively on other people for support and nurturance, and feel helpless in the face of potential abandonment, they appear to have an increased predisposition to depression (Birtchnell, 1984; Zuroff & Mongrain, 1987). Overholser, Kabakoff, and Norman (1989) point out that the criteria for DPD con-tain many traits commonly found in depression, including lack of initia-tive, feelings of helplessness, and difficulty making decisions. In empiri-cal studies, Overholser (1992) found that subjects reporting elevated levels of dependency displayed significantly higher levels of depression, loneliness, and self-criticism and significantly lower levels of self-esteem. Dependent subjects have also been found to show a tendency to attrib-ute happiness to external events and to show absolute expectations for the behavior of themselves and others, as well as showing deficits in social skills and problem-solving abilities (Overholser, 1991). They showed lower levels of problem-solving confidence and a tendency to avoid dealing with problems when they occurred. These differences were found despite equivalence across groups in level of intelligence and severity of depression.

Individuals with DPD also often present with anxiety disorders. In their study of panic disorder, Reich, Noyes, and Troughton (1987) found DPD to be the most frequent Axis II diagnosis, especially in the subgroups with phobic avoidance. Depending on the instrument used, roughly 40% of the subjects with some phobic avoidance met criteria for DPD. In a sample of psychiatric inpatients, Overholser et al. (1989) found dependent patients to display Minnesota Multiphasic Personality Inventory (MMPI) profiles suggestive of anxiety, self-doubt, and social insecurity, regardless of their level of depression. Dependent clients in treatment for anxiety disorders showed better response in terms of decreasing avoidance when exposure was structured and directed by the therapist (Chambless, Renneberg, Goldstein, & Gracely, 1992; Turner, 1987).

Somatic complaints are also common among patients with DPD. In a study of 50 women who were classified as passive–dependent and seen as outpatients, D. Hill (1970) found that all the women reported somatic complaints, usually leading to a great deal of attention from family and professionals. Many of these patients looked to medications as their primary source of potential help. Greenberg and Dattore (1981) found that men who developed a physical disorder (cancer, benign tumors, hypertension, or gastrointestinal ulcers) had significantly higher premorbid scores on dependency-related MMPI scales than did men who remained well over a 10-year period. Similarly, Vaillant (1978) and Hinkle (1961) found a relationship between dependent personality traits and a general predisposition to disease. In a more recent review of the empirical literature, Greenberg and Bornstein (1988) conclude that "an individual with a dependent personality orientation is clearly at risk for a variety of physical disorders, rather than being predisposed to exhibit one particular type of symptom" (p. 132). In addition, they conclude that dependent people are more apt to view their problems in somatic rather than psychological terms, are more likely to seek medical help for their problems, will tend to initiate help seeking earlier, and will follow through on treatment more conscientiously than will independent people.

Women receive DPD diagnoses at significantly higher rates than do men (Bornstein, 1996). Outpatients with DPD were found to be more likely to have a family environment distinguished by low expressiveness and high control than outpatients without DPD or normal controls

(Head, Baker, & Williamson, 1991). A study of family environments of nonclinical subjects found that dependent individuals had families that were low in emphasis on independent function, low in cohesion, and high on control (Baker, Capron, & Azorlosa, 1996).

A study by Beck and his colleagues (Beck et al., 2001) examined whether specific sets of dysfunctional beliefs were differentially associated with five of the personality disorders (dependent, avoidant, obsessive–compulsive, narcissistic, and paranoid) as predicted by Beck's cognitive theory. These researchers found that patients with DPD endorsed sets of beliefs theoretically consistent with dependent personality significantly more frequently than did patients with the other personality disorders and patients without a personality disorder diagnosis.

DIFFERENTIAL DIAGNOSIS

When an individual presents for treatment with low self-confidence and a clearly high need for reassurance, the diagnosis of DPD should be considered.

Debbie was a 45-year-old married woman, referred for treatment by her physician for the treatment of panic attacks. During the evaluation, she appeared to be very worried, sensitive, and naive. She was easily overcome with emotion, cried on and off, and was self-critical at every opportunity. For example, when asked how she got along with other people, she reported that "others think I'm dumb and inadequate," although she could give no evidence as to what made her think that. She reported that she did not like school because "I was dumb" and always felt that she was not good enough. She needed a great deal of reassurance from the therapist before she would even attempt to count backwards from 100 by 7's as part of a mental status examination. In addition to the panic attacks and avoidance, she reported being seriously depressed on and off for at least 5 years and having severe premenstrual syndrome. She reported drinking one to three shots of liquor daily, but she did not see that as a problem.

In diagnosing DPD, it is important to go beyond initial presentation and to assess carefully the patient's relationship history, particularly noting how he or she has responded to the ending of relationships and how other people have said that they perceive the patient. It can be helpful to ask carefully about how decisions are made, exploring everyday decisions as well as major ones. Information should also be gathered about how the patient feels about being alone for extended periods. In addition, it can be useful to ask how the patient handles situations when he or she disagrees with someone else or is asked to do something unpleasant or demeaning. The therapist's own reaction can be helpful in alerting him or her to the possibility that a patient may have a DPD. If the therapist feels tempted to rescue the patient, or makes unusual exceptions due to the patient's neediness, further data should be collected to rule DPD in or out.

Debbie stayed in her first marriage for 10 years, even though "It was hell." Her husband had affairs with many other women and was verbally abusive. She tried to leave him many times but gave in to his repeated requests to return. Eventually, she divorced him, and shortly afterwards she met and married her current husband, whom she described as kind, sensitive, and supportive. Debbie stated that she preferred to have others make important decisions and agreed with other people in order to avoid conflict. She worried about being left alone without anyone to take care of her and reported feeling lost without other people's reassurance. She also reported that her feelings were easily hurt, so she worked hard not to do anything that might lead to criticism.

Dependent features can be a part of a variety of disorders, so it is important to be careful to differentiate DPD from other disorders that share some similar features. For example, although patients with either histrionic personality disorder or DPD may appear childlike and clinging, patients with the latter diagnosis are less flamboyant, egocentric, and shallow than those with the former diagnosis. The individual with DPD tends to be passive, submissive, self-effacing, and docile. This contrasts with the actively manipulative, gregarious, charming, and seductive behaviors of the individual with histrionic personality disorder. The individual with avoidant personality disorder has a strong need for affection from others, like the individual with DPD. However, the avoidant strongly doubts and fears that such affection will be attained, whereas the individual with DPD tends to trust and faithfully rely on others, anticipating that such efforts will be rewarded with affection and nurturance. Agoraphobics are dependent on other people, but specifically to avoid being alone in case of panic attacks. Agoraphobics are generally more insistent in asserting their dependence than individuals with DPD, actively demanding that they be accompanied wherever they go. It is possible, however, to meet the criteria for both panic disorder with agoraphobia and DPD, in which case both diagnoses should be given (on Axis I and II, respectively).

Although Debbie sought treatment for her panic attacks and had showed extensive patterns of avoidance over the past 7 years, she acknowledged that many of her problems existed long before the agoraphobia and panic attacks. She did not like doing things alone long before she had a panic attack, and she had been having thoughts such as "I'm no good" since at least the third grade. She clearly met criteria for both DPD and panic disorder with agoraphobia, as well as major depression.

CONCEPTUALIZATION

DPD can be conceptualized as stemming from two key assumptions. First, these individuals see themselves as inherently inadequate and helpless and, therefore, unable to cope with the world on their own. They see the world as a cold, lonely, or even dangerous place that they could not possibly handle alone. Second, they conclude that the solution to the dilemma of being inadequate in a frightening world is to try to find someone who seems able to handle life and who will protect and take care of them. They decide that it is worth giving up responsibility and subordinating their own needs and desires in exchange for being taken care of. This adaptation, of course, carries adverse consequences for the individual. For one thing, by relying on others to handle problems and make decisions, the individual has little opportunity to learn and master the skills needed for autonomy. Some people never learn the skills of independent living (such as assertiveness, problem solving, and decision making), while others do not recognize the skills they have and therefore do not use them, thus perpetuating their dependency. In addition, the idea of becoming more competent can be terrifying, because dependent individuals fear that if they are any less needy they will be abandoned without being equipped to cope on their own.

This arrangement has several additional disadvantages for the dependent person. He or she always has to be very careful to please the other person and avoid conflict for fear of jeopardizing this all-important relationship and being left to fend for him- or herself. Thus, assertion and expressing one's own opinion clearly are out of the question. Also, the individual with DPD may seem so desperate, needy, and clinging that it can be difficult to find a partner who is willing or able to meet his or her needs for any length of time. If the relationship ends, the individual feels totally devastated and sees no alternatives unless he or she can find someone new to depend on.

Debbie reported that she always had an excellent relationship with her father, saying that "I was his little angel child." He got mad at her only once, over a little matter, but otherwise things were always good between them. She described her mother as more domineering and said that they tended to clash a lot, but "I went to her for everything." It was in school that Debbie learned she was "dumb and not good enough." She used to "read backwards" and the teachers sometimes ridiculed her in front of others. She would get physically sick and throw up at school at times and occasionally avoided going to school.

Debbie married young and moved directly from relying on her parents to relying on her husband, without any period during which she lived on her own. She found it difficult to leave her first husband, even though he was abusive and unfaithful to her, and found it devastating to be without him once they actually separated. She found a new relationship soon after the divorce and felt tremendously relieved once she had a partner to take care of her again.

The main cognitive distortion in DPD is dichotomous thinking with respect to independence. Beliefs basic to DPD may include "I can't survive without someone to take care of me"; "I'm too inadequate to handle life on my own"; "If my spouse (parent, etc.) left me, I'd fall apart"; "If I were more independent, I'd be isolated and alone"; and "Independence means being completely on your own." These individuals believe that either they are completely helpless and dependent or they are totally independent and alone, with no gradations in between. They also show dichotomous thinking regarding their abilities: either they do things "right" or they are completely "wrong." Of course, they generally conclude that they are completely wrong, incapable, and a total failure. They also tend to show the cognitive distortion of "catastrophizing," especially when it comes to the loss of a relationship. They go far beyond the normal level of concern that it would be sad and difficult to lose a relationship; they believe that it would be a total disaster and they would completely and permanently fall apart if a relationship should end.

The basic beliefs and cognitive distortions of the DPD lead to automatic thoughts such as "I can't," "I never would be able to do that," and "I'm much too stupid, weak, etc." When asked to do something, they also have thoughts such as "Oh, my spouse could do that much better," and, "I'm sure they don't really expect me to be able to do that."

When asked to do serial 7's during the initial evaluation, Debbie made comments such as "Oh, I'm no good at math, I'll never be able to do that," and, "Is that really necessary? I can just tell you right now that I can't do it." In the first therapy session, when the therapist outlined the plan for treatment, she said, "Oh, I won't be able to record thoughts," and "I'm sure that may help some people, but I'm too dumb to do that."

TREATMENT APPROACH

It is easy to assume that the goal of treatment with DPD is independence. In fact, many dependent patients' worst fear is that therapy will lead to total independence and isolation, with them facing life completely on their own with no aid or support from others. A better word for the goal of therapy with the DPD would be "autonomy." Autonomy has been described as being capable of acting independently of others, yet capable of developing close and intimate relationships (Birtchnell, 1984). To achieve this, it is necessary to help the patient to learn to become gradually more separate from significant others (including the therapist) and to increase his or her self-confidence and sense of self-efficacy. However, given the common fear that competence will lead to abandonment, this must be done gradually and with some delicacy.

Although it may be obvious to the therapist from the beginning that dependence is the major issue for the patient, it is rarely acknowledged by the patient as being part of the presenting problem. In fact, even the use of the words "dependence," "independence," or "autonomy" can frighten the patient early in the treatment if he or she does not feel ready to explore these issues. Regardless of the specific goals of therapy, the issue of dependence will become obvious to both the therapist and the patient as treatment proceeds, but it may be more natural and less frightening to the patient to let the actual use of these terms come first from the patient when he or she is ready to bring them up.

Although specific words such as "dependence" were not explicitly used in the early treatment sessions, Debbie was able to articulate therapy goals, such as "To increase my self-confidence so I can (1) be more outgoing and initiate contacts, (2) initiate projects, (3) take on things at work, (4) be more comfortable around others, and (5) reduce my fear of failure and give myself more credit for what I do."

Collaboration Strategy

Because the individual with DPD comes into treatment looking desperately for someone to solve his or her problems, engaging the patient in treatment may necessitate initially allowing some dependence in the treatment. Collaboration does not need to always be 50-50, and at the beginning of treatment, the therapist may need to do more than half of the work. However, that pattern needs to change throughout the course of therapy, with the patient gradually being asked to provide his or her own agenda items, homework assignments, and so on, so that the treatment eventually becomes more clearly the patient's own. The therapist needs to work consistently throughout treatment to wean the patient gradually away from dependence and toward autonomy.

It is particularly important to use guided discovery and Socratic questioning when working with patients who have a DPD. These patients are likely to look on the therapist as "the expert" and hang on the therapist's every word, and it can be tempting just to tell them exactly what the problem is and what they need to do, thereby taking on an authoritarian role. Unfortunately, this encourages the patient to become dependent on the therapist rather than to develop autonomy. Initially, some active guidance and practical suggestions by the therapist can facilitate treatment engagement. A totally nondirective approach could be too anxiety provoking for these patients to tolerate for long. However, when the patient asks what to do, the therapist needs to be careful to use Socratic questioning and guided discovery and help the patient reach his or her own solutions rather than make direct suggestions.

Debbie seemed to look to her therapist to come up with the answers, especially when it came to understanding and explaining her own feelings. She would walk into sessions saying, "I felt depressed and discouraged last week. Why?" fully expecting her therapist to sit down and explain it all to her without any effort on her part. Instead, the therapist would ask her questions about how she had felt, when her feelings had seemed to change, and details of specific thoughts and feelings she had had when particularly upset. Through this process of questioning, Debbie was able to arrive at her own increased understanding of what had transpired throughout the week and how her feelings were related to her thoughts.

As long as the therapist persists in using guided discovery to help the patient to explore his or her thoughts and feelings, making use of the interactions between the patient and the therapist in the session can lead to interventions with a particularly strong impact due to their immediacy. To use the relationship between the therapist and the patient as an example of an ongoing pattern of dependent relationships, it is necessary to encourage the patient to explore his or her thoughts and feelings about the therapist as well as about other relationships. These patients may be so focused on other relationships in their lives that it may not occur to them that thoughts and feelings about the therapist are important, or even appropriate, to discuss.

At one point, when the therapist was teaching Debbie to pinpoint and examine her automatic thoughts, Debbie arrived clearly upset, apologizing profusely for not having done her homework. The therapist chose to use her current thoughts and feelings as an example of pinpointing automatic thoughts. Debbie reported experiencing high levels of anxiety and guilt, with her primary automatic thought being, "Tom [the therapist] is going to be so disappointed in me." They were then able to examine this thought more objectively, rerating her anxiety and guilt after their discussion. Debbie felt significantly less upset after the discussion. Using her immediate thoughts and feelings about the therapist as a basis for exploring automatic thoughts not only made a powerful demonstration of how useful the process could be in changing feelings but also gave her explicit permission to openly discuss her feelings toward the therapist.

Another important collaboration strategy is for the therapist to monitor his or her own thoughts and feelings toward the patient. The temptation to rescue the DPD patient is particularly strong, and it can be very easy either to accept the patient's belief in his or her own helplessness or to try to rescue the patient out of frustration with slow progress.

Unfortunately, attempts at rescuing the patient are incompatible with the goal of increasing the patient's autonomy and self-sufficiency. When therapists find themselves making exceptions for a patient (e.g., prescribing medications or doing interventions without the usual thorough evaluation), because it seems so urgent and this clearly "pathetic" patient needed immediate help, it is wise for them to assess whether they are simply accepting a dependent patient's view of his or her own helplessness. Whenever a therapist feels tempted to be more directive and less collaborative with a patient, or to make exceptions, it may be useful to write a Dysfunctional Thought Record to clarify whether the exception is going to be in the best long-term interests of the patient or whether it will serve to foster dependency.

Often, Debbie's therapist would ask her what seemed to be a simple question about her thoughts or feelings, and she would respond by saying, "My mind is blank, I just can't think." After having dealt with these reactions many times, he would have strong feelings of frustration and annoyance at her self-deprecation and apparent helplessness. At these times, he became aware of having thoughts like, "Oh, c'mon! You can do this," "This is really simple stuff," "Maybe she really is stupid," and "Oh, stop acting helpless and just do it!" Instead of impatiently lashing out at her, he was able to respond to his thoughts with challenges like, "She really isn't stupid, she's just used to seeing herself that way. It may seem simple to me, but it clearly isn't simple to her. If I act impatient and aggravated with her, I'll just confirm her belief that she is stupid. I need to just slow this down, and help her look at these thoughts and think it through."

At other points in therapy, her therapist would get frustrated at her slow progress. For example, while doing an *in vivo* driving exposure, the therapist waited on the front steps while Debbie drove on her own to and from work. As he waited, he was struck with frustration and pinpointed automatic thoughts such as, "For Pete's sake, look at what we're doing here! All this fuss over driving 1½ miles to work! What's the big deal to driving a car a stupid 1½ miles! Just get in there and do it!" Rather than staying with his frustration, however, he challenged his automatic thoughts with responses such as, "My goals can't be her goals. I can't make her do what I want her to. She needs to move at her own pace. I just need to lower my sights. What is insignificant to me isn't insignificant to her."

It is crucial to set clear limits on the extent of the therapist's professional relationship with the DPD patient. It is our clinical experience that these individuals are more likely than others to report that they have fallen in love with their therapists. Even if it is part of a therapist's usual style, it is safer to minimize physical contact with these patients (even hand shaking, pats on the back, or a casual hug), and it is vital not to bend the usual rules of maintaining a clearly professional relationship. If exposure to anxiety-provoking situations necessitates the therapist being outside the office with the patient, it is important to be explicit about the goals of the exercise, keep it very professional (e.g., take notes of cognitions and write down anxiety levels at regular intervals), and minimize casual conversation. For example, when Debbie was avoiding doing homework that involved driving due to her anxiety, the therapist went driving with Debbie to help her get over this hurdle. However, they discussed the exercise carefully beforehand and planned out a specific route, and he monitored her anxiety levels and cognitions throughout the drive, so that she did not misinterpret this as just "going for a drive with Tom."

If the therapist notices indications that the patient is beginning to feel romantically or personally involved with the therapist, or if the patient expresses these feelings overtly, thoughtful and careful handling of the situation is crucial. If reactions toward the therapist are regularly discussed, it will be easier and more natural to pinpoint and examine these highly sensitive thoughts and feelings. It is important for the therapist to acknowledge the patient's feelings, and explain how these are reactions that commonly occur in therapy. However, it is also crucial for the therapist to explicitly state that despite these feelings, it is not an option for the relationship to change into a more personal, rather than a professional, relationship. The patient is likely to have strong emotional reactions to the process of discussing these feelings, as well as to the setting of clear limits by the therapist, so that the thoughts and feelings of the patient about this issue will need to be pinpointed and discussed throughout the next several sessions, and possibly throughout the rest of treatment.

Specific Interventions

The structured collaborative approach used in cognitive therapy can be used to help encourage the patient to take a more active role in dealing with his or her problems. Even the setting of an agenda can be an exercise in taking more initiative. It is common for the patient with DPD to try to delegate all the power in the therapy to the therapist, for example, by responding to "What do you want to focus on today?" with statements such as "Oh, whatever you want" and "Oh, how am I supposed to know? I'm sure whatever you have in mind is best." In standard cognitive therapy with most patients, the therapist gives the patient the option of suggesting topics for the agenda but provides topics for the session if the patient has nothing particular in mind. However, with patients with DPD, it is important go one step further, explaining that because this is their therapy, they will be expected to make suggestions each session about how they want to spend the time.

With Debbie, the therapist was able to get her to collaborate in agenda setting by taking whatever she said at the beginning of the session and asking if they should discuss it this session. For example, when, at the beginning of one session, Debbie blurted out, "I didn't do anything this week," the therapist said, "Oh, should we include that on our plan for this week and discuss that?" even though she had not originally offered that as an explicit agenda item. Part of the written homework assignment for the week for patients with DPD can include jotting down some ideas for topics for the following session. By making it clear that they are expected to contribute items to the agenda, continuing to ask at the beginning of each session even if they repeatedly offer no suggestions, and waiting until they do offer some suggestions before moving on, the therapist may be able to foster active involvement in the treatment. Because these patients tend to be so eager to please, they generally try to do what is expected of them. Eventually, Debbie brought her own agenda items (e.g., "feeling down" and "problems with daughter") into each session.

Clear, specific goals and progress toward them can be used as powerful evidence to challenge the dependent person's underlying assumption that he or she is helpless. After all, one of the best ways to challenge the belief that one is helpless is to collect concrete evidence of personal competence. With agoraphobia as her main presenting problem, Debbie's goals included the following:

1. Being able to drive
2. Going to the grocery store alone
3. Going to shopping malls alone
4. Sitting any place I want at church

Doing graded exposure to these anxiety-provoking situations provided an excellent challenge to Debbie's belief in her helplessness. When Debbie was able to go to a grocery store alone, do her shopping, and write a check, she was very proud of herself and felt a bit more capable. The patient does not need to be working on an anxiety hierarchy, however, to collect systematic evidence of competence. The accomplishment of any concrete goal will achieve the same purpose. When Debbie was able to complete a sewing project, she had more confidence that she could try things even if they were somewhat challenging. As outlined in Turkat and Carlson's (1984) case example of treatment of an individual with DPD, the therapist and patient can collaboratively develop a hierarchy of increasingly difficult independent actions. For example, a hierarchy of decision making could range from what type of fruit to have for lunch to decisions regarding jobs and places to live. Every decision made can increase the patient's belief that he or she can do at least some things independently.

Regardless of the specific interventions used in therapy, the patient's DPD is likely to impede progress toward his or her goals. At times at which this is occurring, the patient's automatic thoughts can become a productive focus for intervention.

In the second session, when the concept of a hierarchy was introduced, Debbie had difficulty understanding the idea and became very self-critical. She decided that it was much too complicated to rate her anxiety from 0 to 100, so she and the therapist agreed to use a scale from 0 to 10 instead. When the idea of relaxation training was introduced in the third session, she reported thoughts such as "I won't be able to do it," "It's too complicated," and "I'll fail."

In particular, automatic thoughts regarding inadequacy are likely to interfere with trying homework assignments between sessions. Therefore, these thoughts need to be elicited and evaluated very early in treatment. Behavioral experiments in the session can be very useful in challenging some of these ideas.

When the idea of monitoring and challenging automatic thoughts was introduced, Debbie responded with her typical thoughts of "I can't do it." Rather than taking an authoritarian role and just plunging forward anyway, the therapist helped her to write a list of the advantages and disadvantages of doing Dysfunctional Thought Records. As they explored the pros and cons, she reported the thought, "I can't comprehend anything written." The therapist was able to set up a behavioral experiment to challenge this thought by pulling a book out of his bookshelf, opening it to a random page, and asking Debbie to read the first sentence aloud. He then asked her to explain to him what the sentence meant. When she was, in fact, able to do this, they were able to write a convincing rational response to her automatic thought, stating that "It's true that it's hard for me to understand some things that are written, but if I work at it I usually can."

Considering the dependent patient's underestimation of competence, it makes sense to practice new tasks and potential homework assignments in the session before expecting the patient to do it at home alone. For example, with most patients it is possible to demonstrate the first three columns of a Dysfunctional Thought Record and then send the patient home to pinpoint thoughts between sessions. With Debbie, however, it was necessary for her and her therapist to agree to work together on pinpointing thoughts in the session until she felt comfortable trying it on her own. They gradually worked on giving Debbie more responsibility for doing the thought sheets in the office, and it was not until after several sessions of practice that she was actually writing out thoughts and responses during the session and felt ready to begin doing them on her own. Although she denigrated her first attempt to do a Dysfunctional Thought Record on her own at home, it was no worse than many patients' initial efforts (see Figure 12.1). After some suggestions by the therapist, her second attempt at homework was much improved (see Figure 12.2).

When planning interventions, it is not safe to assume that the patient actually has skill deficits even when he or she appears to be quite unable to function effectively in the world. Some patients have many of the skills needed to function independently and successfully but either do not recognize this or fail to use the skills they have. When there is, in fact, a skill deficit, the patient can be trained in such skills as assertion (e.g., Rakos, 1991), problem solving (Hawton & Kirk, 1989), decision making (Turkat & Carlson, 1984), and social interaction (Liberman, De Risis, & Mueser, 1989) in order to increase his or her competence.

Debbie had relied on others for so long that she did have genuine skill deficits; thus, she needed training in a variety of coping skills in addition to help in challenging her negative thoughts about her own abilities. In dealing with her anxiety, she needed thorough training in relaxation skills (e.g., Bernstein & Borkovec, 1976; Bourne, 1995). When discussing differing ways to deal with her husband and daughter, she needed some explicit training in assertiveness. Even in concrete areas of life, her skill level could not be taken for granted. In doing graded exposure to driving situations, it was necessary to do more than just reduce her anxiety. She had for so long been convinced that she was incapable of driving that she had questions about how to make basic driving decisions (e.g., how do you decide when to stop at a yellow light?), and these needed to be addressed in addition to her anxiety.

Situation	Emotion(s)	Automatic thoughts	Rational response
Came into work and panicked	Anxious Stomach churning Shaky	Too many people. Eat slow because of stomach. Calm down. Relax	Don't know how to finish. Stomach upset for 2 hours. Calmed down about 3 o'clock.

FIGURE 12.1. Debbie's initial attempt at using the Dysfunctional Thought Record.

Situation	Emotion(s)	Automatic thoughts	Rational response
Banquet dinner	Anxious Scared Angry Sad 100	People I don't know. 100 I'm going to say something stupid. 100 I hope they don't have soup. 100 Everybody will see me shake if I eat it. 100 I'll make a bad impression and they'll wonder what's wrong with me. 100	I have good qualities even if I'm not the most educated. Most people won't notice me. Some might, some might not.

FIGURE 12.2. Debbie's second attempt at using the Dysfunctional Thought Record.

In addition to training dependent patients in a variety of general coping and problem-solving skills, Overholser (1987) recommends that dependent patients be taught self-control skills such as those originally developed by Rehm (1977) for the treatment of depression. Training in self-control includes three basic components: self-monitoring, self-evaluation, and self-reinforcement. Self-monitoring involves teaching the patient to record the frequency, intensity, and duration of specific behaviors, including the antecedents and consequences of the behaviors. Learning to keep such concrete data can be useful to help the patient see definite changes and improvement, rather than working simply for the therapist's approval. Self-evaluation involves comparing one's observed performance with one's standard for performance. Dependent people (such as Debbie) can have unrealistically high standards for performance or can be so focused on other people's standards that they do not have a clear image of standards for themselves. Training in more appropriate self-evaluation can help dependent patients develop such standards and learn to distinguish when a request for assistance is necessary, not merely a sign of their own uncertainty. Self-reinforcement involves providing appropriate consequences based on one's performance in relation to one's standards. Teaching the dependent individual to reinforce his or her own desirable behavior is probably the most important aspect of self-control, because dependent people tend to rely exclusively on other people to provide all their reinforcement. Initial self-reinforcers may include concrete rewards for desirable behavior (e.g., tokens to be redeemed for a wanted gift, going for a pleasant walk, and reading a chapter of a novel) but also need to include building in positive cognitive reinforcers (e.g., "Hey, I really followed through and did a good job!").

Although the patient with DPD is generally cooperative and eager to please in the beginning of treatment, there may be a problem with following through on homework assignments. This can result from the patient's belief that he or she is not capable of doing the homework or from skill deficits, but it can also occur if the patient becomes frightened by moving too quickly in therapy, advancing too markedly toward his or her goals. If so, it can be useful to list the advantages and disadvantages of changing, seriously exploring the disadvantages of achieving the patient's goals. Often, when first asked about the disadvantages of improving in therapy, the patient will be surprised and insist that it would be completely positive to achieve his or her goals. On careful examination, however, there are disadvantages to making any type of change. Exploring reasons not to change can put the patient in the position of trying to convince the therapist that change is worthwhile, and that can increase motivation to complete homework.

Several months into treatment, Debbie did her first *in vivo* exposure session, which was driving with the therapist in the car. Although the exposure went very well, her anxiety came down as expected, and she was able to drive further than anticipated, she was not sure how she felt at the end of the session and reported "a lot of mixed feelings." It was addressed in the next session as follows:

THERAPIST: Even though the driving *in vivo* went quite well, you had some mixed feelings about it. What are your thoughts about it this week?

DEBBIE: I'm not sure how I feel about last week. I'm so confused. I've even thought about quitting therapy.

THERAPIST: That's a little surprising to me. On the one hand, the driving went well, and your anxiety dropped quickly, but on the other hand you suddenly have thoughts about dropping out of therapy. What do you think is going on here?

DEBBIE: I don't know. Something happened to me last week. Am I fighting it because I know I can do it? Am I afraid I'm going to be independent? I like George [husband] taking care of me.

THERAPIST: This seems pretty important. Help me understand this. Does driving mean that you could become more independent, and that concerns you?

DEBBIE: Maybe.

THERAPIST: What might happen if you became more independent?

DEBBIE: Well, then I could fail.

THERAPIST: What do you mean?

DEBBIE: Independent people do things. And I might fail. I guess if I lean on George, then I can't fail.

THERAPIST: So if you're able to drive that will mean you're more independent, and if that happens you could be more open to failing at some things.

DEBBIE: I think so.

THERAPIST: OK. There's a lot to talk about here, but it helps me to understand what you're going through. It looks a little like your success frightened you because it challenged how you see yourself. Can we spend some time discussing this, to try to understand better what it's all about?

DEBBIE: Yes, I'd like to, because it all seems so confusing to me.

[Later, following exploration of network of cognitions regarding independence . . .]

THERAPIST: OK, to summarize, it looks a little like you weren't quite ready for all the changes greater independence could bring. I'm wondering if it would make some sense to slow things down a bit so you can feel more in control of your change and do it at a pace you can handle.

DEBBIE: You mean we can do that? I'm feeling more comfortable now. I'm starting to relax.

THERAPIST: Can you think of ways to slow your progress to a rate that's more acceptable to you?

Sometimes, an exploration of the advantages and disadvantages of changing will reveal that change really does not seem worthwhile to the patient.

Mary, a housewife in her early 20s, sought treatment for depression. She had always been extremely dependent on her mother and never learned to do things on her own. She rigidly believed that she could not do anything successfully on her own and was therefore terrified to try anything new because of certain miserable failure. She had married her high school sweetheart and was upset when they had to move out of the state due to changes in his job. Following the move, Mary immediately became very depressed. She felt overwhelmed by her expectations of being a wife and helpless to handle her new responsibilities without her mother nearby. She ruminated about her inadequacies and believed everything would be fine again if she could only be back in her hometown.

As treatment progressed, she revealed that if she became less depressed and learned to accept life away from her hometown, she was concerned that her husband would have no incentive to move back. When she acknowledged that her main goal was to convince her husband to move back to her hometown, it became clear why she had been noncompliant in treatment. In fact, her mood did not improve until her husband agreed that they could move back within the year.

Thus, there often are some compelling reasons for the dependent person to be ambivalent about changing. Although the person struggling with helplessness may feel that he or she has no power, taking the helpless role can actually be very powerful and reinforcing (as with Mary), and this role can be difficult to give up. If the patient can identify what would be lost if he or she were less helpless, it may be possible to find a more constructive substitute. For example, Debbie was concerned that her husband would not spend time with her if she did not need him to go shopping with her, so she scheduled a weekly "date" with him. This allowed time with her husband, without needing to be helpless.

The patient's dichotomous view of independence is a crucial area to explore. When the patient believes that one is either totally dependent and helpless or that one is totally independent, isolated, and alone, any movement toward autonomy at all can seem like a commitment to complete and permanent alienation. Drawing a continuum from dependence to independence with the patient can be very useful (Figure 12.3). Small steps toward independence are less frightening when one can see that there are many steps in between the extremes of total dependence and total independence. Another useful illustration is to point out how even independent, well-functioning adults take steps to be sure that assistance

Totally Dependent		Totally Independent
	0 1 2 3 4 5 6 7 8 9 10	
Doesn't do anything alone		Does everything alone
Has someone else make all decisions		Makes her own decisions without considering anyone else
Does whatever she's told		Does whatever she wants
Agrees with what is said		Expresses opinions no matter what anyone thinks
Has someone else always there to handle problems		Handles all problems on her own
Completely helpless		Totally competent
Subservient, docile		Doesn't need anyone
Like a puppy, always acting happy and pleased		Outspoken, aggressive, brash Isolated and alone

FIGURE 12.3. A typical continuum of independence developed jointly with a dependent client.

is available when needed (e.g., by joining automobile clubs); thus, no one needs to be totally independent at all times and it is no disgrace to admit that one might need help from time to time.

Debbie's dichotomous thinking led her to conclude that she was "stupid" or a "dope" whenever she perceived that she was less than perfect (e.g., if she made even a small, simple mistake). Challenging this cognitive distortion through highlighting the double-standard inherent in her approach was very helpful to her. When asked if she would draw the same conclusions if a friend made the same mistake, she was able to see that she was setting totally different standards for herself from those she would see as appropriate for other people. Keeping her dichotomous thinking in mind when setting homework assignments, the therapist specifically assigned her to do imperfect Dysfunctional Thought Records deliberately (e.g., use poor spelling, messy writing, not include all thoughts, and put some items in the wrong column). This was explained to Debbie as an attempt to short-circuit her tendency to begin a task, quit as soon as she saw it as not coming out perfectly, and conclude she is stupid.

At some point in the treatment, dependent patients will need to explore the belief that if they become more competent they will be abandoned. One useful way to challenge this is by setting up specific behavioral experiments in which they behave a bit more competently and observe the reaction of others. This type of assignment involves other people, so it is truly an "experiment" in the sense that neither the patient nor the therapist can be certain what the results will be. Although it may be irrational to believe that one will end up totally abandoned and alone forever if one is assertive, the therapist really does not know if more autonomy will, in fact, lead to abandonment by any particular individual. Without having met Debbie's husband George, her therapist had no way of knowing how he would react to changes in Debbie. Many people are attracted to dependent individuals, so it is possible that a spouse (parent, etc.) will react negatively if the patient begins to change by becoming more assertive and independent. The dependent behavior may be actively reinforced by significant others, and attempts to change may be punished. However, it is also possible that the spouse could react well to these changes, even if the patient feels certain that the spouse will react negatively. By starting with small steps, one can usually observe the spouse's reaction without risking serious or permanent consequences.

Debbie was very concerned about how her husband would react to her increasing independence. His first wife had had an affair and he many times expressed fear that she, too, would have an affair. He seemed to facilitate her dependence in many ways, by accompanying her to stores, offering to do things that she could do by herself, and worrying if he did not know exactly where she was at any time. Although Debbie was concerned about his reactions, she had been doing graded exposure to increasingly anxiety-provoking situations, including going to grocery stores and driving on her own. She tried to stay aware of her husband's reactions and to her surprise she did not perceive anything but positive reactions to her progress. Her therapist had offered to meet with Debbie and her husband for a few conjoint sessions if that seemed necessary, but when Debbie was able to look at the situation objectively, she realized that he could handle her progress and couple sessions would not be necessary.

In cases in which the spouse's reaction to increased assertiveness is, in fact, negative, it may be necessary to explore other options for treatment. Marital or family therapy can often help both spouses adjust to the changes in the identified patient—and sometimes even change together. If, however, either the patient or the spouse is not willing to pursue conjoint treatment, the patient may need to explore the advantages and disadvantages of a variety of options, including maintaining his or her current approach to relationships, modifying assertiveness to be more tolerable to the spouse, and even possibly ending the relationship. Even though the idea of ending the relationship may be very frightening to the patient, it may need to be acknowledged as one of many possible options.

Whether the person decides to stay in the relationship and work toward change, stay in it and accept it as it is, or get out of the relationship, the therapist will eventually need to discuss the possibility that the relationship may end and challenge the patient's catastrophic thinking in regard to the loss of relationships. Even if the patient insists that things are wonderful in the dependent relationship, accidents are always possible, and no one can absolutely count on another person always being there. Of course, the therapist would never try to minimize the grief involved in losing an important relationship. The goal is not to try to convince dependent patients that other people are unimportant but to help them to see that even though it may be very upsetting, they could and would survive the loss of the relationship.

MAINTAINING PROGRESS

It is possible to foster the progression in therapy from dependence to autonomy by changing the structure of therapy itself. Moving from individual to group therapy can help to reduce the patient's dependence on the therapist and serve to dilute the relationship. In a group setting, the patient can still get a great deal of support but can begin to derive more support from peers than from the therapist. This serves as a good first step toward finding more natural means of support for autonomy in the patient's circle of family and friends. Modeling has been found to help increase independent behavior (Goldstein et al., 1973), and in group therapy the other patients can serve as models for the development of many skills. In addition, the group therapy setting provides a relatively safe place to practice new skills, such as assertion.

The termination of therapy may be extremely threatening for the person with a DPD, because he or she may believe it impossible to maintain progress without the therapist's support. Rather than trying to challenge this belief through strictly verbal means, the process of "fading" sessions by scheduling them less frequently can serve as a behavioral experiment to test out this belief. For example, once the patient sees that he or she can function well over 2 weeks instead of 1, monthly sessions can be tried. If the patient is not able to maintain progress over the course of 2 weeks, it is possible that he or she is not yet ready for termination, and it may be appropriate to return to weekly sessions until further problems are resolved. If patients can be given a great deal of control over the spacing of the sessions, this is likely to leave them feeling less threatened and more willing to try some fading, because the choice is not irrevocable. The therapist can fade sessions further and further, offering to meet every month, every 3 months, or even every 6 months. When given this type of free choice, however, patients usually come to realize that if they can go a full month without therapy, they really no longer need to be in treatment.

Another strategy that can make termination easier for the person with a DPD is the offer of booster sessions when necessary. Whenever terminating therapy with a patient, the therapist can explain that if the patient experiences any difficulties in the future, either with issues already discussed or new ones, it is a good idea to recontact the therapist for one or two booster sessions. Such booster sessions get patients "back on track" by encouraging them to resume the interventions that had helped in the past. Simply knowing that they have the option of recontacting the therapist helps to make the transition to termination easier for many patients. Allowing the dependent patient to achieve more autonomy may mean that he or she makes independent decisions, making treatment take a different course than the therapist had anticipated. At times, it may be necessary to let go of the patient to allow him or her to be more independent.

Later in the treatment, Debbie had gone for several sessions where her motivation seemed to be waning and she was not following through on homework assignments. Her thoughts and feelings about the assignments had been discussed at length over a number of sessions. As she came into this session, Debbie said, with great hesitation:

DEBBIE: I don't want to do this anymore.

THERAPIST: Help me understand. I thought you wanted to be able to drive further.

DEBBIE: I do, but not right now. I feel like you're pushing me.

THERAPIST: You almost sound a little angry.

DEBBIE: (*after a pause*) Well, maybe I am. Guilty too.

THERAPIST: Guilty?

DEBBIE: Like maybe I should do more and you'll be upset if I don't.

THERAPIST: What do you want?

DEBBIE: (*adamantly*) I want to work on driving at my own pace.

THERAPIST: Sounds like you're pretty clear about it. What's wrong with that?

DEBBIE: Well, nothing, I guess. But then I wonder if I've made any progress.

THERAPIST: Would you like to spend some time reviewing progress, so we can see what the evidence tells us and what that means for where we go from here?

DEBBIE: Yes. That's a really good idea. I feel relieved already. I thought you were going to be mad at me.

THERAPIST: You felt some pressure to please me?

DEBBIE: Yes, but I guess it was coming from me and not you. [Discussion proceeds to review Debbie's progress. Debbie felt she'd made important progress on seven of her eight goals.] I feel a lot more relaxed now. I didn't realize I'd come so far.

THERAPIST: The evidence would seem to say that you have. So where do you see yourself wanting to go from here?

DEBBIE: I just want to work on the driving by myself. I know that I need to just do it.

THERAPIST: Then would you like to spend some time discussing how you'll do that, and looking at what could get in the way of continued progress? [15 minutes of discussion on Debbie's plan for driving.] OK. So now it looks like you've got a clear plan for how to continue your progress, as well as some ideas for what to do if problems crop up. How's that feel to you?

DEBBIE: Really good. I thought I was going to leave here upset today. But I know this is what I want.

THERAPIST: So you expected that if you were clear on what you wanted with me that it would be a disaster. What did you discover?

DEBBIE: Just the opposite. And that it's OK to decide on what I want.

THERAPIST: And of course you know that if you decide you want more assistance, or show signs of sliding backwards, it would make good sense to call me so we can figure out what the best course of action would be.

CONCLUSION

Although treatment of DPD can be a slow, process, arduous and frustrating at times, it can be rewarding as well. As demonstrated by Turkat and Carlson (1984) in their case study of a patient with DPD, recognition of the disorder, a comprehensive case formulation, and strategic planning of interventions based on this formulation is likely to make the treatment more effective and less frustrating than symptomatic treatment alone. With the proper conceptualization and careful strategic planning throughout treatment, the therapist may have the opportunity to watch the patient blossom into an autonomous adult, providing satisfaction that is remarkably similar to that of watching a child grow up.

CHAPTER 13

Avoidant Personality Disorder

Most people use avoidance at times in their life, especially to relieve anxiety or when faced with difficult life choices or situations. Avoidant personality disorder (APD) is characterized by pervasive behavioral, emotional, and cognitive avoidance, even when personal goals or wishes are foiled by such avoidance. Cognitive themes that fuel avoidance in APD include self-deprecation, beliefs that unpleasant thoughts or emotions are intolerable, and an assumption that exposure of the "real self" to others or assertive self-expression will be met with rejection.

People with APD express a desire for affection, acceptance, and friendship yet frequently have few friends and share little intimacy with anyone. In fact, they may experience difficulty even talking about these themes with the therapist. Their frequent loneliness, sadness, and anxiety in interpersonal relationships are maintained by a fear of rejection, which inhibits the initiation or deepening of relationships.

A typical person with APD believes, "I am socially inept and undesirable," and "Other people are superior to me and will reject or think critically of me if they get to know me." As the therapist elicits thoughts and uncomfortable feelings stemming from these beliefs, patients frequently begin to avoid or "shut down" by changing the topic, standing up and walking around, or reporting that their minds have "gone blank." As therapy proceeds, the therapist may find that this emotional and cognitive avoidance is accompanied by cognitions such as "I can't handle strong feelings, " "You [therapist] will think I'm weak," "Most people don't have feelings like this," and "If I allow myself to experience negative emotion, it will escalate and go on forever." People with APD have a low tolerance for dysphoria both in and out of the therapy session and use a variety of activities including substance abuse to distract themselves from negative cognitions and emotions.

People with APD may initially present in therapy with depression, anxiety disorders, substance abuse, sleep disorders, or stress-related complaints, including psychophysiological disorders. They may be attracted to cognitive therapy because it is a brief therapy and they (erroneously) believe this form of therapy requires little self-disclosure or revelation of personal history.

HISTORICAL PERSPECTIVES

Millon (1969) first coined the term "avoidant personality." Millon's formulation of APD is largely based on social learning theory. He described this personality as consisting of an "active–detached" pattern representing "a fear and mistrust of others."

> These individuals maintain a constant vigil lest their impulses and longing for affection result in a repetition of the pain and anguish they have experienced with others previously. Only by active withdrawal can they protect themselves. Despite desires to relate, they have learned it is best to deny these feelings and keep an interpersonal distance. (Millon, 1981a, p. 61)

A more cognitive perspective can be found in the writings of Karen Horney (1945), who described an "interpersonally avoidant" person more than 40 years before the DSM-III-R (American Psychiatric Association, 1987) formulation: "There is an intolerable strain in associating with people, and solitude becomes primarily a means of avoiding it. . . . There is a general tendency to suppress all feeling, even to deny its existence" (pp. 73–82). In a later book, Horney (1950) wrote a description of such an avoidant person that is consistent with cognitive formulations:

> On little or no provocation he feels that others look down on him, do not take him seriously, do not care for his company, and, in fact, slight him. His self-contempt . . . make[s] him . . . profoundly uncertain about the attitudes of others toward him. Being unable to accept himself as he is, he cannot possibly believe that others, knowing him with all his shortcomings, can accept him in a friendly or appreciative spirit. (p. 134)

Until recent years, little had been written about APD from a cognitive perspective. In this chapter we demonstrate how examination of the automatic thoughts, underlying assumptions, and core beliefs of APD patients can lead to a parsimonious conceptualization that describes the development and maintenance of this disorder. Following this conceptualization, clinical strategies are suggested that can help modify the problematic thoughts and behaviors, as well as the underlying assumptions and core beliefs that maintain the disorder.

RESEARCH AND EMPIRICAL DATA

Most of the published research on cognitive therapy for APD has consisted of uncontrolled clinical reports and single-case-study designs (Beck, Freeman, & Associates, 1990; Gradman, Thompson, & Gallagher-Thompson, 1999; Newman, 1999). There is only one published outcome study that used a cognitive intervention with social skills training (not a full course of cognitive therapy per se) with APD patients. These patients experienced decreased social anxiety and increased social interaction, as did those who received social skills training alone (Stravynski, Marks, & Yule, 1982).

A number of researchers (Heimberg, 1996; Herbert, Hope, & Bellack, 1992) have argued that APD is simply a qualitatively more severe form of generalized social anxiety and studies do demonstrate the effectiveness of cognitive therapy for generalized social phobia, albeit with lower treatment response rates than found for nongeneralized social phobics (Brown, Heimberg, & Juster, 1995; Chambless & Hope, 1996). However, until there is more widespread agreement that these two diagnoses are the same, this research should be considered as only tentative support for the efficacy of cognitive therapy with APD.

Additional outcome studies, using a robust cognitive therapy treatment, are needed. If this therapy is found to be efficacious, a number of other important avenues should be explored. For example, this chapter describes social and cognitive factors that seem relevant in the developmental history of patients with this disorder. Research studies are needed to examine whether these interpersonal experiences and the concomitant beliefs held by patients are a critical part of the development of APD. Determination of etiology can also be an important step toward developing programs to prevent or to identify and treat this disorder in children.

DIFFERENTIAL DIAGNOSIS

Table 13.1 summarizes the DSM-IV-TR criteria (American Psychiatric Association, 2000) for APD. It is apparent that features of this disorder overlap with other diagnostic categories, most notably generalized social

TABLE 13.1. DSM-IV-TR Diagnostic Criteria for Avoidant Personality Disorder

A pervasive pattern of social inhibition, feelings of inadequacy, and hypersensitivity to negative evaluation, beginning by early adulthood and present in a variety of contexts, as indicated by four (or more) of the following:

(1) avoids occupational activities that involve significant interpersonal contact, because of fears of criticism, disapproval, or rejection
(2) is unwilling to get involved with people unless certain of being liked
(3) shows restraint within intimate relationships because of the fear of being shamed or ridiculed
(4) is preoccupied with being criticized or rejected in social situations
(5) is inhibited in new interpersonal situations because of feelings of inadequacy
(6) views self as socially inept, personally unappealing, or inferior to others
(7) is unusually reluctant to take personal risks or to engage in any new activities because they may prove embarrassing

Note. From American Psychiatric Association. (2000, p. 721). Copyright 2000 by the American Psychiatric Association. Reprinted by permission.

phobia; panic disorder with agoraphobia; and dependent, schizoid, and schizotypal personality disorders. To make a differential diagnosis it is important that the therapist inquire about the beliefs and meanings associated with various symptoms as well as the historical course of avoidant patterns.

Social phobia shares many of the features of APD. Most people with social phobia experience social anxiety in a few specific situations (e.g., public speaking or signing checks in public) whereas APD is marked by anxiety across all social situations. In this way, the generalized type of social phobia is similar to APD and when generalized social phobia is diagnosed, an additional diagnosis of APD should be considered.

People with panic and agoraphobia often show similar behavioral and social avoidance to those with APD. However, the reasons for this avoidance are quite different. Avoidance seen in people with panic and agoraphobia is fueled by fears of a panic attack, sensations associated with panic attacks, or distance from a safe place or person who can "rescue" them from personal disaster (physical or mental). Avoidance in APD is fueled by fears of criticism or social rejection in relationships.

Dependent personality disorder and APD are marked by similar self-views ("I am inadequate") but are differentiated by their views of others. Those with Dependent personality disorder see others as strong and able to care for them. Those with APD see others as potentially critical and rejecting. Thus, people with dependent personality disorder seek close relationships and feel comforted by them; people with APD are often fearful of establishing close relationships and feel vulnerable within them.

People with APD are often socially isolated, as are those with schizoid personality disorder and schizotypal personality disorder. The main differences between these personality disorders and APD is that people with APD desire acceptance and close relationships. People diagnosed with schizoid personality disorder or schizotypal personality disorder prefer social isolation. Those with schizoid personality disorder are indifferent to criticism or rejection from others. Those with schizotypal personality disorder may react to negativity from others but more often from paranoia ("What are they up to?") rather than the self-deprecation common to APD.

As mentioned previously, patients with APD often seek treatment for related Axis I disorders. It is important that proper diagnosis of APD be made early in therapy because these Axis I disorders can be treated successfully with standard cognitive therapy methods as long as the therapist includes strategies to overcome the characteristic avoidance that otherwise might cause roadblocks to treatment success.

Somatoform disorders and dissociative disorders may also accompany APD, although less commonly. Somatoform disorders may develop when physical problems provide a reason for social avoidance. Dissociative disorders occur when the cognitive and emotional avoidance patterns of patients are so extreme that they experience a disturbance in identity, memory, or consciousness.

CONCEPTUALIZATION

Patients with APD wish to be closer to other people yet they generally have few social relationships, particularly intimate ones. They are fearful of initiating relationships or of responding to others' attempts to initiate relationships with them, because they are certain they will be rejected and view such rejection as unbearable. Their social avoidance is usually apparent. Less obvious is their cognitive and emotional avoidance, in which they avoid thinking about things that lead to dysphoric feelings. Their low tolerance for dysphoria also leads them to distract themselves behaviorally from their negative cognitions. This section explains social, behavioral, cognitive, and emotional avoidance from a cognitive perspective. A Cognitive Conceptualization Diagram (J. Beck, 1995) provides an example of an APD patient, showing the relationship between her early experiences and the emergence of her negative beliefs and coping strategies—and how these core beliefs, assumptions, and behavioral patterns influence her reaction to current situations (Figure 13.1).

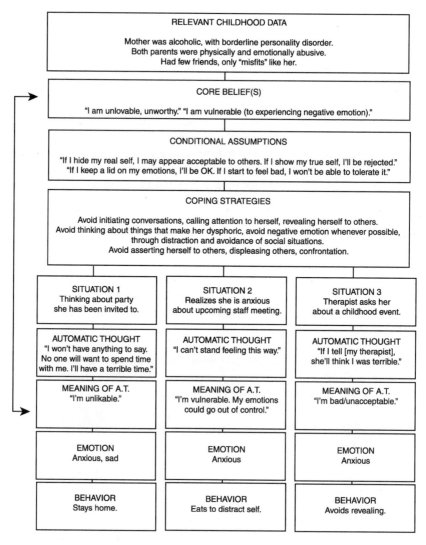

FIGURE 13.1. Cognitive Conceptualization Diagram.

Social Avoidance

Core Beliefs

Avoidant patients have several long-standing dysfunctional beliefs that interfere with social functioning. These beliefs may not be fully articulated but reflect patients' understandings of themselves and others. As children, they may have had a significant person (parent, teacher, sibling, peer) who was highly critical and rejecting of them. They develop certain schemas from interactions with that person, such as "I'm inadequate," "I'm defective," "I'm unlikable," "I'm different," "I don't fit in." They also develop negative beliefs about other people: "People don't care about me," "People will reject me."

Underlying Assumptions

Not all children with critical or rejecting significant others become avoidant. People with APD make certain assumptions to explain negative interactions: "If this person treats me so badly, then I must be a bad person," "If I don't have friends then I must be different or defective," and "If my parents don't like me, how could anyone?"

Fear of Rejection

As children, and later as adults, people with APD make the error of assuming that others will react to them in the same negative fashion as the critical significant person did. They continually fear that others will find them lacking and will reject them. They are afraid they will not be able to bear the dysphoria that they believe will arise from the rejection. Thus they avoid social situations and relationships, sometimes severely limiting their lives, to avoid the pain they expect to feel when someone inevitably (in their judgment) rejects them.

This prediction of rejection causes dysphoria which itself is extremely painful. But the prospect of rejection is even more painful because the avoidant person views others' negative reactions as justified. Rejection is interpreted in a very personal manner, as being caused solely by personal deficiencies: "He rejected me because I'm inadequate," "If she thinks I'm unintelligent [unattractive, etc.], it must be true." These attributions are generated by negative self-beliefs and, in turn, reinforce these dysfunctional beliefs, leading to more feelings of inadequacy and hopelessness. Even positive social interactions do not provide a safe haven from expectations of rejection, "If someone likes me that means he/she doesn't see the real me. As soon as he/she gets to know me, I'll be rejected. It is better for me to withdraw now before that happens." Thus, people with avoidant personality seek to avoid dysphoria by avoiding relationships, both positive and negative ones.

Self-Criticism

Avoidant patients experience a string of self-critical automatic thoughts, both in social situations and when contemplating future encounters. These thoughts produce dysphoria but are rarely evaluated, as patients assume them to be accurate. They arise from the negative beliefs described previously. Typical negative cognitions are "I'm unattractive," "I'm boring," "I'm stupid," "I'm a loser," "I'm pathetic," "I don't fit in."

In addition, both before and during social encounters, people with APD have a stream of automatic thoughts that predicts—in a negative direction—what will happen: "I won't have anything to say," "I'll make a fool of myself," "He won't like me," "She'll criticize me." Patients initially may or may not be fully cognizant of these thoughts. They may primarily be aware of the dysphoria that these thoughts evoke. Even when recognized, cognitions are accepted as valid and are not tested for accuracy. Instead, people with APD actively avoid situations that they believe may engender self-critical cognitions and dysphoria.

Underlying Assumptions about Relationships

Avoidant personality beliefs also give rise to dysfunctional assumptions about relationships. People with APD believe that they are basically unlikable but that if they can hide their true selves, they may be able to deceive others, at least a little or for a while. They believe they cannot let anyone get close enough to discover what they "know" to be true about themselves—that they are inadequate, unlikable, and so on. Typical underlying assumptions are as follows: "I must put on a façade for others to like me," "If others really knew me, they wouldn't like me," "Once they get to know me, they'll see I'm really inferior," and "It's dangerous for people to get too close and to see the real me."

When they do establish relationships, people with APD make assumptions about what they must do to preserve the friendship. They may go overboard to avoid confrontation and may be quite unassertive. Typical assumptions are as follows: "I must please her all the time," "He'll like me only if I do whatever he wants," and "I can't say no." They may feel as if they're constantly on the brink of rejection: "If I make a mistake, he'll change his whole view of me," "If I displease him in any way, he'll end our friendship," and "She'll notice any imperfection in me and reject me."

Misevaluation of Others' Reactions

Avoidant patients have difficulty evaluating others' reactions. They may misread neutral or positive reactions as negative. Like social phobics, some APD patients are likely to focus on their own internal negative thoughts, feelings, and physiological reactions, more than on the facial expressions and body language of those with whom they are interacting. They hope to elicit strongly positive reactions from people whose opinions are irrelevant to their lives, such as store clerks or bus drivers. It is very important to them that no one thinks badly of them, because of the belief: "If anyone judges me negatively, the criticism must be true." It seems dangerous to be in positions in which they can be evaluated, because (their perception of) negative or even neutral reactions from others confirm beliefs they are unlikable or defective. They lack inner criteria with which to judge themselves in a positive manner; instead, they rely solely on their perception of others' judgments.

Discounting Positive Data

Even when faced with evidence, incontrovertible to others, that they are accepted or liked, people with APD discount it. They believe they have deceived the other person or that the other person's judgment is faulty or based on inadequate information. Typical automatic thoughts include: "He thinks I'm smart, but I've just fooled him," "If she really knew me, she wouldn't like me," "He's bound to find out I'm really not very nice."

Case Example

Jane exemplifies someone with APD. Her mother was alcoholic, had borderline personality disorder, and abused Jane verbally and physically. As a child, Jane made sense of her mother's abusive treatment by believing that she (Jane) must be an intrinsically unworthy person to be treated so badly. She could not explain the abuse by accounting for it by her own bad behavior; in fact, she was an extremely well-behaved child who tried desperately to please her mother. Therefore, Jane concluded that her mother treated her so badly because she (Jane) was bad at heart. (She never thought to attribute her mother's behavior to problems within her mother.) As an adult in her late 20s, Jane constantly expected rejection because she believed others would eventually find out she was inherently unworthy and bad.

Jane had a host of automatic thoughts before every social encounter. She was highly self-critical and predicted she would not be accepted. She thought that people would not like her, that they would see she was a loser, and that she would not have anything to say. It was important to Jane that everyone she met should respond to her positively. She became upset if she perceived that someone in even the most fleeting encounter was reacting negatively or neutrally. If a newspaper vendor failed to smile at her or a salesclerk was slightly curt, Jane automatically thought it must be because she (Jane) was somehow unworthy or unlikable. She then felt quite sad. Jane even discounted positive feedback from a friend. She believed she was putting on a façade, and her friend would cut off the relationship as soon as she discovered what Jane was really like. As a result, Jane had few friends and certainly no close ones.

Cognitive, Behavioral, and Emotional Avoidance

In addition to social avoidance, most people with APD also demonstrate cognitive, behavioral, and emotional avoidance. They avoid *thinking* about matters that produce dysphoria and behave in ways that permit them to continue this avoidance. A typical pattern emerges:

1. Avoidant patients become aware of a dysphoric feeling. (They may or may not be fully aware of the thoughts that precede or accompany the emotion.)
2. Their tolerance for dysphoria is low so they do something to distract themselves and feel better. They may discontinue a task or fail to initiate a task they had planned to do. They may turn on the television, pick up something to read, reach for food or a cigarette, get up and walk around, and so forth. In short, they seek a diversion in order to push away uncomfortable thoughts and feelings.
3. This pattern of cognitive and behavioral avoidance is reinforced by a reduction in dysphoria and so it eventually becomes ingrained and automatic.

Patients acknowledge their behavioral avoidance, at least to some extent. They invariably criticize themselves in global, stable terms: "I'm lazy," or "I'm resistant." Such pronouncements reinforce beliefs about being inadequate or defective and lead to hopelessness. Patients do not see avoidance as their way of coping with uncomfortable emotions. They generally are not aware of their cognitive and emotional avoidance until such a pattern is made clear to them.

Attitudes about Dysphoric Moods

Avoidant patients often have dysfunctional attitudes toward dysphoric emotions: "It's bad to feel bad," "I shouldn't have to feel anxious," "I should always feel good," "Other people rarely feel scared or embarrassed or bad." Avoidant patients believe that if they allow themselves to feel dysphoric, they will be engulfed by the feeling and never be able to recover: "If I let my feelings get unbottled, I'll be overwhelmed," "If I start feeling a little bit anxious, I'll go to my worst point," "If I start feeling down, it'll get out of control and I won't be able to function."

Excuses and Rationalizations

Avoidant patients have a strong desire to reach their long-term goal of establishing closer relationships. In this respect, they differ from schizoid patients, for whom a lack of intimacy with others is egosyntonic. Avoid-ant patients feel empty and lonely and want to make closer friends, get a better job, and change their lives. Even when aware of what they must do to realize their desires, though, the short-term cost of experiencing negative emotions seems too high. They make a myriad of excuses for not doing what is necessary to reach their goals. "I won't enjoy doing it," "I'll be too tired," "I'll feel worse [more anxious, bored, etc.] if I do it," "I'll do it later," "I don't feel like doing it now." When "later" co-mes, they invariably use the same excuses, continuing their behavioral avoidance. In addition, avoidant patients may not believe they are capa-ble of reaching their goals. They make certain assumptions: "There's nothing I can do to change my situation," "What's the use of trying? I won't be able to do it anyway," "It's better to lose by default than to try and inevitably fail."

Wishful Thinking

Avoidant patients may engage in wishful thinking about their future. They may believe that one day the perfect relationship or perfect job will effortlessly arise from out of the blue. In fact, they often do not believe they will be able to reach their goals through their own efforts: "One day I'll wake up and everything will be fine," "I can't improve my life by myself," "Things may get better, but it won't be through my own ef-forts."

Case Example

Jane, the patient described earlier, worked at a level below her capabili-ties. She avoided taking the steps that could result in a better position: talking to her boss about a promotion, investigating other job opportu-nities, networking with others. She continually clung to the hope that something would happen to propel her out of her current situation. Atti-tudes such as these pervaded therapy as well. Jane expected the therapist would "cure" her with little or no effort on Jane's part. In fact, Jane be-lieved that the "cure" had to come from the outside, as she was com-pletely ineffectual in making changes herself.

Conceptualization Summary

Avoidant patients hold deep-seated negative beliefs about themselves, others, and unpleasant emotional experiences. These beliefs often stem from childhood interactions with rejecting and critical significant per-son(s). They see themselves as inadequate and worthless, others as criti-cal and rejecting, and dysphoric emotions as overwhelming and intolerable. Socially, they avoid situations in which other people could get close and discover the "real" them. Behaviorally, they avoid tasks that would engender thoughts that make them feel uncomfortable. Cognitively, they avoid thinking about matters that produce dysphoria. Their tolerance for discomfort is quite low, and they rely on distractions whenever they begin to feel anxious, sad, or bored. They are unhappy with their current state but feel incapable of changing through their own efforts.

TREATMENT APPROACH

Collaboration Strategy

Two barriers to collaboration that can be expected with APD patients are their fear of rejection and distrust of others' expressions of caring. They often have a host of negative cognitions about the therapy relationship, just as they do about other relationships. Identifying and testing these dysfunctional thoughts during therapy is essential to forming an active collaborative relationship and can serve as a model for doing so in other relationships.

Even when avoidant patients are aware of automatic thoughts about the therapist or therapy relationship, they are usually unwilling at first to reveal them. They often infer criticism ("You must think I didn't do the homework very well") and disapproval ("You must be disgusted with me when I cry like this"). Avoidant patients may also discount the therapist's direct expression of approval or caring: "You like me only because you're a therapist and you're trained to like everybody," or "You may think that I'm OK now, but if I told you about my relationship with my mother, you'd dislike me."

The therapist can elicit these automatic thoughts when patients display a change of affect ("What is running through your mind right now?"), in the midst of discussions ("Are you predicting what you think I must be feeling or thinking now?"), or toward the end of a session ("Were you aware of making any assumptions about my [the therapist's] thoughts and feelings during our session today? . . . How about when we discussed your difficulty completing this week's assignment?").

Once elicited, automatic thoughts can be evaluated in several ways. Initially, the therapist can tell patients directly what he or she [the therapist] was thinking. It is helpful for patients to rate how much they believe the therapist's feedback (using 0–100% scale) and to monitor changes in their degree of belief as their trust in the therapist grows. After several such direct expressions, patients can be encouraged to evaluate their negative beliefs about the therapy relationship in light of these past experiences with the therapist ("Do you remember how I reacted the last time you didn't complete the assignment?").

Patients can also test out their automatic thoughts by engaging in small experiments. As the following example demonstrates, patients can be asked to describe an experience they are certain the therapist will find unacceptable and to evaluate the validity of this belief in small stages.

Jane felt certain that the therapist would judge her negatively if she revealed how abusively her mother had treated her as a child. This therapy excerpt demonstrates how the therapist worked with Jane's automatic thoughts and then shifted the discussion to identifying and evaluating Jane's assumption about the therapeutic relationship.

JANE: I can't tell you this part.

THERAPIST: You don't have to but I wonder what you are afraid will happen if you do?

JANE: You won't want to see my any more.

THERAPIST: And if you don't tell me, then you think I will?

JANE: Well, it's complicated but I don't want you to know this bad thing about me.

THERAPIST: Can you think of any other possible responses I might have—other than not wanting to see you any more? Is it possible, for example, that what you are afraid to tell me might actually help us understand you better?

[Jane and the therapist explore this for a few minutes. Jane decides, based on history, that the therapist may have a reaction other than rejection, although this is hard for her to imagine. They agree she will test this out by revealing the information in small steps.]

JANE: Well, you see, I had a pretty terrible childhood.

THERAPIST: Oh.

JANE: And my mother . . . Well, she hit me a lot.

THERAPIST: Oh, I'm sorry. Can you tell me a little more about it?

[In small steps, Jane reveals some of the obviously unprovoked physical and emotional abuse she suffered and then bursts into tears.]

JANE: So now you can see how bad I really was. (*Bursts into tears.*)

THERAPIST: I'm confused. You say you were a bad kid? And you *deserved* all that abuse?

JANE: Yes. I must have. Why else would she [mother] have treated me like that?

THERAPIST: Well, I suppose that could be why. On the other hand, I wonder if maybe your *mother* had a serious problem. . . . In any case, even if you were a bad child, why would I want to stop seeing you?

JANE: (*pause*) Well, you wouldn't like me any more.

THERAPIST: Oh, that's interesting. But isn't it possible that knowing about your difficult childhood could make me want to help you even *more*?

JANE: (*softly*) I don't know.

THERAPIST: How could you find out?

JANE: I don't know.

THERAPIST: You could ask me.

JANE: (*tentatively*) Do you want to stop seeing me?

THERAPIST: No, of course not! In fact, the opposite! I'm so glad you trusted me enough to tell me about what happened to you. Now it's starting to be more understandable why you see yourself so negatively. . . . Now, how much do you believe that?

JANE: I'm not sure . . . Maybe 50-50?

THERAPIST: That's pretty good. Maybe we can work on this a little bit each session, until you are more certain that I understand and want to help. Would that be okay?

JANE: OK.

In this example and the dialogue that continued, the therapist was able to help Jane recognize that even though she viewed herself as bad and likely to be rejected, her therapist did not share this view. The therapist was able to persuade her to reveal her past abuse in small parts and to directly test her fears of rejection. Doing so in therapy served as a model when Jane later agreed to do the same with her closest friend— and provided yet another opportunity to find out that her fears of rejection were unfounded. Indeed, her revelations increased her friend's sense of intimacy and caring toward Jane.

Because avoidant patients are reluctant to say things that they believe may lead the therapist to think badly of them, it is important for the therapist occasionally to ask directly whether a patient has been afraid to reveal something. Unless patients with APD do express these suppressed topics, they may continue to believe that the therapist would reject them (or at the very least, view them negatively) if this piece of information were known. The therapist might say, for example, "You know sometimes patients are reluctant to tell me certain things because they predict they'll feel too upset or that I'll react negatively to it. Do you ever sense that maybe there is something you're holding back? You don't have to tell me what it is, if you don't want, but it would help me to know if there is something you haven't said."

Avoidant patients often assume that once they establish a relationship, they must continually try to please the other person. They believe that if they assert their own desires the other person is bound to sever the relationship. In therapy, this can lead to extreme compliance and unwillingness to give the therapist negative feedback.

One way to encourage patient assertiveness in therapy is the use of a therapist feedback form at the end of the session. Patients can rate the therapist on a checklist of qualities including process (e.g., "The therapist listened well and seemed to understand me today") and content (e.g., "The therapist explained the homework clearly enough"). In the next session the therapist can review the ratings and discuss relatively low ratings. By taking a nondefensive stance and discussing possible changes in session content and process, the therapist can reward patients for assertive criticism, correct legitimate dissatisfactions, and demonstrate the change potential of relationships. Later, patients can be encouraged to give more direct verbal feedback. Experiments can be designed for practicing assertiveness within other relationships. Role-playing assignments and guided-imagery practice are very helpful prior to *in vivo* assertiveness.

Specific Interventions

Standard cognitive therapy approaches (Beck, Rush, Shaw, & Emery, 1979; J. Beck, 1995; Greenberger & Padesky, 1995; Padesky, 1995; Salkovskis, 1996) can be used with APD patients to help them manage depression, anxiety disorders, substance abuse, and other Axis I problems. Guided discovery using standard cognitive-behavioral methods for testing automatic thoughts and underlying assumptions can help them begin to counter self-criticism, negative predictions, maladaptive assumptions, and misevaluations of others' reactions. Special techniques, outlined below, can help APD patients overcome the cognitive and emotional avoidance that otherwise may hamper these standard approaches.

Overcoming Cognitive and Emotional Avoidance

Although patients with APD experience a range of dysphoric moods, it is not desirable simply to teach them to eliminate depression and anxiety. One of the complications that can interfere with standard cognitive therapy treatment is that these patients avoid thinking about things that cause unpleasant emotions. They also, as described earlier, have many negative assumptions about experiencing negative emotions. Because cognitive therapy *requires* a patient to experience such emotions and to record the thoughts and images accompanying various emotional experiences, this cognitive and emotional avoidance can prove a serious impediment to treatment.

Avoidant patients not only avoid experiencing negative emotions between sessions (e.g., they often fail to start or complete therapy assignments) but also avoid feeling dysphoric during therapy sessions (e.g., they may fail to report negative thoughts or change the subject). It is desirable to diagram the process of avoidance so that patients can examine how the avoidance operates and how they can intervene to stop it. Figure 13.2 illustrates a typical example; patients should be encouraged to discover similar patterns on a daily basis. It is helpful, when applicable, to reframe patients' notions of themselves as "lazy" or "resistant" (qualities that are more trait-like and can seem more difficult to modify). Rather, in evaluating themselves in light of the diagram, they can see that they avoid situations in which they have automatic thoughts that engender unpleasant emotions. Together therapist and patient can evaluate these negative cognitions and increase the patient's tolerance for dysphoria.

Before embarking on the process of increasing such tolerance, it is helpful to provide a rationale. Through guided discovery, patients can confirm the disadvantages of avoidance, such as the improbability of their reaching their goals and the likelihood that positive emotions, like negative emotions, will not be fully experienced. If applicable, the therapist and patient can explore the origin of the avoidance of dysphoria. Often such avoidance was initiated in childhood, when a patient may indeed have been more vulnerable and less able to cope with unpleasant or painful feelings.

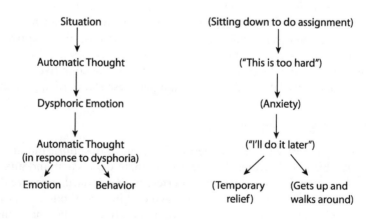

FIGURE 13.2. Avoidance pattern diagram.

One of the best ways to begin increasing emotional tolerance is to evoke emotions in the session by discussing experiences about which patients report discomfort. As they begin to react strongly, some cognitive avoidance may be initiated (e.g., patients may change the topic, get up and walk around, or experience their minds "going blank"). The therapist can direct them back to the feelings in order to begin to identify and test the beliefs leading to the avoidance. A therapy excerpt illustrates this process.

JANE: *(in the middle of an imagery exercise)* I don't want to talk about this anymore.

THERAPIST: What are you feeling right now?

JANE: Depressed . . . and scared—real scared.

THERAPIST: What do you think will happen if you keep feeling this way?

JANE: I'll freak out—go crazy. You'll see just what a basket case I am.

THERAPIST: As we've discussed before, these feelings you avoid may lead to some useful information. Try staying with them for now. Continue imagining yourself in the restaurant with your friend. Tell me what happens. *(long pause)*

JANE: *(sobbing)* He's going to be angry with me. I'm a rotten person for making him so unhappy.

In this portion of the session, the therapist helped the patient become aware of and "stay with" her distressing thoughts and images. At the same time, she was able to test out her belief that she would "go crazy" and get out of control if she allowed herself to experience strong emotions. The therapist reminded her of this prediction and allowed the patient time to reflect on how she did experience strong emotions but never really got "out of control."

Repeated experiences such as this one may be necessary to build tolerance for dysphoria and erode patients' dysfunctional beliefs about experiencing uncomfortable emotions. To desensitize patients, a hierarchy may be constructed that outlines increasingly painful topics to discuss in therapy. The therapist can elicit patients' predictions of what they fear will happen before they discuss each succeeding topic, test out the predictions, and accumulate evidence to contradict their faulty beliefs (e.g., "It'll be too painful to discuss," "If I start feeling bad, the feeling will never end," etc.). Patients can also construct hierarchies for assignments outside therapy to increase tolerance for negative emotions. Such assignments can be labeled "emotional tolerance practice" or "overcoming avoidance." They may involve initiating certain behaviors ("Work on your thesis for 30 minutes without a break") or structured reflection

("Think about telling your boss you want more time off"). Again, it is helpful for patients to predict what they fear will happen if they engage in an assigned activity, and to test out and modify these ideas.

Avoidant patients often have difficulty identifying automatic thoughts for homework (or even in the therapy session itself). Usually, asking patients in the session to imagine and minutely describe a situation as if it were happening right then helps identify thoughts. A second technique, if applicable, involves role play. Patients play themselves, and the therapist takes on the part of the other person involved in a specific situation. While reenacting an upsetting situation, patients are instructed to capture their automatic thoughts. If these more standard techniques are unsuccessful, the therapist can compile a checklist of hypothesized thoughts, based on a specific patient's previously identified thoughts and beliefs and on the case conceptualization. Patients can be instructed to review the checklist to see if any of these thoughts occurred in the situation. They can also use the checklist to identify cognitions while still in a distressing situation.

For patients able to identify their thoughts but who fail to do homework assignments, it may be useful to plan and rehearse homework using imagery, as in the following example:

THERAPIST: We've agreed that you're going ask your boss to leave work early on Friday. I'd like you to take a minute to imagine yourself a few minutes before you walk into his office and see if there's anything that might get in the way of your doing that.

JANE: (*pause*) OK. I'm in my office and I think, "I'll go later."

THERAPIST: And how are you going to answer that thought?

JANE: I don't know. I probably won't answer that. I'll probably just not go.

THERAPIST: Will not going help you fulfill your goal of leaving early for your trip?

JANE: No.

THERAPIST: What could you do or say to make it more likely that you will ask him?

JANE: I could read the card we wrote today that reminds me that every time I avoid I strengthen my old habits, and every time I follow through with my plans, I strengthen my new, better habits.

THERAPIST: OK. Imagine yourself picking up the card. What happens next?

[Jane continues describing process of gaining the courage to meet with her boss and specific interfering automatic thoughts. Together they devise responses to each thought to support action rather than avoidance.]

If necessary, the therapist can employ a point–counterpoint approach at this time. First, patients argue with their "emotional" voice why they do not have to undertake the assignment, while the therapist answers with (and models) an "antiavoidance" voice. Then they switch roles so the patients have practice using the antiavoidance responses. Finally, patients may write down their predicted automatic thoughts on index cards, with the antiavoidance responses in their own words on the back. They may read these cards daily—especially before undertaking an assignment that they are likely to avoid.

The experiences in and between therapy sessions such as those described earlier will aid patients in identifying dysphoric thoughts and tolerating negative feelings. As such tolerance grows, they may begin to change in the way they relate to family members (e.g., they may become more assertive). They also may experience more intense sadness, fear, or anger as they bring into awareness memories and reactions they have avoided for so many years. At this point, it is helpful to teach them cognitive and behavioral approaches to manage these moods.

The therapist can point out that even though the patient now understands the importance of negative feelings and is willing to tolerate them, it is not necessary or desirable to experience intense feelings all the time. Patients can be instructed to keep diaries of feelings and thoughts when they occur, and then to use automatic thought records to test out the "hot thoughts" most closely connected to their feelings (cf. Greenberger & Padesky, 1995). If they have not yet learned cognitive restructuring methods, they can use distraction after writing the thoughts and feelings and can then bring the diary to therapy for assistance in testing out thoughts.

At this point, it may also be helpful to do couple or family therapy if the patient is in a relationship or living with parents. Therapy sessions can provide a safe forum for patients to test the validity of relevant beliefs and thoughts. One patient, for example, feared that her husband had been angry with her for some time because she did not work outside the house. In one of their couple's sessions, the therapist encouraged her to ask if this was true. In the course of the session, her husband denied this yet revealed other situations that did distress him. These difficulties were then resolved through joint problem solving.

Couple or family therapy may also be indicated when avoidant patterns are supported by the patient's social system. For example, the husband of another patient had his own negative assumptions about the expression of emotion ("Expressing feelings leads to conflict and irreparable harm"). Therapy with the family can help deal with dysfunctional assumptions held by family members and can provide a forum for teaching constructive skills for communication and problem solving (e.g., Beck, 1988; Dattilio & Padesky, 1990).

Skill Building

Sometimes patients with APD have skill deficits because of impoverished social experiences. In these cases, skill-training exercises should be included in the therapy, so the patient has a reasonable chance of success in social interactions designed to test beliefs. For some, social skills training will begin with nonverbal cues (e.g., eye contact, posture, and smiling.) Patients can practice in therapy sessions, at home, and then in low-risk social situations. Patients with meager social experience may need educational information to evaluate experiences more accurately (e.g., "If you wait until the last minute on weekends to make plans, most people will already be busy"). More advanced social skills training may include instruction regarding conversational methods, assertiveness, sexuality, and conflict management.

Patients' negative beliefs about themselves may create obstacles to trying out newly developed skills. They may need to be encouraged to act "as if" they possessed a certain quality. For example, one patient had the thought "I won't be able to make small talk at the party. I'm not confident enough." The patient was encouraged to act as if she were confident; indeed, she discovered that she could appropriately engage in conversation. During behavioral skills training, it is critical to elicit automatic thoughts, especially ones in which patients disqualify their progress or the training itself: "These exercises are teaching me to fool people so they don't see my inadequacy," "Only a real loser has to learn how to talk at this age." Therapist and patient can then work together to test the validity and utility of these beliefs.

Identifying and Testing Maladaptive Beliefs

A major portion of the therapy involves helping patients identify and test the cognitive underpinnings of avoidant patterns. To do this, therapist and patient first gain an understanding of the developmental roots of the negative beliefs, paying particular attention to how these beliefs might have been helpful at some earlier time in the patient's life. Next, alternative new beliefs can be identified (Mooney & Padesky, 2000; Padesky, 1994) that the patient wishes were true (e.g., "I'm likable," "Other people will be understanding if I make a mistake."). Old and new beliefs are tested through experiments, guided observation, and role-play reenactments of early schema-related incidents. Finally, patients are directed to begin to notice and remember data about themselves and their social experiences that support the new, more desirable beliefs. A case example illustrates these points.

At age 24, Jane had little dating experience and only one friend. After several months of therapy in which she learned to do cognitive restructuring, gained basic skills, and even succeeded in beginning a steady relationship with a man she met at work, Jane still strongly held the belief "I'm unlikable." The therapist and Jane agreed to focus on testing the validity of this belief, as it seemed to be the core theme of her negative automatic thoughts. First, the therapist and Jane reviewed the developmental origins of this belief. She had believed she was unlikable as long as she could remember, and her abusive mother underscored this conclusion by frequently yelling, "You're so bad! I wish you were never born!"

One powerful method that can be used when a patient recalls such vivid childhood scenes is psychodrama. First, Jane played herself, and the therapist acted as her mother. Jane was asked to reexperience her childhood feelings as if she was 6 years old and then to describe the experience to the therapist. Next, Jane was asked to act as the mother, and the therapist played the part of the 6-year-old Jane. Again, Jane reported her emotional and cognitive experience.

In this case, Jane was able to empathize with her mother and recognize how unhappy and bad her mother felt when her father abandoned her. For the first time, Jane realized her mother was feeling terrible about herself yet blamed Jane, an easy target. Once Jane had better understanding of the whole situation, she was able to speculate that she might not have been quite so unlikable as her mother implied.

A third psychodrama allowed Jane to "try on" this new viewpoint. The therapist and Jane first discussed how a healthier mother would have handled the loss of her husband. Next, they discussed how almost any child in Jane's situation might have drawn negative, invalid conclusions about herself. After planning responses Jane could make to her mother, Jane role-played 6-year-old Jane again; however, this time she assertively defended herself:

MOTHER: [played by the therapist] You're no good! I wish you were never born! The only reason your father left us was that he didn't want you.

JANE: Don't say that, Mommy. Why are you so angry?

MOTHER: I'm angry because you're such a bad child!

JANE: What did I do that was so bad?

MOTHER: Everything. You're a burden. You're too much to take care of. Your father didn't want you around.

JANE: I'm sad Daddy left. Are you sad, too?

MOTHER: Yes. Yes, I am. I don't know how we're going to get by.

JANE: I wish you didn't get so mad at me. I'm only a kid. I wish you would get mad at Daddy, instead. He's the one who left. I'm the one who's staying with you.

MOTHER: I know. I know. It wasn't really your fault. Daddy isn't living up to his responsibilities.

JANE: I'm really sorry, Mommy. I wish you didn't feel so bad. Then maybe you wouldn't yell at me so much.

MOTHER: I guess I do yell at you because I'm unhappy.

Once Jane understood that her mother's harsh treatment stemmed from her mother's personal unhappiness, rather than representing valid judgments of young Jane she was able to consider that perhaps her belief that she was totally unlikable warranted closer examination. At this point, Jane and her therapist began a historical test of her belief (Padesky, 1994; Young, 1984). Using one page for every few years of her life, Jane and the therapist gathered historical evidence for and against the proposition Jane was totally unlikable. Jane predicted that if this belief were true, there would be few items in the "evidence against" column and an increasing number of facts in the "evidence for" column as she grew older.

In fact, Jane discovered that evidence for her likability was greater than she had realized (e.g., she had a best friend in elementary school, people at work were friendly toward her, her housemate often invited her to do things, and her cousins seemed very happy every time they saw Jane or spoke to her by phone). Also, the balance tipped toward likability after Jane had left home and begun therapy. She began to understand how her self-imposed isolation led to few opportunities for people to know her.

A historical review of a negative core belief does not remove the power of a core belief, even with evidence such as in Jane's case. Because Jane had lived her entire life interpreting (and misinterpreting) experiences to support her belief, she had no positive belief to replace the "unlikable" belief. Another important part of therapy, therefore, involved helping Jane construct and validate a more positive belief: "I am okay."

Some helpful techniques at this stage of therapy were prediction logs, positive-experience logs, and imagery rehearsal of new behaviors. In prediction logs, Jane recorded her expectations for different social experiences (e.g., "I'll try to talk to three people at the party tomorrow night but no one will want to talk to me") and actual outcomes ("Two people were really friendly and one was okay"). Keeping track of what actually happened in many situations over time helped Jane see that her negative core belief did not predict her current experiences well at all.

In addition, Jane kept a list of social interactions that supported the new belief. This positive experience log required Jane to shift her attention from rejection experiences to ones involving acceptance or social enjoyment. When she became self-critical, and the negative core belief was activated, she reviewed this log to help reactivate the more positive core belief.

Finally, as Jane began changing her beliefs about her likability, she became willing to enter more social situations (e.g., enrolling in a photography course and making a special effort to talk to classmates each week, inviting coworkers to lunch, and arranging a party for her roommate's birthday). She prepared for these new experiences through imagery rehearsal with her therapist. In imagery, she concretely imagined the experiences and reported to the therapist any difficulties or embarrassment encountered. They then discussed possible solutions to these social dilemmas, and Jane rehearsed the desired behavior and conversations in imagery before *in vivo* practice.

Treatment Summary

Treatment of APD patients involves the establishment of a trusting therapy alliance fostered by the identification and modification of patients' dysfunctional thoughts and beliefs regarding this relationship, especially expectations of rejection. The therapy relationship serves as a laboratory for testing beliefs prior to the APD patient testing out beliefs in other relationships. It also provides a safe environment to try out new behaviors (e.g., assertiveness). Mood management techniques are employed to teach patients to manage their depression, anxiety, or other disorders.

The goal is not to eliminate dysphoria altogether but to increase patients' tolerance for negative emotion. A schematic diagram to illustrate the process of avoidance and a strong rationale for increasing tolerance of emotions help patients agree to experience negative feelings in the session—a strategy that may be implemented in hierarchical fashion. Tolerance of negative affect within sessions may have to precede "emotion tolerance" or "antiavoidance" practice outside therapy. An important key to increasing tolerance is the continual testing of beliefs concerning what patients fear will happen if they experience dysphoria.

Couple or family therapy may be indicated, as well as social skills training. Finally, treatment also encompasses the identification and modification of maladaptive core beliefs through interventions involving imagery, psychodrama, historical review, and prediction logs. More positive beliefs may have to be constructed and validated through a variety of techniques, such as positive-experience diaries described previously.

Therapist Reactions

Some therapists may experience considerable frustration with patients with APD because progress is usually quite slow. In fact, it can be a challenge to keep avoidant patients in therapy as they may begin to avoid therapy, too, by canceling appointments. It is helpful for therapists to realize that patients' avoidance of behavioral assignments, or of therapy itself, provides an opportunity to uncover the automatic thoughts and attitudes associated with avoidance.

If such avoidance is present, the therapist (and patients, too) may begin to feel hopeless about therapy. It is important to anticipate and to undermine hopelessness by focusing on progress made in sessions. A functional way to deal with avoidance of homework assignments is to focus on the thoughts that interfered with undertaking or completing a task, to help patients test out and answer those thoughts in the future.

Typical therapist cognitions about the avoidant patient may include the following: "The patient isn't trying." "She won't let me help her." "If I try really hard, she'll drop out of therapy anyway." "Our lack of progress reflects poorly on me." "Another therapist would do better." The therapist thinking these types of thoughts may begin to feel helpless, unable to assist the patient in effecting significant change. When these beliefs occur, the therapist can test them by reviewing what has transpired in therapy. It is important to keep realistic expectations for progress and to recognize achievement of small goals.

Finally, therapists need to distinguish between real obstacles and patients' rationalizations for avoidance. Jane, for example, claimed she could not go to her aunt and uncle's anniversary party because she could get lost and because she did not want them to have to pay for her dinner. She also rationalized that they would not miss her anyway. After evaluating her specious reasoning in therapy, Jane realized that her aunt and uncle probably did want her to come—they had always acted warmly toward her, had invited her to many family functions in the past, and made an effort to spend one-on-one time with her. After this discussion, Jane was willing to make the trip. It is likely that therapists who fail to confront avoidant patients' excuses will feel hopeless and helpless, as their patients do.

MAINTAINING PROGRESS

The final phase of therapy involves developing a plan to maintain progress as patients with APD can easily become avoidant again. Progress maintenance involves work in both the behavioral and cognitive realms. Ongoing behavior goals often include activities such as the following: establishing new friendships; deepening existing relationships; taking on more responsibility at work (or change jobs); expressing opinions and acting in an appropriately assertive way with others; tackling previously avoided tasks at work, school, or home; trying new experiences; taking a class; pursuing a new hobby; volunteering; and so on.

These goals may feel risky to the patient. If thinking about them engenders distress, the anxiety can be framed in a positive way. Emergence of anxiety signals the reactivation of dysfunctional attitudes that could derail the patient from achieving personally important goals. Thus, anxiety is used as a spur to look for automatic thoughts and underlying assumptions that interfere with the ability to achieve goals. The patient can review what helped in therapy to devise a system to recognize and respond to these negative cognitions and attitudes after therapy is terminated.

It is important for patients to attenuate their residual dysfunctional attitudes, and to strengthen their new, more functional beliefs. On a daily or weekly basis, they should review the evidence against the old beliefs and the evidence supporting the new ones. One way to achieve this goal is to encourage patients to keep a daily log in which they record their experiences, both positive and negative, during the period when these beliefs are active. They then develop arguments to undermine the dysfunctional belief and to strengthen the functional belief.

Two typical entries in Jane's log were as follows:

9/27—Two people from work invited me to go with them to hear some blues at a club. I talked to them and they seemed fine about my being there with them. This is evidence against my old belief and evidence for my belief that I'm okay.

10/1—My roommate seemed disappointed when I said I didn't want to go out to dinner. I felt bad and thought, "I shouldn't have said that." According to my old belief, I would consider myself bad—I'm bad if I make others feel bad. According to my new belief, I'm not bad. It's inevitable that other people will get disappointed sometimes, and it has nothing to do with my worth as a person. It's not good to always put others first. It's good to assert my desires, too.

It is particularly important for patients to remain viligant of situations they are avoiding and to become aware of cognitions that foster the avoidance. They can use either the kind of log described above or a thought record to uncover dysfunctional attitudes behind the desire for avoidance and to develop or strengthen more functional attitudes. One of Jane's typical avoidance entries was as follows:

10/24—Thinking about asking boss for time off. Feeling very anxious. A.T. [automatic thought]: "He'll get mad at me." Dysfunctional attitude: "It's terrible for people to get mad. Functional attitude: It's OK if he gets mad. He may not even get mad, but if he does, he won't be mad forever. This is good practice for me to act assertively. I'll never get what I want if I let my attitude get in the way. The worst that will happen is he'll say no.

A belief that is particularly troublesome for the avoidant patient is, "If people really knew me, they'd reject me." This belief is likely to be activated as patients begin to develop new relationships and to reveal more of themselves to others. If relevant, it is often helpful for patients to review their initial fears of revealing themselves to their therapist and how they think about this now. They can experiment with others by disclosing a relatively "safe" but previously unrevealed statement about themselves and examining what transpires. They can continue to do so in a hierarchical fashion, gradually disclosing more about themselves to others.

In addition to daily belief logs and thought records, daily or weekly review of specially prepared index cards is also helpful. Patients record a troublesome belief on one side of a card, with evidence against it beneath. On the other side is the more functional attitude with supportive evidence. Patients can rate their degree of belief in each attitude on a regular basis. A significantly increased degree of belief for a dysfunctional attitude or a significantly decreased degree of belief for a new attitude indicates that patients need to work in that area.

Toward the end of therapy, the therapist should assess the benefits of spacing out sessions. Avoidant patients often need encouragement to reduce the frequency of therapy sessions, taking more time to engage in new experiences between sessions and to test out their fears. On the other hand, some avoidant patients may desire and feel prepared to terminate, but may fear hurting the therapist's feelings by making such a suggestion.

Finally, it is helpful for therapists and avoidant patients jointly to develop a plan for the patients to continue therapy on their own when formal therapy is terminated. Patients might, for example, set aside at least a few minutes each week to do activities aimed at continuing the progress made in therapy. During this time they can review self-assigned homework progress, examine any situations they avoided, investigate obstacles, look ahead to the coming week predicting which situations may be troublesome, and devise a way to deal with likely avoidance. They can review relevant notes or thought records from therapy. And, finally, they can self-assign homework and schedule their next self-therapy session.

An important goal of progress maintenance is to predict likely difficulties in the period following termination. Once predicted, patients can be encouraged and guided to devise a plan to handle these troublesome situations. Patients may find it useful, for example, to compose paragraphs to address the following difficulties:

What can I do if I find myself starting to avoid again?

What can I do if I start believing my old beliefs more than my new
beliefs?
What can I do if I have a setback?

Review of these paragraphs at relevant times can help maintain progress.

CONCLUSION

A cognitive formulation for APD is parsimonious and there are clinical
reports and single-case-design studies suggesting that cognitive therapy
can be efficacious. If cognitive therapy continues to be demonstrated as
effective in controlled outcome studies, further research to determine
which dysfunctional attitudes are most central to the maintenance of
APD could help strengthen and streamline the therapy. The conceptualization provided here suggests cognitive themes that are likely topics for
such research.

CHAPTER 14

Obsessive–Compulsive Personality Disorder

If it's worth doing, it's worth doing well.

A stitch in time saves nine.

A place for everything, and everything in its place.

The obsessive–compulsive personality style is common in contemporary Western culture, particularly among males (American Psychiatric Association, 2000). This may be partially due to the high value that society places on certain characteristics of this style. These qualities include attention to detail, self-discipline, emotional control, perseverance, reliability, and politeness. However, some individuals possess these qualities in such an extreme form that they lead to either functional impairment or subjective distress. Thus, the individual who develops obsessive–compulsive personality disorder (OCPD) becomes rigid, perfectionistic, dogmatic, ruminative, moralistic, inflexible, indecisive, and emotionally and cognitively blocked.

The most common presenting problem of persons with OCPD is some form of anxiety. Compulsives' perfectionism, rigidity, and rule-governed behavior predispose them to the chronic anxiety that is characteristic of generalized anxiety disorder. Many compulsives ruminate about whether they are performing well enough or doing the wrong thing, which often leads to the indecisiveness and procrastination that are frequent presenting complaints. The chronic anxiety may intensify to the point of panic disorder if these individuals find themselves in a severe conflict between their compulsiveness and external pressures. For example, if a compulsive individual is approaching the deadline for a project but is progressing very slowly due to perfectionism, his or her anxiety may escalate. The compulsive then may catastrophize about his or her physical symptoms, such as rapid heartbeat and shortness of breath. This may lead to the vicious cycle often seen in patients with panic disorder, in which worry leads to increased physical symptoms, which lead to further increased worry, and so on.

Individuals with OCPD also suffer from specific obsessions and compulsions more than average. Rasmussen and Tsuang (1986) found that 55% of a sample of 44 individuals with obsessive or compulsive symptoms also had OCPD.

Another common presenting problem in OCPD is depression. This may take the form of dysthymic disorder or unipolar major depressive episode. Compulsives often lead rather flat, boring, unsatisfying lives and suffer from chronic mild depression. Some will become aware of this over time, although they may not understand why it is occurring and will come to therapy complaining of anhedonia, boredom, lack of energy, and not enjoying life as much as others appear to. Sometimes they will be pushed into therapy by spouses who view them as depressed and depressing. Due to their rigidity, perfectionism, and strong need to be in control of themselves, their emotions, and their environment, compulsives are very vulnerable to becoming overwhelmed, hopeless, and depressed. This may happen when they experience their lives as having gotten out of control and their usual coping mechanisms as being ineffective.

Compulsives often experience a variety of psychosomatic disorders. They are predisposed to developing such problems because of the physical effects of their chronically heightened arousal and anxiety. They frequently suffer from tension headaches, backaches, constipation, and ulcers. They may also have Type A personalities and thus are at increased risk for cardiovascular problems, particularly if they are frequently angry and hostile. Patients with these disorders are often referred to psychotherapy by physicians, because compulsives usually view these disorders as having physical causes. Getting them to understand and work on the psychological aspects of these problems can be quite difficult.

Some patients with OCPD present with sexual disorders. The compulsive's discomfort with emotion, lack of spontaneity, overcontrol, and rigidity is not conducive to a free and comfortable expression of his or her sexuality. Common sexual dysfunctions experienced by the compulsive are inhibited sexual desire, inability to have an orgasm, premature ejaculation, and dyspareunia.

Finally, compulsives may come to therapy due to problems other people are having in coping with them. Spouses may initiate couple therapy because of their discomfort with the compulsive's lack of emotional availability or workaholic behavior resulting in little time spent with the family. Families with a compulsive parent may come for therapy due to the rigid, strict style of parenting, which can lead to chronic fighting between the parent and children. Employers may send compulsive employees to therapy because of their continual procrastination or their inability to function effectively in interpersonal relationships on the job.

HISTORICAL PERSPECTIVES

The obsessive–compulsive personality has been one of the primary areas of interest in the mental health field since the early 20th century. Freud (1908/1989) and some of the other early psychoanalysts (Abraham, 1921/1953; Jones, 1918/1961) were the first to develop an explicit theory and form of treatment for these individuals. Some confusion developed around the terms "obsession" and "compulsion," because they were used by the early analysts to refer both to specific symptomatic, pathological behaviors and to a type of personality disorder. Both the Axis I diagnosis of obsessive–compulsive disorder and the personality disorder, OCPD, were hypothesized to have originated during the anal stage of development (ages 1–3) due to inappropriate toilet training.

Sullivan (1956) wrote about OCPD from the perspective of interpersonal psychoanalysis, a theory he developed. Sullivan thought that the primary problem in individuals with OCPD was their extremely low level of self-esteem. He hypothesized that this occurred when a child grew up in a home environment in which there was much anger and hatred, which were hidden behind superficial love and "niceness." Because of this, Sullivan hypothesized that compulsives learned "verbal magic," where words are used to disguise or excuse the true state of affairs. An example of this would be, "This spanking will hurt me more than it will hurt you." His view was that compulsives learn to rely primarily on words and external rules to guide their behavior. He theorized that they do not tend to develop emotional and interpersonal skills and usually avoid intimacy because of their fear of letting others know them.

More recently, Millon (1996; Millon, Davis, Millon, Escovar, & Meagher, 2000) has written about OCPD from the perspective of his biopsychosocial–evolutionary theory. Millon has stated that the compulsive style is well suited to the demands of developed societies. He identifies the "pure compulsive" as well as a number of variants of the compulsive personality, ranging from the relatively normal to the more pathological. Millon sees the compulsive personality as one of two interpersonally conflicted styles whose fundamental struggle is between obedience and defiance.

According to Beck's model (e.g., Beck, Rush, Shaw, & Emery, 1979), cognitive theory "is based on the underlying theoretical rationale that an individual's affect and behavior are largely determined by the way in which he structures the world. His cognitions . . . are based on attitudes or assumptions . . . developed from previous experiences" (p. 3).

David Shapiro was the first theorist to write extensively about OCPD from a primarily cognitive point of view. Shapiro, who was trained as a psychoanalyst, developed his concepts out of his dissatisfaction with the psychoanalytic theory of personality disorders. Shapiro delineated the structure and characteristics of a number of what he referred to as "neurotic styles." Shapiro (1965) wrote that a person's "general style of thinking may be considered a matrix from which the various traits, symptoms, and defense mechanisms crystallize" (p. 2).

Shapiro, although not presenting a comprehensive theory of OCPD, discussed what he saw as three of its primary characteristics. The first characteristic was a rigid, intense, sharply focused style of thinking. Shapiro found compulsives to have a "stimulus-bound" quality to their cognition, comparable in certain ways to that of brain-damaged people. By this, he meant that they are continually attentive and concentrating and rarely seem to just let their attention wander. Thus, they tend to be good at detailed, technical tasks, but are poor at discerning more global, impressionistic qualities of things, such as the tone of a social gathering. Shapiro referred to compulsives as having "active inattention." They are easily distracted and disturbed by new information or external events outside their narrow range of focus, and they actively attempt to keep this distraction from occurring. As another consequence of this, they are rarely surprised.

The second characteristic Shapiro discussed is the distortion in the obsessive–compulsive's sense of autonomy. Unlike normal self-direction based on volition and choice, the compulsive deliberately and purposefully self-directs each action. Thus, the compulsive exerts a continuous willful pressure and direction on himself as if by an "overseer" and even exerts "an effort to direct his own wants and emotions at will" (Shapiro, 1965, pp. 36–37). The fundamental aspect of the compulsive's experience is the thought, "I should." Compulsives experience any relaxation of deliberateness or purposeful activity as improper and unsafe. They invoke morality, logic, social custom, propriety, family rules, and past behavior in similar situations to establish what the "should" is in a given situation, and then act accordingly.

The final characteristic identified by Shapiro was the obsessive–compulsive's loss of reality or sense of conviction about the world. Because compulsives are cut off from their wants, preferences, and feelings to a large degree, their decisions, actions, and beliefs tend to be held much more tenuously than those of most people. This leads to alternations between doubt and dogmatism, which Shapiro saw as reciprocal attempts to deal with this conflict.

Guidano and Liotti (1983) have also written about OCPD from a cognitive perspective. Their position is that perfectionism, the need for certainty, and a strong belief in the existence of an absolutely correct solution for human problems are the maladaptive components underlying both OCPD and the ritualistic behavior of obsessive–compulsive disorder. They theorized that these beliefs lead to excessive doubting, procrastinating, overconcern for detail, and uncertainty in making decisions. Guidano and Liotti have found, as did Sullivan (1956) and Angyal (1965), that compulsives have usually grown up in homes in which they are given mixed, contradictory messages by at least one of their parents.

RESEARCH AND EMPIRICAL DATA

There has been little definitive research on OCPD. To date, most of the knowledge about this disorder has been derived from clinical work. However, there is considerable evidence that OCPD does exist as a separate entity. Several factor-analytic studies have found that the various traits hypothesized to comprise OCPD do tend to occur together (A. Hill, 1976; Lazare, Klerman, & Armor, 1966; Torgerson, 1980). However, there is little evidence that OCPD stems from inadequate toilet training, as psychoanalytic theory proposes (Pollock, 1979). Adams (1973), in working with obsessive children, did find that the children's parents had a number of obsessive traits, including being strict and controlling, overconforming, unempathic, and disapproving of spontaneous expression of affect. It has not yet been determined what percentage of children with obsessive–compulsive personality traits develops into adults with OCPD.

There has been some research into the genetic and physiological bases of OCPD. A study by Clifford, Murray, and Fulker (1984), found a significantly higher correlation of compulsive traits, as measured by the trait scale of the Layton Obsessive Inventory, in a sample of monozygotic twins than in a sample of dizygotic twins. In another study, Smokler and Shevrin (1979) examined compulsive and histrionic personality styles in relation to brain hemiphericity as reflected by lateral eye movements. The authors found that the compulsive subjects looked predominantly to the right when responding to experimental tasks, which they interpreted as showing a higher degree of left-hemisphere activation, while the histrionic subjects looked predominantly to the left. Because the left hemisphere has been associated with language, analytic thinking, and reason, it was expected to be predominant in compulsive subjects. The right hemisphere has been associated with imagery and synthetic thinking.

In a recent study, Beck and his colleagues (Beck et al., 2001) investigated whether dysfunctional beliefs discriminated among personality disorders, including OCPD. In their study, a large number of psychiatric outpatients (mean age 34.73 years) completed the Personality Belief Questionnaire (PBQ) at intake and were evaluated for personality disorders using a standardized clinical interview. The subjects also completed the Structured Clinical Interview for DSM-IV (SCID-II; First, Spitzer, Gibbons, & Williams, 1995) Self Report Questionnaire. Their findings showed that patients with OCPD (as well as patients with avoidant, dependent, narcissistic, and paranoid personality disorders) preferentially endorsed PBQ beliefs theoretically linked to their specific disorders. Beck et al. (2001) interpreted their results as supporting the cognitive theory of personality disorders.

Although many clinicians report success in treating OCPD with cognitive therapy (e.g., Beck, Freeman, & Associates, 1990; Freeman, Pretzer, Fleming, & Simon, 1990; Pretzer & Hampl, 1994), the definitive outcome research has not yet been conducted. However, there have been a few recent studies that tend to support the use of cognitive interventions with compulsive traits and OCPD.

Hardy and his colleagues (Hardy, Barkham, Shapiro, Stiles, Rees, & Reynolds, 1995) examined the impact of Cluster C personality disorders on outcomes of contrasting brief psychotherapies for depression. Twenty-seven of their 114 depressed patients obtained a DSM-III diagnosis of Cluster C personality disorder, that is, obsessive–compulsive, avoidant, or dependent personality disorder, whereas the remaining 87 did not. All patients completed either 8 or 16 sessions of cognitive-behavioral or psychodynamic–interpersonal psychotherapy. On most measures, personality-disordered patients began with more severe symptomatology than patients without personality disorders. Among those who received psychodynamic–interpersonal therapy, personality-disordered patients maintained this difference posttreatment and at 1-year follow-up. Among those who received cognitive-behavioral therapy, posttreatment differences between those with and without personality disorders were not significant. The length of treatment did not influence these results. It should be noted, however, that Barber and Muenz (1996) found that individuals with compulsive personality did better with interpersonal psychodynamic therapy than with cognitive therapy.

In a study comparing cognitive therapy to medication, Black, Monahan, Wesner, Gabel, and Bowers (1996) examined abnormal personality traits in patients with panic disorder. Cognitive therapy was associated with a significant reduction in abnormal personality traits, as measured by the Personality Diagnostic Questionnaire—Revised (Hyler & Reider, 1987). This was true for compulsive, as well as for schizotypal, narcissistic, and borderline personalities.

McKay, Neziroglu, Todaro, and Yaryura-Tobias (1996) examined changes in personality disorders following behavior therapy for obsessive–compulsive disorder (OCD). Twenty-one adults who were diagnosed with OCD participated. At pretest, the mean number of personality disorders was approximately four, whereas the posttest number was approximately three. Their analyses suggest that this change, although apparently small, was clinically relevant, because change in number of personality disorders was significantly related to treatment outcome. Although treatment was successful in reducing OCD symptoms, obsessive–compulsive personality was more resistant to change.

DIFFERENTIAL DIAGNOSIS

Table 14.1 presents the DSM-IV-TR diagnostic criteria for OCPD. Assessment and diagnosis of OCPD are not usually difficult if the clinician is aware of and watchful for its various manifestations. At the first telephone contact with the compulsive, the therapist may detect signs of ri-

---

TABLE 14.1. DSM-IV-TR Diagnostic Criteria for Obsessive–Compulsive Personality Disorder

A pervasive pattern of preoccupation with orderliness, perfectionism, and mental and interpersonal control, at the expense of flexibility, openness, and efficiency, beginning by early adulthood and present in a variety of contexts, as indicated by four (or more) of the following:
(1) is preoccupied with details, rules, lists, order, organization, or schedules to the extent that the major point of the activity is lost
(2) shows perfectionism that interferes with task completion (e.g., is unable to complete a project because his or her overly strict standards are not met)
(3) is excessively devoted to work and productivity to the exclusion of leisure activities and friendships (not accounted for by obvious economic necessity)
(4) is overconscientious, scrupulous, and inflexible about matters of morality, ethics, or values (not accounted for by cultural or religious identification)
(5) is unable to discard worn-out or worthless objects even when they have no sentimental value
(6) is reluctant to delegate tasks or to work with others unless they submit to exactly his or her way of doing things
(7) adopts a miserly spending style toward both self and others; money is viewed as something to be hoarded for future catastrophes
(8) shows rigidity and stubbornness

Note. From American Psychiatric Association (2000, p. 279). Copyright 2000 by the American Psychiatric Association. Reprinted by permission.

gidity or indecisiveness in arranging the first appointment. Indecisiveness in the compulsive will be based on the fear of making a mistake rather than the fear of displeasing or inconveniencing the therapist, as might be seen in a patient with dependent personality disorder.

Upon first meeting, the clinician may notice that the compulsive patient is rather stilted and formal and not particularly warm or expressive. In trying to express themselves correctly, compulsives often ruminate a great deal about a topic, making sure that they tell the therapist all the details and consider all the options. Conversely, they may speak in a slow, hesitating manner, which is also due to their anxiety about not expressing themselves correctly. The content of the compulsive's speech will consist much more of facts and ideas rather than of feelings and preferences. In obtaining historical and current life information, possible indicators of OCPD include the following:

1. The patient was raised in the rigid, controlling type of family discussed earlier.
2. The patient lacks close, self-disclosing interpersonal relationships.
3. The patient is in a technical, detail-oriented profession such as accounting, law, or engineering.
4. The patient either lacks many leisure activities or has leisure activities that are purposeful and goal-directed and not merely pursued for enjoyment.

Formal psychological testing may be helpful at times in diagnosing OCPD. The Millon Clinical Multiaxial Inventory (Millon, Davis, & Millon, 1996) was specifically designed to diagnose personality disorders and is often useful in understanding the various manifestations of OCPD. Typical responses on projective tests are a large number of small-detail responses on the Rorschach, and long, detailed, moralistic stories on the Thematic Apperception Test. The therapist will need to consider whether the time and money spent on projective tests are worthwhile, because an accurate diagnosis and understanding of the patient can probably be obtained without them.

The simplest and most economical way to diagnose OCPD is usually just to ask patients directly, in a straightforward, noncritical manner, whether the various DSM-IV-TR criteria apply to them. Most compulsives will quite readily admit to such criteria as not feeling comfortable expressing affection, being perfectionistic, and having difficulty throwing old things away. However, they might not understand the connection between such characteristics and their presenting problems for therapy.

OCPD has a number of elements in common with other Axis I and II disorders that may need to be ruled out for accurate diagnosis (American Psychiatric Association, 2000). The difference between OCPD and OCD is relatively easy to determine. Only OCD has true egodystonic obsessions and compulsions, whereas OCPD does not. However, if diagnostic criteria are met for both disorders, both diagnoses should be made.

OCPD and narcissistic personality disorder (NPD) tend to share perfectionism and the belief that other people cannot do things as well as they can. An important difference is that individuals with OCPD are self-critical, whereas those with NPD think they have achieved perfection. Both individuals with NPD and antisocial personality disorder lack generosity but will indulge themselves. However, individuals with OCPD are stingy with themselves as well as others. OCPD shares with schizotypal personality disorder an apparent formality and social detachment. In SPD, this results from a fundamental lack of capacity for intimacy, whereas in OCPD, this results from discomfort with emotions and excessive devotion to work.

On occasion, OCPD may also need to be differentiated from personality change due to a general medical condition, such as the effect of a disease process upon the central nervous system. OCPD symptoms may also need to be differentiated from symptoms that may have developed in association with chronic drug use (e.g., cocaine-related disorder not otherwise specified).

CONCEPTUALIZATION

The conceptualization of OCPD used in this chapter integrates the views given above and follows Freeman et al. (1990) and Pretzer and Hampl (1994). The driving schemas are considered to be: "I must avoid mistakes at all costs," "There is one right path/answer/behavior in each situation," "Mistakes are intolerable." Most of the problematic aspects of OCPD are seen here as resulting from the strategies these patients use to avoid mistakes: "I must be careful and thorough;" "I must pay attention to details;" "I must notice mistakes immediately so they can be corrected"; and "To make a mistake is to deserve criticism. The goal of compulsive individuals is to eliminate mistakes, not merely to minimize them. This results in a desire for total control over themselves and their environment.

An important characteristic distortion of these individuals is dichotomous thinking. This is shown in the belief, "Any departure from what is right is automatically wrong." Beyond the many intrapersonal problems described previously, such beliefs lead to interpersonal problems because relationships often involve strong emotions and do not have unambiguously correct answers. Relationships are also problematic because they threaten to distract these individuals from work and thus to promote mistakes. The compulsives' solution is to avoid both the emotions and the ambiguous situations.

Another prominent cognitive distortion in OCPD is magical thinking: "One can prevent disasters/mistakes by worrying about them." If the perfect course of action is unclear, it is better to do nothing. Therefore, compulsive patients tend to avoid mistakes of commission but not omission. They tend to catastrophize changing their approach to life, believing that nothing except their compulsivity stands between them and sloth or promiscuity.

The following composite case study will be used to demonstrate various aspects of the cognitive approach to OCPD.

Mr. S was a 45-year-old white engineer who was married, with a school-age son. He came for cognitive therapy after a recent exacerbation of a chronic and severe muscular pain in his back, neck, and shoulders. Mr. S had suffered from this condition since his late 20s. Because he originally considered his pain to be a physical problem, Mr. S sought treatment from physical therapists, chiropractors, and massage therapists and he took various muscle relaxants and anti-inflammatory medications. These treatments helped somewhat, but Mr. S had a severe episode of pain in his late 30s when he had to miss 3 weeks of work. At that time he was working on an important and complicated project. He then began seriously considering that his neck and back pain might be related to the degree of psychological stress that he was experiencing.

Mr. S had been born in a medium-size city in the United States and was raised in a conservative, religious, middle-class family. He was the younger of two children, with a sister 7 years older. Mr. S described his father as being a nice, somewhat anxious man with whom Mr. S had a good but not very close relationship. He was much closer to his mother and stated that he was always concerned about her opinion of him. His mother was very involved with Mr. S when he was a child. He liked the attention but also experienced her as being a critical, judgmental woman who had many rules about the way that people are supposed to behave. Mr. S remembered one particular incident, when he was in first grade, in which a friend had gotten a citizenship award and he had not. Although she did not explicitly state it, he got the impression that his mother was dissatisfied with him and was thinking, "Your friend earned an award, so why can't you?"

Mr. S reported feeling reasonably happy during his childhood. By sixth grade, however, he started becoming concerned about his grades and popularity. In school, he coped with this by either working very hard to do well (while always worrying that he was not doing well enough) or else by procrastinating and trying not to think about what he was supposed to be doing. Socially, he became introverted, avoidant, and emotionally constricted. By being less involved and expressive, the less chance it seemed to him that he had of being criticized or rejected. These patterns of behavior gradually increased throughout his adolescence.

During his second year of college, Mr. S experienced a great deal of anxiety over his inability to perform academically up to his expectations. It became harder to complete written assignments, because he was concerned that they would not be good enough. In addition, Mr. S felt very lonely and isolated due to his being away from home and his inability to develop friendships or romantic relationships. He became increasingly pessimistic about himself and his future. This culminated in a major depressive episode, during which he lost interest in most activities and spent the majority of his time sleeping. This episode lasted a couple of months and led to Mr. S dropping out of school and joining the army. The increased structure and companionship in the army were helpful, and he functioned well for the 3 years he was in the service. He then returned to school and obtained his engineering degree.

Mr. S had worked as an engineer since his late 20s and had been moderately successful in his career. At the time he sought treatment, he was performing some administrative and supervisory duties, which were less comfortable for him than the more structured, technical, detail-oriented engineering work on which he spent most of his time.

Mr. S was never comfortable or very successful with dating. In his early 30s, he was reintroduced to a woman he had met briefly several years before. She remembered him—which surprised and flattered him—and they started dating. They married 1 year later, and 2 years after that had a child. Mr. S described the marriage as being good but not as close as he would like. He felt emotionally and sexually restrained with his wife, and he realized this was part of his problem. Mr. S did not have any close friends but was marginally involved with various church and civic groups.

The cognitive therapist can begin to form a conceptualization of Mr. S using this information. A number of themes emerge, suggesting possible schemas. Mr. S repeatedly expresses a sense of his own inadequacy. This is shown in his description of the interaction with his mother when he was in first grade. His sense of himself as inadequate in comparison to others is suggested by his lifelong pattern of avoidance and isolation. He states that the less involved and expressive he is, the less chance he has of being criticized or rejected. This leads to another theme in Mr. S's history. He seems to have a strong expectation of criticism by others, from his mother and his childhood peers to his current supervisor. Mr. S's strong sense of inadequacy and expectation of criticism seem to stem from his perfectionism. He worries about making mistakes even when his performance is fine, and he can never believe that he is doing well enough. This can be seen as early as grade school and continuing into his current job. Because Mr. S. shows a number of characteristics of OCPD, the therapist will keep the possibility of this disorder in mind as treatment continues. Additional information will influence the therapist's emerging cognitive conceptualization of Mr. S.

TREATMENT APPROACH

In addition to teaching patients the cognitive theory of emotion, it is important at the beginning of cognitive therapy to establish therapeutic goals. These obviously relate to the presenting problems and may, for the compulsive, include such things as "getting assignments or work done on time," "reducing the frequency of tension headaches," or "being able to have orgasms." It is important to be specific in listing goals; general goals such as "not being depressed" are harder to work with. If the patient is mainly concerned with depression, it is necessary to break that down into its various aspects, such as not being able to get up in the morning or not being able to accomplish anything, to be able to work effectively with the depression.

After goals have been established that the patient and therapist agree are relevant and workable, the goals are ranked in the order they are to be worked on, as it is difficult and often nonproductive to try to work on them all at once. Two criteria to use in ranking the goals are the importance of each problem and how easily solvable it is. It is often helpful to have rapid success early in therapy to heighten the patient's motivation and belief in the therapeutic process. After the problem areas have been established, it is important to identify the automatic thoughts and schemas that are associated with them.

Early in the course of cognitive therapy, it is vital to introduce the patient to the idea that feelings and behaviors are based on the perceptions of, thoughts about, and meanings given to life events. The cognitive model can be demonstrated by watching for an affective shift in the session and then asking the patient what he or she had been thinking just before. Another way to demonstrate this would be to describe a situation such as waiting for a friend who is late and listing the various emotions that the person waiting may be experiencing, such as anger, anxiety, or depression, and relating these feelings to thoughts that were probably producing them: "How dare he make me wait for him," "Maybe he was in an accident," or "This just proves that nobody likes me."

Generally, the problem being worked on is monitored each week between sessions, usually on a Dysfunctional Thought Record (Beck et al., 1979). The Dysfunctional Thought Record allows patients to list what the situation is, how they are feeling, and what their thoughts are when the problem occurs. Thus, a compulsive working on procrastination might become aware that when he or she is doing a task at work, he is feeling anxious, and thinking, "I don't want to do this assignment because I won't be able to do it perfectly." After a number of similar examples of automatic thoughts have been gathered, it becomes apparent to the compulsive that much of the anxiety and procrastination is due to perfectionism. It is then crucial to determine the assumptions or schemas underlying the various automatic thoughts. In the example of perfectionism, the underlying assumption may be, "I must avoid mistakes to be worthwhile." It is often helpful at this point to assist the patient in understanding how he or she learned the schema. Usually it developed out of interactions with parents or other significant figures, although sometimes the schemas are based more on cultural norms or developed in more idiosyncratic ways. Therapy then consists of helping the compulsive patient to identify and understand the negative consequences of these assumptions or schemas and then to develop ways of refuting them so that they no longer control the patients' feelings and behavior and lead to the problems that brought him or her to therapy.

Mr. S's goal in therapy was to eliminate, or at least greatly diminish, the pain he experienced in his back and neck. Unlike many psychosomatic patients, he had already come to accept that psychological factors played a major part in his pain. The therapist discussed the cognitive model with Mr. S, and Mr. S. was quite receptive to it. The homework assignment for the first few weeks was to monitor his pain on the Weekly Activity Schedule. This consisted of ranking the severity of his pain from 1 to 10 on an hour-by-hour basis while also noting what he was doing. At first, Mr. S noticed that the pain was most severe in the evening, when he was home with his family. This was difficult for him to understand, as usually he enjoyed his evenings at home and found them relaxing. Through data gathering, Mr. S realized that he distracted himself from the pain as it was building during the day. At times, distraction is a useful technique for compulsives, particularly with their nonproductive, ruminative thinking. In Mr.S' case, however, distraction interfered with the assessment of the problem. As he became more aware of his pain, he noticed that it would start as a type of tingling, sunburn-like feeling and then progress from mild to a more severe pain. Under prolonged stress, the muscles in his back and neck would spasm, and he would have to spend a couple of days at home in bed.

Collaboration Strategy

Compulsives enter therapy for a variety of reasons; however, they rarely ask for help with their personality disorder. Sometimes they are aware that certain aspects of their personality, such as being perfectionistic, contribute to their psychological problems.

The general goal of psychotherapy with OCPD patients is to help them alter or reinterpret the problematic underlying assumptions so that behaviors and emotions will change. Cognitive therapists are generally much more willing to accept patient's complaints at face value than are psychodynamic therapists (who focus their attention much more on unconscious factors). Thus, when a patient initially complains of anxiety, headaches, or impotence, this is frequently the problem that is addressed. Sometimes the compulsive's complaints are more externalized—for example, "My supervisors are very critical of my work with no good reason." This type of problem presentation can be more difficult to work with. The therapist can still directly address the presenting complaint, however, by clearly establishing that because the supervisor's behavior cannot be directly changed through the therapy, the goal will need to be to change the patient's behavior in ways that may lead to the supervisor's acting differently.

As in all therapies, it is important at the start to establish a rapport with the patient. This can be difficult with compulsive patients because of their rigidity, discomfort with emotion, and tendency to downplay the importance of interpersonal relationships. Cognitive therapy with the compulsive tends be even more businesslike and problem-focused than usual, with less emphasis on emotional support and relationship issues. Usually, rapport is based on the patient's respect for the therapist's competence and a belief that the therapist respects and can be helpful to the patient. Trying to develop a closer emotional relationship than the compulsive is comfortable with early in therapy can be detrimental and may lead to an early termination. See Beck's (1983) article on the treatment of autonomous depression for a further discussion of this point.

Compulsives can elicit a variety of emotional reactions from therapists. Some therapists find these patients to be somewhat dry and boring because of their general lack of emotionality and their tendency to focus more on the factual aspects of events rather than the events' affective tones. They can also be experienced as exasperating because of their slowness and focus on details, particularly to therapists who value efficiency and goal-directedness. Therapists who tend to like the idealization and dependency that many patients develop in therapy often find compulsive patients less rewarding, as they tend not to form this kind of therapeutic relationship. Some compulsives act out their needs for control in the therapy in either a direct or a passive–aggressive manner. For example, when given a homework assignment, they might directly tell the therapist that the assignment is irrelevant or stupid, or else agree to do it but then forget or not have the time to get the assignment done. These patients can elicit anger and frustration from therapists and bring up conflicts related to the therapists' own need to be in control.

Another problematic situation may occur when the therapist's schemas are also compulsive. As noted early in this chapter, subclinical compulsive characteristics can be conducive to success in Western culture. The cognitive therapist may have achieved his or her academic and professional success through conscientiousness, attention to detail, self-discipline, perseverance, reliability, and so on. If the therapist is also perfectionistic, rigid, overly controlled, and lacking in insight, he or she may also be blind to the patient's pathology. Such therapists may buy into their patients' perspective uncritically and therefore miss opportunities to help them.

Therapists' reactions to compulsive patients can provide valuable information about the patients and the sources of their difficulties. However, therapists should avoid trying to make changes in the patient based on their own values rather than the patient's needs and presenting problems. For example, Mr. S may have been less emotionally expressive than his therapist would prefer, but this was not a source of significant impairment or subjective distress for him and therefore not a focus of treatment.

Specific Techniques

Within the broad general structure of cognitive therapy, a number of specific techniques are helpful with obsessive–compulsive patients. It is important to structure the therapy sessions by setting an agenda, prioritizing the problems, and using problem-solving techniques. This is useful in working with a number of characteristics, including indecisiveness, rumination, and procrastination. Structure forces the patient to pick out and work on a specific problem until it improves to an acceptable level. If the compulsive has difficulty working with the structure, the therapist can have the patient look at his or her automatic thoughts about it and relate this difficulty to the general problems of indecisiveness and procrastination. The Weekly Activity Schedule (Beck et al., 1979), a form on which patients can schedule activities on an hourly basis, can also help them add structure to their lives and become more productive while exerting less effort.

The therapist must be prepared for the compulsive patient to use these or other specific techniques in a perfectionistic manner. For example, it is not unusual for patients with OCPD to bring a thick stack of flawlessly typewritten Dysfunctional Thought Records to session as their homework for the week. Although this conscientiousness might at first appear to be helpful for their progress in therapy, it is usually better seen as a sample of their problematic behavior. Compulsive patients often display their typical vacillation and rumination in their use of the Dysfunctional Thought Record. They may bounce back and forth between the automatic thoughts and rational response columns, never reaching a balanced conclusion. This may be seen as a sample of the thinking process in which they engage privately. It therefore provides an opportunity to address the process as well as the content of their cognitions.

Because of compulsives' frequent problems with anxiety and psychosomatic symptoms, relaxation techniques and meditation are often helpful. Compulsives frequently have difficulty using these techniques at first, due to their belief that they are wasting time by taking half an hour off to relax or meditate. A cognitive therapy technique that is useful in addressing these issues is to list advantages and disadvantages of a specific behavior or belief. A disadvantage to relaxation techniques for the compulsive may be that they take time; an advantage might be that then the patient can actually get more done because he or she is more refreshed and less anxious.

It is often useful to conduct a behavioral experiment with OCPD patients. For example, instead of directly trying to dispute a certain belief held by a compulsive, the therapist can take a neutral, experimental attitude toward it. Thus, if a compulsive individual claims not to have time to relax during the day, the therapist may suggest an experiment to test this claim. The patient may compare productivity on days he uses relaxation techniques in contrast to the days he does not. Compulsives tend to value pleasure much less than productivity. It is often therapeutic to help them become aware of this and to evaluate with them the assumptions behind their value system concerning the place of pleasure in their lives.

Several cognitive and behavioral techniques can be useful in helping compulsive patients cope with chronic worrying and ruminating. Once patients agree that this is dysfunctional, they can be taught thought-stopping and refocusing techniques to redirect their thought processes. If they continue to believe that worrying is helpful or productive, they may agree to limit it to a certain time period during the day. This at least manages to free them from worrying for the rest of the day. Graded task assignments, in which a goal or task is broken down into specific definable steps, are often helpful. These steps serve to counter patients' dichotomous thinking and perfectionism by demonstrating that most things are accomplished by degrees of progress, rather than by being done perfectly or in their entirety right from the beginning.

After Mr. S learned to monitor his pain more consistently, he discovered that three types of situations were associated with his muscular tension. These included (1) having tasks or assignments to do; (2) having procrastinated and thereby having many things not completed; and (3) being expected to participate in social situations with new people. Mr. S and his therapist decided to work initially on the first situation, as it occurred much more often than the third, and tended to cause the second. For example, he once noticed that he was experiencing a moderate degree of back pain while standing and rinsing off the dishes before putting them in the dishwasher. He was thinking that the dishes needed to be perfectly clean before putting them in the dishwasher. This thought was making the task stressful and take much longer than it should. Collecting a number of similar examples helped Mr. S see that his perfectionism resulted in numerous tasks each day becoming sources of stress that produced pain. He then began to look for the general assumptions or schemas underlying his automatic thoughts. Mr. S. developed the diagram shown in Figure 14.1 as a model of his behavior.

The therapist and Mr. S then further discussed the meaning of this pattern of thinking and behavior.

THERAPIST: So you find that you experience a lot of stress when having to do a task because you believe that no matter how well you do it, it won't be acceptable?

PATIENT: Yes, and I think that's why I tend not to make decisions or to procrastinate so I don't have to deal with these feelings.

THERAPIST: So you avoid and procrastinate in order to reduce your stress?

PATIENT: Yes, I think so.

THERAPIST: Does that actually work for you as a way of reducing stress?

PATIENT: No, putting things off usually just make it worse. I like to think I'm a pretty responsible person, and it really bothers me not

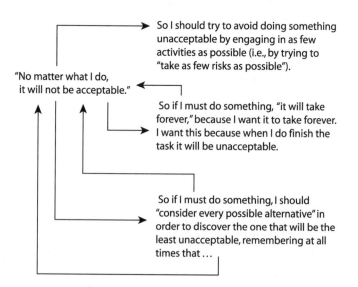

FIGURE 14.1. Mr. S's model of his behavior.

to be getting things done. I've had some of my worst back pain after I've been procrastinating all week.

THERAPIST: You wrote on the diagram that you believe what you do won't be acceptable. What if you did something that wasn't acceptable to certain other people? What about that would upset you?

PATIENT: What do you mean?

THERAPIST: Do you think it's possible for someone to do something that someone else would consider unacceptable, yet not get upset about it?

PATIENT: Yes, I've known some people like that. I guess for me, though, I feel like I am personally unacceptable or deficient if I don't function up to a certain level, which often seems impossible for me to do.

Thus, Mr. S's core schema or belief was that if he did not always function perfectly, then he was personally unacceptable. Given there was little chance that he could perform well enough to be acceptable, his primary symptoms were a form of anxiety (i.e., the physical stress in his back). At times, though, Mr. S would give up and conclude that no matter what he did would be unacceptable. At these times, such as during college, he would become hopeless and depressed.

After uncovering Mr. S's core belief, the focus in therapy was to change it, as the belief was the primary source both for Mr. S's current symptoms and for his OCPD. As the therapist and Mr. S discussed his belief over the next few sessions, he came to understand better how he had internalized the very high standards he believed his mother had for him. In addition, he became very self-critical, as he had experienced his mother to be when he did not meet her expectations; he also expected others to be very critical of him.

The therapist and Mr. S started examining the validity of his beliefs by first looking at whether they appeared to be accurate interpretations of the past. For one homework assignment, Mr. S listed all the times he could remember in the past that others had been very critical of him, and also listed possible alternatives as to why they might have acted that way. Mr. S did have the thought that probably others had been disapproving of him on many occasions but just had not said so. The therapist and Mr. S then discussed what he could do about this belief.

THERAPIST: So it still seems to you that most others are disapproving of you, even though you can think of very few times when you have had clear evidence that this was true?

PATIENT: Yes, I still often think that others aren't pleased with what I am doing, and then I am very uncomfortable around them.

THERAPIST: How do you think you could find out if these thoughts are accurate or not?

PATIENT: I don't know.

THERAPIST: Well, in general, if you wanted to know what someone was thinking, what would you do?

PATIENT: I guess I would ask them.

THERAPIST: Would that be possible for you? Do you think you could ask for feedback the next time you believe someone is disapproving of you?

PATIENT: I'm not sure. They might not like my asking them or they might not tell me the truth.

THERAPIST: That is a possibility and we maybe we can think of a way to determine that later on. In the meantime, what if we start with someone you believe to be pretty honest and nonjudgmental? Who do you think would fit that description?

PATIENT: My boss is a decent guy and I'd really like to not have to worry that he is judging me all the time.

THERAPIST: Can you think of a relatively safe way you could ask your boss how he is feeling about you or your work?

PATIENT: I suppose I could say something like this: "Jack, you seem to be concerned about something. Is anything bothering you about the way my project is going?"

THERAPIST: That sounds pretty good. Would you be willing to accept that as your homework for next week? Would you be willing to ask your boss his thoughts once this week when you think he is disapproving of you and record both what you expect him to say and what he actually says?

PATIENT: OK, I'll try that.

This was an example of setting up a behavioral experiment to test out a specific dysfunctional belief. Over the next couple of weeks, Mr. S did, on several occasions, ask others what they were thinking when he thought that they were evaluating him critically. He found that on all but one occasion, he had misinterpreted what others were thinking about him. On that occasion, one of his bosses at work was mildly annoyed with him, but this was due to Mr. S being late in getting him some work. The patient realized from this that his procrastination caused more problems and dissatisfactions for him than his level of performance.

Mr. S, like many compulsives, had the belief that it was often functional to put things off because this enabled him to perform better. The therapist had him evaluate this belief in a homework assignment by rating his level of performance from 1 to 10 on a variety of tasks. He then compared the average level of performance on those tasks he had done immediately. He found that his average level of performance was slightly higher on tasks that he did without procrastinating. Mr. S attributed this to the increased stress he would feel about tasks he avoided.

Another technique that proved helpful to Mr. S was having him compare the values and standards he had for himself to those he had for others. He came to realize that he was much more critical and demanding of himself than he was of others, and he agreed that it did not make much sense to have two different sets of values. The therapist then built on this understanding by having him note when he was being self-critical and ask himself what he would be thinking if he observed someone else performing at the same level. Mr. S found that this technique helped him to be more understanding and less critical of himself. This technique does not work with many compulsives, however, because compulsive patients are frequently as critical and demanding of others as they are of themselves.

The therapist and Mr. S also identified the primary cognitive distortions and maladaptive modes of thought that Mr. S frequently used. These included:

1. Dichotomous thinking ("If I don't do this task perfectly, I have done it terribly");
2. Magnification ("It is horrible if I don't do this well");
3. Overgeneralization ("If I do something poorly, it means I am an unacceptable person");
4. "Should" statements ("I should do this perfectly").

Mr. S monitored the use of these thought patterns on Dysfunctional Thought Records, and identified how they increased his stress level and often lowered his level of performance.

MAINTAINING PROGRESS

For most patients it is easy to slip back into familiar but dysfunctional cognitive and behavior patterns. This is particularly true with personality-disordered patients, as their problems are so ingrained. Cognitive therapy has advantages over some other forms of therapy in coping with this. Patients become very conscious of the nature of their problems, and they learn effective ways of coping. They learn how to use tools such as the Dysfunctional Thought Record, which they can use outside the therapy context to work on problem areas.

It is crucial when nearing the end of therapy to warn patients about the possibility of relapse, and to have them watch closely for minor recurrences of the problems that brought them to therapy. These are indications that the patients need to do some more work—either by themselves with the tools they learned in therapy, or with the therapist. It is important that patients realize it is common to need occasional booster sessions so they will not be ashamed to get help if a problem recurs. Most cognitive therapists build this into the therapy by scheduling periodic booster sessions after the main part of the therapy has been completed.

As Mr. S learned to recognize and understand the distortions in his thought processes, he became increasingly effective at responding rationally to his automatic thoughts. This helped Mr. S break the habitual cognitive and behavioral patterns that led to his muscular pain. A couple of sessions were spent in working on his social anxiety, which was also related to his perfectionism and fears of being unacceptable. As a result of the progress he had already made in these areas, Mr. S found that he was experiencing less social anxiety. He also found he was able to continue making progress by using the same techniques he had learned to help with his anxiety about doing tasks.

After 15 sessions over a 6-month period, Mr. S was experiencing little back pain, and when he did, he was generally able to recognize the source of his stress and his dysfunctional automatic thoughts, and then modify them. At a 6-month follow-up session, Mr. S reported having remained relatively pain-free. He had one difficult weekend before he had to make a speech, but he had been able to cope with this and prepare the speech, and the presentation went well.

CONCLUSION

Based on considerable clinical experience and some research support, cognitive therapy appears to be an effective and efficient treatment for OCPD. Compulsives often respond particularly well to certain aspects of cognitive therapy. These include its problem-focused nature, its use of homework assignments, and its emphasis on the importance of thought processes. Individuals with OCPD seem to prefer therapeutic approaches that are more structured and problem-focused to approaches that focus primarily on the therapeutic process and the transference relationship as the means of change (Juni & Semel, 1982).

CHAPTER 15

Passive–Aggressive Personality Disorder (Negativistic Personality Disorder)

. . . they see the dark lining in the silver cloud.
—MILLON (1969, p. 288)

The current diagnostic criteria for passive–aggressive personality disorder (PAPD) have progressed from a conglomerate of oppositional behaviors directed toward authority figures to incorporate a more dimensional personality construct, the negativistic personality (DSM-IV-TR, 2000; Millon, 1969, 1981).[1] Specific characteristics of PAPD form a pervasive pattern of antagonistic neglect of external demands for the individual's adequate social and occupational performance. Evidence of this passive resistance and oppositional style includes persistent, deliberate procrastination, resistance to authority, argumentativeness, protests, and obstruction. Deadlines are nearly impossible to meet, and missing them is fre-

---

[1]Both the diagnostic classification and the placement of this disorder changed from DSM-III-R to DSM-IV-TR. Passive–aggressive personality was listed in the text as a personality disorder in DSM-III-R. In DSM-IV-TR, the disorder is revised to passive–aggressive personality disorder (negativistic personality disorder), and placed in an appended section of proposed diagnoses for further study. For the sake of brevity, in this chapter we refer to the current diagnostic construct simply as PAPD.

quently externalized so that the missed deadline may be blamed on "forgetfulness," unreasonable demands, or the "authorities" having unrealistic expectations, or even a lack of "fairness" in setting deadlines to begin with (Ottaviani, 1990). The largely passive nature of these resistant behaviors evokes tremendous frustration in others, straining personal, social, and vocational relationships. Unmet obligations and expectations are often defining issues that provoke others to confront this individual. Worsening the situation, the individual with PAPD may solicit others' help and guidance, all the while thwarting and sabotaging the suggestions given.

Millon's construct of negativistic personality added phenomenological, intrapsychic, and biophysical domains to the diagnosis. These additional clinical domains further pinpointed characteristics typically associated with the PAPD disorder, including resentfulness, an interpersonally contrary style, a cognitively skeptical view, a discontented self-image, vacillating objects, poor displacement mechanisms, a divergent disorganization, and an irritable mood. Associated with these domains are feelings of being misunderstood, an intense ambivalence, and sullenness (Millon & Davis, 1996) (Table 15.1). The dimensional approach to this disorder permits better diagnostic discrimination and a holistic assessment, key for clinically informed treatment plans.

Significant social impairment is evident in the entitled, inconsistent, angry, and contrary interpersonal style of patients with PAPD. They may seek out others for company, but due to their intense ambivalence, may reject and alienate the very company they seek. They may demonstrate their anger through passive or active means. For example, they may show up for a meeting an hour late or, more subtly, arrive consistently late for work by 15 minutes. They may offer to stay 15 minutes later to make up the time and wonder what the problem is that others do not accept the "compromise." Patients with PAPD may express ambivalence within the therapeutic process through obstructionism, defiance, procrastination, verbal sparring, and treatment noncompliance.

Clinicians can easily recognize the core features of the PAPD as a chronic unwillingness to fulfill expectations (Wetzler & Morey, 1999), beyond simply being angry about a life situation (Ottaviani, 1990). As the diagnostic term implies, the passive–aggressive expresses hostility through a covert or passive medium of argumentativeness, cantankerousness, refusal to conform, and irritability. Passive–aggressive patients also present as sullen, moody, and ambivalent (Millon, 1969). Malinow (1981) states, "The term itself, passive–aggressive, is ambivalent and suggests paradox" (p. 121). Millon's (1981; Millon & Davis, 1996) description of the active ambivalent defines and embodies the vacillating nature of the patient with PAPD. On one hand, the patient wants someone to take care of him or her and make life gratifying. On the other hand, he or she does not want to lose

TABLE 15.1. Clinical Domains of the Negativistic (Passive–Aggressive) Prototype

Behavioral level

(F) Expressively resentful. Resists fulfilling expectancies of others, frequently exhibiting procrastination, inefficiency, and obstinacy, as well as oppositionalism and irksome behaviors; reveals gratification in demoralizing and undermining the pleasures and aspirations of others.

(F) Interpersonally contrary. Assumes conflicting and changing roles in social relationships, particularly dependent and contrite acquiescence and assertive and hostile independence; conveys envy and pique toward those more fortunate, as well as acting concurrently or sequentially obstructive and intolerant of others, expressing either negative or incompatible attitudes.

Phenomenological level

(F) Cognitively skeptical. Is cynical, doubting, and untrusting, approaching positive events with disbelief, and future possibilities with pessimism, anger, and trepidation; has a misanthropic view of life, whines and grumbles, voicing disdain and caustic comments toward those experiencing good fortune.

(S) Discontented self-image. Sees self as misunderstood, luckless, unappreciated, jinxed, and demeaned by others; recognizes being characteristically embittered, disgruntled and disillusioned with life.

(S) Vacillating objects. Internalized representations of past comprise a complex of countervailing relationships, setting in motion contradictory feelings, conflicting inclinations, and incompatible memories that are driven by the desire to degrade the achievements and pleasures of others, without necessarily appearing so.

Intraspsychic level

(F) Displacement mechanism. Discharges anger and other troublesome emotions either precipitously or by employing unconscious maneuvers to shift them from their instigator to settings or persons of lesser significance; vents disapproval by substitute or passive means, such as acting inept or perplexed, or behaving in a forgetful or indolent manner.

(S) Divergent organization. A clear division in the pattern of morphologic structures such that coping and defensive maneuvers are often directed toward incompatible goals, leaving major conflicts unresolved and full psychic cohesion often impossible because fulfillment of one drive or need inevitably nullifies or reverses another.

Biophysical level

(S) Irritable mood. Frequently touchy, temperamental, and peevish, followed in turn by sullen and moody withdrawal; is often petulant and impatient, unreasonably scorns those in authority and reports being annoyed easily or frustrated by many.

Note. (F), functional domain; (S), structural domain. From Millon and Davis (1996, p. 550). Copyright 1996 by John Wiley & Sons, Inc. Reprinted by permission.

autonomy or freedom, and he or she resents the direction and power of those in authority or those on whom he or she depends. Trapped somewhere between this intense dependence and demand for autonomy, the patient with PAPD experiences an exquisite anguish of never feeling content or satiated. It is this ever-present lack of contentment which can emulate symptoms of an ill-tempered depressive as defined by Schneider (1958). The pervasive skepticism of the passive–aggressive has a narcissistic flair in that life's woes and negative turns are somehow connected and directed toward the patient with PAPD, and external demands are predictably viewed as a personal affront and are therefore offensive. The pervasive negativism of PAPD is self-defeating, and due to its very nature becomes self-fulfilling (Stone, 1993a).

Strongly held, powerful schema will dictate that direct assertion is potentially catastrophic. This is due to believing a loss of autonomy is risked through disagreement, rejection, or refusal from others. Thus, to avoid being controlled and ever-resentful of authority, patients with PAPD respond to external demands in a passive, provocative, and indirect manner. Ever pessimistic and fearful of assertion and confrontation, the patient with PAPD is enveloped within a pattern of self-defeat. This pattern starts and stalls their way through life creating a path of "unfinished business" (Wetzler & Morey, 1999, p. 57). Stone (1993a) writes, "They may refuse to work, stage impasses, refuse stubbornly to progress in any direction, etc.-all of which ultimately defeats their own cherished hopes and ambitions" (p. 362). If directly confronted about passive behaviors, the patient typically responds with incredulous resentment, all the while proclaiming innocence and justification of his or her actions. Some responsibility for his or her dilemmas may be evident, but the patient will construct counterarguments to nullify any positive suggestion or idea, such that no lasting beneficial change occurs (Stone, 1993a).

The passive–aggressive typically presents for treatment as a result of complaints by others when he or she is unable to finish tasks, complete assignments, or meet expectations (Freeman, 2002; Ottaviani, 1990). An authority figure or supervisor in a vocational role may instigate the referral through an employee assistance program due to the individual not meeting deadlines, following directions, or dissolving morale among the other employees. A romantic partner or spouse may also pressure the individual to seek treatment due to his or her lack of contributing to the household, childrearing, or even the relationship. The personal pressure may be demands to get a job, to enroll in a course, be responsible for child care, or to do something at home (Stone, 1993a). Everyday responsibilities such as paying bills, responding to requests for additional information, and difficulties with other persons perceived to be in positions of authority (e.g., physicians, therapists, and professors) cause ongoing problems. For example, one patient with PAPD resented the obligation of taking his daily antihypertensive medications and stated, "I don't want to carry all these pills around, and certainly don't want to be held hostage." Not only did he refuse to take his medications, he also refused to allow the therapist to collaborate with the treating physician, and he refused to return for a follow-up visit. In another case, the patient's wife threatened to leave the relationship if the patient did not enter treatment. This patient had spent at least 11 years attempting to complete a doctoral program, at least 5 years of which were spent disputing university policies and procedures.

HISTORICAL PERSPECTIVES

Although the form of expressing hostility either directly or indirectly is conclusively a feature of PAPD as identified in early DSMs, only the pre-World War II literature captures the holistic clinical domains that Millon proposes in the more contemporary negativistic personality disorder (Millon & Davis, 1996). Relevant early literature describes forerunners of the diagnosis, including the cognitive, interpersonal, self-image, and affective components neglected within the initial versions of the DSMs. These early formulations were retrospectively defined as the cyclothymic, ill-tempered depressive, oral sadistic melancholic and masochist, highly neurotic and low in conscientiousness (dutifulness), and socially maladaptive personality types (cited in Millon & Davis, 1996).

Historically, the diagnosis of PAPD existed within the main text of the original DSM-I (American Psychiatric Association, 1952) through the DSM-III-R (American Psychiatric Association, 1987). Although the terms passive-dependent and passive–aggressive character or styles had been referred to in early psychoanalytic writings, their formal origins are traced to World War II, where the *zeitgeist* of the times compelled military personnel to identify or label those recruits who had difficulty following standard protocol and rules (Malinow, 1981). Recruits needed to ". . . adapt to a wide range of cultural and social conditions and to the many roles that he would be called on to perform" (Malinow, 1981, p. 122), especially combat. The military demanded the recruit to receive and follow direction and orders and have an understanding of the universal need to cooperate with one another. The War Department formalized these behaviors and the associated personality pattern in conjunction with prevalent psychoanalytic terms in a technical bulletin shortly after World War II (Millon & Davis, 1996). The passive–aggressive constellation of symptoms was classified as an immaturity (neurotic) reaction to military stress. This stress was associated with helplessness, obstructiveness, angry and aggressive outbursts, passivity, and inadequate behaviors. This was the template for all passive–aggressive personality diagnoses and definitions (Malinow, 1981). The passive–aggressive label remained in use through 1951 by the Standard Veterans Administration Classification (Millon & Davis, 1996). The army noted that 6.1% of all psychiatric admissions to military facilities were diagnosed with this disorder. Shortly, thereafter, DSM-I (American Psychiatric Association, 1952) included the diagnosis of passive–aggressive as a personality disorder and syndrome (Malinow, 1981).

While attempting to formulate revision of DSM, researchers continued to express doubt as to the validity of the PAPD diagnosis, suggesting that as a discrete category, it was not to be included in the first draft of DSM-III. Several theorists considered this group of behaviors as merely a defensive type reaction for some individuals when they are in a relatively weak position, such as those in the military, rather than a personality syndrome (Malinow, 1981). This may also include those patients in a psychiatric hospital setting or presenting for a psychiatric evaluation who may, as a result of being in a position of relative weakness, adopt a passive–aggressive style (Frances, 1980). Challenged by those who were proponents, the DSM-III Task Force later adopted the diagnosis.

Millon argued for the PAPD to be expanded to a more comprehensive construct, negativistic personality disorder, which added related characteristics rather than focusing primarily on the narrow behavior of resisting authority. Millon included in the more comprehensive construct for the proposed new disorder, negativistic personality disorder (NPD), four new aspects: irritable affectivity; cognitive ambivalence; discontented self-image; and interpersonal vacillation (Millon & Davis, 1996). Millon attempted to include not only the aspects of passiveness of aggression but also to include the active ambivalence often subjectively experienced by patients with PAPD. An intense conflict between ideas of dependence and the need for self-assertion contributes to an impulsive and quixotic emotionality. Personal relationships are fraught with wrangles and disappointments, provoked often by the characteristic fretful, complaining, and negativistic behaviors (Millon & Davis, 1996).

DSM-IV retained the categorical diagnostic system and placed the diagnosis of PAPD (NPD) into the Appendix to await further research and validation as a diagnosis. The DSM-IV Axis-II Work Group agreed to reassess the original proposed criteria and personality disorder from Millon's draft in 1975. The Task Group, recognizing that fundamental changes needed to occur, made the decision to include the diagnosis as the reformulated NPD, to be included within the Appendix. The disorder, categorized as passive–aggressive (negativistic) personality disorder, is listed as such so as not to appear as a radical departure from the original diagnosis of PAPD. Within the DSM-IV-TR (American Psychiatric Association, 2000), the diagnosis PAPD (NPD) awaits further research to determine its validity as a personality disorder diagnosis and its discriminative ability.

RESEARCH AND EMPIRICAL DATA

Little empirical research has been completed with the PAPD as the primary focus. However, both McCann (1988) and Millon (1993) state that this is largely due to the restrictive criteria of the original PAPD diagnosis. Until recently, only two studies specifically examined the patient with PAPD.

The first study to specifically address PAPD was completed by Whitman, Trosman, and Koenig (1954). The authors examined the operational use and potential comorbidity in a psychiatric outpatient clinic of the then new diagnostic category, PAPD. Using the DSM-I (American Psychiatric Association, 1952) criteria, the authors examined a total of 400 outpatients who presented to an outpatient clinic for psychotherapy. The PAPD diagnosis was the most frequently occurring personality disorders, with 92 patients having passive–aggressive or passive-dependent personality. In addition, the patients with PAPD broke contact or terminated treatment after one return visit more frequently than any other personality type.

Characteristics of PAPD were assessed in a longitudinal study of psychiatric patients (Small, Small, Alig, & Moore, 1970). From the 100 probands selected, passive–aggressive patients were more often male, and represented 3% of the total (3,682 subjects). At follow-up after 7 and 15 years, compared to 50 matched controls with other psychiatric diagnoses, the passive–aggressive group was still "in the process of completing their education and had not yet qualified for other than casual employment" (p. 975). Small et al. (1970) noted several common attributes among the patients with PAPD at both intervals including alcohol abuse, interpersonal strife, verbal aggression, emotional storms, impulsivity, and manipulative behavior.

Within the past few years, additional studies have been completed to either validate the diagnosis or examine its characteristics. The incidence of PAPD was demonstrated higher in a study by Fossati et al. (2000) than in prior studies. Of a sample of 379 in- and outpatients admitted to the Medical Psychology and Psychotherapy Unit of the Scientific Institute H San Raffaele of Milan, 47 subjects (12.4%) received a DSM-IV PAPD diagnosis. Of those patients, 89.4% received an additional personality disorder diagnosis. In particular, the authors noted a significant correlation with narcissistic personality disorder, the only personality disorder to significantly coincide with PAPD. Characteristics such as grandiosity and interpersonal exploitation of others were features most strongly associated with PAPD. The authors conclude that PAPD may be more of a subtype of narcissistic personality disorder rather than its own distinctive personality disorder.

Vereycken, Vertommen, and Corveleyn (2002) investigated the personality style of young men with chronic authority conflicts using the Millon Clinical Multiaxial Inventory-I (MCMI-I; Millon, 1983). The authors compared the diagnoses of young men with chronic and acute authority conflicts with a normal control group. Chronic authority conflict was frequently associated with PAPD (28 of 41 patients) and was not associated strongly with other personality disorders, providing some evidence that PAPD is a distinct diagnosis.

DIFFERENTIAL DIAGNOSIS

Currently, if a patient meets criteria for PAPD, the diagnosis is formally categorized within the personality disorder not otherwise specified category (see Table 15.2). Although many patients present with behaviors considered to be passive–aggressive (e.g., tardiness, treatment noncompliance, and resentfulness), the passive–aggressive patient approaches life and all its challenges in this same pattern. The traits are not reactive and transient but, rather, chronic, inflexible, and maladaptive.

It is difficult to complete a diagnostic interview with passive–aggressive patients due to their confusing, evasive answers. For example, a patient who is asked a direct question such as, "Is the sky blue?" answers in a truthful but cantankerous way, "Not where I'm sitting." If asked about work status, this patient may respond, "How do you define work?" This can lead to tangential discussions defining particular words or constructs. The assessment yields a frustrating puzzle of incomplete

---

TABLE 15.2. DSM-IV-TR Research Criteria for Passive–Aggressive Personality Disorder (Negativistic Personality Disorder)

A. A pervasive pattern of negativistic attitudes and passive resistance to demands for adequate performance, beginning by early adulthood and present in a variety of contexts, as indicated by four (or more) of the following:

    (1) passively resists fulfilling routine social and occupational tasks
    (2) complains of being misunderstood and unappreciated by others
    (3) is sullen and argumentative
    (4) unreasonably criticizes and scorns authority
    (5) expresses envy and resentment toward those apparently more fortunate
    (6) voices exaggerated and persistent complaints of personal misfortune
    (7) alternates between hostile defiance and contrition

B. Does not occur exclusively during Major Depressive Episodes and is not better accounted for by Dysthymic Disorder.

Note. From American Psychiatric Association (2000, p. 791). Copyright 2000 by the American Psychiatric Association. Reprinted by permission.

answers laden with inconsequential details. A typical assessment can quickly become argumentative as the patient poses additional questions that demonstrate resentfulness at being asked to supply an answer (external demands), such as, "why is that important?" and "how is this important to the evaluation?" Fighting a subordinate or dependent position, the passive–aggressive retains autonomy by avoiding direct answers and therefore does not acquiesce to the authority figure.

Unlike the depressive style of the individual with PAPD, the individual with depression has more self-deprecating thoughts, is more likely to blame him- or herself for misfortune, and exhibits a negative view of the future. Depression is possible in the patient with PAPD, so evaluation for associated high-risk behaviors such as suicidality, homicidality, or substance abuse should not be overlooked. Additional Axis I problems may include anxiety disorders. Anxiety symptoms are likely to present during times that directly challenge the patient to be assertive, respond to an external demand, or when forced to choose a specific course of action.

Narcissistic and borderline characteristics are quite similar and may overlap with PAPD. Narcissism is manifested in the individual's considerable focus on their own plight and misfortune, attitudes of grandiosity and entitlement, and potent inability to empathize with others. Differentiation can be made between the two disorders as the narcissist is typically more active and directly aggressive, and if in disagreement with an authority figure or external demand, will not hesitate to assert dominance. Narcissists believe themselves to be an authority, whereas the passive–aggressives believe they are victims of authority. Millon and Davis (1996) write that although borderline patients also demonstrate severe ambivalence and vacillation, borderline personality disorder is more severe in terms of cognitive polarities, shifts in affectivity, and behavioral impulsivity.

CONCEPTUALIZATION

The cognitive profile of the patient with PAPD includes core beliefs, conditional assumptions, and compensatory strategies that are consistent with negativism, ambivalence, resistance, an unwillingness to meet the expectations of others, and an overarching goal of retaining autonomy. Automatic thoughts reflect their unrelenting skepticism and pessimism. This pervades how they view themselves, others, and the world and all its challenges. The desire to be in favor with those in power (dependency and acknowledgement) remains in direct contradiction to their belief that to remain autonomous they must circumvent or ignore rules or expectations. As a means of managing this ambivalence, independence is maintained through passive behavior that does not directly confront or challenge the authority. They retain control and autonomy by avoiding conflict and potential disapproval.

Clinical Example

Mr. Allen was a 47-year-old banker referred by his supervisor because he was missing banking data deadlines, resisting supervision from senior staff, and worse, negativistic with customers. His behavioral presentation suggested symptoms of depression, anxiety, and severe irritability. He described the management at the bank as terribly unfair and believed that they misunderstood his intentions. He was convinced he had created a more efficient means of logging data and was frustrated that his repeated attempts to alter the bank's procedures were largely ignored. To prove his position, he superficially complied with expectations while continuing to process banking data through his own method. He was completely without insight that his continued refusal to conform to the bank's policies and procedures were deemed an infraction. Mr. Allen was enraged that his supervisor had referred him to treatment. He reveled in the fantasy of the time when his supervisor would finally recognize his superior acumen of accounting procedures.

Consistent with his current problems, Mr. Allen had a history of chronic problems with authority figures, supervisors, and rules in general. He was largely a "loner" with few friends, social relationships, or outside interests. He easily alienated others through abrasive, contrary, and caustic interactions and had limited insight as to the impact these actions had on others. He would set long-term goals and projects for himself, but these would invariably fall by the wayside. This was due to the many potential pitfalls, arguments with associated members, and heated discussions regarding what he saw as arbitrary rules and regulations.

When asked if he had other issues he wished to address in psychotherapy, Mr. Allen spoke of global, ambiguous goals such as "finding direction in life" and "finding out who I really am." He described a lonely childhood, filled with frequent moves and changes. His parents were divorced and his mother was the primary caretaker. He had no contact with his father. His emotional memories focused on feeling angry, resentful, and frustrated. He remembered difficulty completing homework but managed to pass all his exams. Social situations were disastrous. He stated that no one really understood him, and girls were somewhat of a mystery to him. He had few dates and never married. His mother recently passed away, causing him to question his life's future direction. He had imagined that he would care for his mother until he was well into his 70s, and now, without her caretaking responsibilities, stated he had absolutely no idea what to do.

Core Beliefs

The patient's core beliefs and related automatic thoughts emanate themes of control and resistance (e.g., "No one should control me" and "To conform means I have no control"). Compliance is synonymous with a loss of control, freedom, and autonomy, a position this patient is unable to tolerate. This difficulty or conflict with accepting influence from others is a fundamental aspect of the intense ambivalence that creates such social impairment. Passivity or superficial compliance is the means of maintaining distance from the demands of a person or situation. They often view themselves as long-suffering and unrecognized for their unique contributions. Table 15.3 lists typical core beliefs.

Mr. Allen's core beliefs of control led him to thwart rules to protect his independence. However, as a means to remain in favor with management and avoid confrontation, he superficially agreed to comply (following bank procedures) when in reality he continued to work in his own way. Omnipresent through his belief system were themes of victimization: Being taken advantage of, being misunderstood, and that no one, even authority, should tell him what to do. He maligned the management's style with coworkers, pressing them to agree with his ideas. He would ask for colleague's opinions and then become argumentative and abrasive if they disagreed with him.

Conditional Beliefs

Conditional PAPD beliefs support superficial compliance and magnify their personal means of handling situations as the best, obvious, and most unique way. Thus, successful management of a situation requires shallow acquiescence, and covert insertion of the "better" PAPD approach. Table 15.3 lists typical conditional beliefs.

Despite direct feedback to the contrary, Mr. Allen remained convinced that if he continued to process the data in the way he believed was most efficient, in time, management would grasp that his way was the right way and the only way. In addition, he maintained the belief that if he told colleagues and supervisors that he would follow directions, confrontation would be avoided in the short run, but eventually the wisdom of his ways would be acknowledged and recognized. Mr. Allen did not appreciate that his superficial compliance was essentially a form of dishonesty, and to the surprise of his colleagues, he remained completely oblivious to the consequences of his actions.

TABLE 15.3. Core, Conditional, and Compensatory Beliefs

Core beliefs

"No one should tell me what to do!"
"I can't depend on anyone."
"To conform means I have no control."
"Expressing anger may cause me difficulty."
"Rules are limiting."
"People do not understand me."
"Others should not question me."
"People will take advantage of me if let them."

Conditional beliefs

"By resisting demands, I remain independent."
"If I follow the rules, I lose my freedom."
"If someone knows information about me, I am vulnerable."
"If I depend upon someone, I have no say."
"If I do what I think is right, others will be convinced it is right."
"By not asserting myself directly, I stay in favor with others."

Compensatory beliefs

"I must circumvent the rules to remain free."
"I must not follow the path of others."
"I will superficially go along with others to avoid conflict."
"I must assert myself indirectly so that I will not be rejected."
"I do not receive the credit I'm due because others can't appreciate me."
"I have unique means of doing things which few understand."

Compensatory Beliefs

Compensatory beliefs of the patient with PAPD largely include themes of remaining in favor of the authority figure by superficially conforming. However, if superficial conformity becomes problematic in any situation, patients with PAPD then rely on the belief that an extreme injustice has occurred. They are convinced they are not being recognized or appreciated for the unique and special contribution they are making, nor are others capable of understanding them. There is a narcissistic quality to their compensatory strategies that can almost appear as a protective mechanism to avoid or avert rejection. However, the intense rage that accompanies these beliefs somewhat contradicts the notion that these beliefs are protective in their function, but rather the result of a narcissistic injury. Table 15.3 lists typical compensatory beliefs.

Mr. Allen's compensatory beliefs consisted of distorted ideas related to his perceived rejection by his supervisor. The rejection, however, was not, in his mind, caused by his insubordination, but rather, due to his supervisor's inability to acknowledge and recognize his unique ideas. He expressed intense anger, disappointment, and frustration at the "system's" inability to "think outside the box." The greater the supervisor's pressure for compliance, the more entrenched he became in his conviction to change the process. He was intensely resentful and at times even undermining of any colleague who received recognition. As others progressed within the bank hierarchy, Mr. Allen became even more convinced that he was being overlooked and neglected.

TREATMENT APPROACH

Beck, Freeman, and Associates (1990) suggest that, in the cognitive-behavioral treatment of PAPD, a collaborative approach be used to identify automatic thoughts and schema related to dysfunctional behaviors and inappropriate expressions of anger. The major focus of the treatment is to challenge basic beliefs and thought patterns of how the self, others, and the world are perceived and that by modifying these irrational beliefs, a change in emotion or affect states will occur, and behavioral change is possible.

Collaboration Strategy

Collaboration is an essential component to treatment with the PAPD patient, although the core beliefs will present unique difficulties in a cooperative therapeutic exchange. As the primary core belief of the patient with PAPD is to resist the dictates of an authority figure, the very therapeutic process is challenged. The patient may believe that the therapist is trying to tell him or her what to change, and how he or she should go about it. It is therefore imperative that the patient make the commitment to the therapeutic process, and become actively involved in its progress. This requires ongoing diligence by the therapist to ensure that the patient maintains some of the control within the therapeutic relationship. Frequent checking and soliciting feedback from the patient is crucial to ensure that he or she does not feel "railroaded" by the therapist's requests. If the patient assumes that the therapist is controlling the session or demanding compliance, the patient may passively resist the process, such as "forgetting" to do homework, no showing, or canceling the session. The patient with PAPD typically resists treatment, as Stone (1993b) writes, "Many quit treatment (a passive–aggressive act in itself) before any positive changes can occur" (p. 308).

Automatic thoughts must be consistently identified both within the session and between sessions, especially in response to affective shifts. The therapist must be able to challenge the patient's distorted beliefs related to being controlled by providing evidence that the patient has collaborated throughout the process and has not been requested or dictated to do something. The therapist and patient must then work together to identify those cognitions that are blocking or preventing task completion (Ottaviani, 1990).

The assessment process with Mr. Allen was lengthy and difficult to complete due to his incomplete and evasive answers. Mr. Allen was not able to articulate clear, specific goals for treatment. Throughout treatment, he was resistant to the suggestions made by the therapist, and on many occasions he was not able to move beyond the setting of the agenda. He would alternately seek answers to ambiguous questions (e.g., "Who am I?") while demanding answers from the therapist. When the therapist offered suggestions, he responded in an angry despondent manner. In an attempt to establish collaboration, the therapist sought his opinion about the subject matter and direction to take in treatment. The therapist was met with responses such as, "Isn't it your job to tell me what to do?" and "How should I know, you're the doctor." Mr. Allen would become argumentative and caustic when discussing the proposed schedule. Any and all suggestions to enhance the quality of his life were refused, disputed, or generally discarded. Yalom's description of the "help-rejecting complainer" summarized many of the interactions between the therapist and Mr. Allen (Yalom, 1985).

In an effort to establish collaboration, the therapist attempted to identify his ambivalence and distorted beliefs related to being controlled. To begin, the therapist and the patient identified several potential goals that could be included within the agenda. Mr. Allen was then encouraged to select and formally list those areas he agreed to address. This written list was signed by both the patient and the therapist to assist in collaborative treatment planning. For example, the following potential goals were listed: improving work relationship with supervisor, examining his contribution to the situation, improving social skills, examining origins of depressive symptoms, anger management and appropriate discharge of anger, and identifying long-term posttreatment goals. By encouraging the patient to choose what he wished to work on, the therapist not only challenged the very passivity that caused problems but encouraged an assertive approach to the setting of the agenda and related goals. In addition, any distortions related to the therapist attempting to control the process could then be disputed:

THERAPIST: So, you agree with the goals that we've listed? (The therapist asked after the patient selected three specific areas to work on).

MR. ALLEN: This appears to be an appropriate course of action. However, I may change my mind later.

THERAPIST: That's fine, as long as we're able to discuss the changes, and how that will affect our schedule of sessions.

MR. ALLEN: You mean your schedule of sessions?

THERAPIST: I'd like to take a moment. I'm confused. I thought the list that we made was what you had agreed to?

MR. ALLEN: Yes it is.

THERAPIST: Would you like to revisit this list or are you feeling unsure about something?

Managing Confrontation

In the foregoing situation, the therapist was able to identify the defiance, while, importantly, not overwhelming the patient with intense confrontation. Beck et al. (1990) note that the therapist must avoid challenging dysfunctional beliefs and behaviors too aggressively or prematurely as direct confrontation may activate compelling core schema related to authority figures and the automatic resistance of influence to maintain control and autonomy. The therapist was later able to connect Mr. Allen's ambivalence with his aggressive verbal responses and defiance. For example, if he disagreed with his own choices within the agenda, the therapist was able to identify this ambivalence as empirical evidence of the patient's inability to comply, even when it was with his own suggestions.

A core feature and belief of the patient with PAPD is ambivalence between "submission to others and gratification of self-needs" (Millon & Davis, 1996, p. 570). Mr. Allen portrayed this fundamental conflict of dependency versus oppositionalism in all manners of communication. In a dependent manner, he sought all the answers from the therapist. When these questions were redirected in an attempt to encourage self-discovery and examine his own needs and to consider more concrete goals, Mr. Allen's contriteness and impatience was further piqued. Angry at his growing dependency he responded in an oppositional manner. He dismissed any and all suggestions, options, or recommendations through passive–aggressive means of communicating, such as using lengthy detail-laden sentences, a loud voice, argumentativeness, sullenness, and verbal aggressiveness. Mr. Allen, within the therapeutic microcosm, demonstrated his inability to appropriately express himself. His verbosity, combined with his hostility, precluded direct communication. Specific goals were difficult to attain and required consistent honing and redirection from the amorphous, detail-laden statements. Mr. Allen was aware that his personality style was at times offensive and alienating to others. However, he continued to demonstrate ambivalence about changing his interaction style despite understanding that it would be beneficial to him. In this situation, the therapist attempted to disseminate the ambivalence by creating a middle ground between dependence (learning new interaction styles with the therapist) and remaining steadfastly oppositional to change. Socratic questioning, providing evidence that change is beneficial, and a related cost-benefit analysis provided the middle ground needed to create a balance between the polarities of dependence and oppositionalism:

THERAPIST: Would you want to talk more about different ways you can interact?

MR. ALLEN: Yes. Those and many others.

THERAPIST: But to do one thing at a time is the only way to focus on something. Do you agree?

MR. ALLEN: Yes, I agree with that but the thought that goes through my mind is subconsciously do I really want to change?

THERAPIST: What parts would you want explore?

MR. ALLEN: The parts that would improve relations with other people.

THERAPIST: How do you want to see yourself relating to others?

MR. ALLEN: I want to be the best person I can be, but I'm having trouble identifying the person I want to be. I want to work on it and I know you're trying to help but I think I'm sort of sliding away, and it's not intentional.

THERAPIST: What do you mean by sliding away?

MR. ALLEN: Because I think you're having a hard time pinning me down.

THERAPIST: Why am I having a hard time pinning you down?

MR. ALLEN: I don't know, but it comes in me, and it may be that although I say that I'm willing to change I'm actually unwilling to change.

THERAPIST: We keep leading back to the relationship issues. Right? The interactions, would you agree?

MR. ALLEN: Yes.

THERAPIST: What would be the positives if you changed the way you interact?

MR. ALLEN: It would open up new associations that might very well be pleasant. It would probably mean getting through life a little easier.

THERAPIST: How might they be more pleasant?

MR. ALLEN: Well, I think that in our society we generally get along better with people if we have manners and if you're friendly. If you're polite it's just a little easier to get along in life rather than if you go around with stickles and prickles always looking for a fight.

THERAPIST: How would it benefit you directly or indirectly to change that?

MR. ALLEN: I don't see how it could fail to benefit me directly.

THERAPIST: Then why am I having a hard time pinning you down?

Avoiding Power Struggles

Covert expressions of resistance within the treatment may include being silent; rationalizing failures to comply with treatment recommendations; responding to confrontation increasingly with feelings of shame, humiliation, resentment and blame; increasing passive resistance to therapy and change which includes oppositional behaviors and purposefully failing or becoming more symptomatic; increasing the amount of help-rejecting complaining and anger toward the therapist and the therapist's apparent inability to help; and talking about or suggesting other treatments or consultations with different therapists (American Psychiatric Association, 1989). Stone (1993b) notes, "These attitudes quickly become apparent, manifesting themselves typically as a need to prove the therapist incompetent" (p. 308). As a means of avoiding struggles with the patient regarding forgetfulness in payment for services, clear written rules of therapy should be outlined for scheduling, billing, and time frames of treatment (Reid, 1988). This should be completed early in the therapy, and most important, the therapist needs to consistently adhere to the limitations that have been set. Again, this process (list) must be completed in a collaborative process, checking with each point that the patient understands and agrees to the structure and limits of the therapeutic process. Passive–aggressive behaviors such as showing up late for a session due to automatic thoughts related to the idea that "Nobody is going to tell me when to arrive or what to do" provide ample *in vivo* opportunity to address, challenge, and dispute these distortions. For example, the therapist can work with the patient to express a more direct means of defiance (e.g., requesting a different time of the session) (Ottaviani, 1990).

Consistency and Empathy

Throughout treatment, the therapist must remain consistent, objective, and empathic with PAPD patients. It is easy to get caught in an almost impossible battle that is waging within such patients that presents as "please help me/screw you" behaviors. Their caustic interactions can prove to be tiring and at times are offensive. The patient's continued ambivalence causes frequent starts and stops through the therapy. As the patient slowly becomes more comfortable (dependent) with suggestions from the therapist, underlying ambivalence can cause an erratic shift, leading to a rejection or setback of the treatment process (oppositional). The therapist needs to consistently identify the dysfunctional thoughts related to these shifts and forge ahead challenging these distortions. Although it can appear that such patients revel in their misery, they experience great discomfort, angst, and sadness in their plight. Rather than personalizing the patient's negativism and becoming offended, the therapist can remember to also conceptualize these actions as learned maladaptive behaviors.

Specific Interventions

Assertiveness Training

Assertiveness training can help patients with PAPD make covert expressions of anger overt and more functional (Hollandsworth & Cooley, 1978; Perry & Flannery, 1982). In Mr. Allen's case, assertion training was used as a means to help him express his frustration with the bank's management in a prosocial manner (e.g., outlining and making a formal presentation vs. covert sabotage). Within the treatment session, the therapist was sure to allot time for feedback as to the direction that the therapy was going, and to solicit any changes that the patient felt they needed to make. This provided ample opportunity for Mr. Allen to appropriately assert his disagreements with the therapeutic process in a positive, structured way. In response, the therapist provided a balance between consistent limits (e.g., length of sessions) and receptiveness to Mr. Allen's requests (e.g., topics for the agenda).

Self-Monitoring and Other Monitoring

Patients with PAPD typically present with an antagonistic, acerbic, and disgruntled style, which sometimes takes the form of transforming him or her into conspiring curmudgeon, as the patient attempts to engage the therapist in a cynical assessment of the world at large. Unaware of their offensive chronic complaining, such patients tire those around them and alienate those they wish to move closer to or seek approval from. By becoming aware of the affective shifts they experience (self-monitoring) in reaction to others, associated automatic thoughts related to being taken advantage of, being misunderstood, or attempting to be controlled are more easily identified and therefore challenged. Identifying how anger, disappointment, and other emotional states actually feel (e.g., physiological reactions) provide a valuable gateway to their associated automatic thoughts and their underlying core beliefs. Homework assignments should include documenting and collecting automatic thoughts, particularly after experiencing an intense emotion. To encourage compliance with these assignments, dysfunctional thought recording should be presented as a "no lose" assignment (Ottaviani, 1990). Not only does the assignment allow for a connection between their thoughts and how they may feel, but it can identify those areas which contribute to any depression or anxiety.

Keeping in mind that those with PAPD have problems with assertion, appropriate monitoring of self-expression of anger can be helpful. This could include monitoring their posture, voice inflections (e.g., yelling), body language (e.g., pointing), eye contact (intense vs. avoidant), or use of biting words within an interaction (Prout & Platt, 1983). Other monitoring could involve helping patients move beyond their own experience to attempting to understand how others may perceive their often loud, mordant, and offensive style. This could include monitoring others for signs of taking offense or disinterest (loss of eye contact, body posture change, verbal cues, etc.). Respect for the personal rights of others is an important component of assertiveness, and this must be explicitly discussed with the patient. This includes the right of another to (predictably) to become peeved or angry with the patient's offending behavior and to take steps to avoid or protect themselves.

Social Skills and Communication Training

Impaired social and communication skills are vital treatment targets with PAPD. Interactions of the patient with PAPD are fraught with negativism, poor boundaries, caustic exchanges, and a controlling style that alternates between garrulousness and simmering silence. Conversely, patients with PAPD frequently lack good listening skills, reciprocation, or sensitivity to feedback or influence from others. For Mr. Allen, lack of connectedness and difficulty with social relationships was due in part to his poor perception of social limits and interpersonal cues. For example, he recounted a heated argument with a neighbor. Mr. Allen had spent an inordinate amount of time asking the neighbor about his 16-year-old daughter and her future college plans. Initially asking appropriate questions, he quickly escalated to a personal agenda of providing mentorship to the girl. He was insistent that he possessed a great knowledge on handling school committees, which he stated are typically biased and poorly organized. Mr. Allen did not recognize that he violated a significant boundary when he asked the girl out to dinner to discuss her plans.

Social skills training helped Mr. Allen better understand the concept of different interpersonal boundaries, warning signs from others that he may be violating their boundaries, and how to express himself in a respectful manner. Lists were made collaboratively identifying what good interaction skills might include and subsequently which areas he wished to develop. He agreed that he needed to learn to communicate a disagreement with someone in an appropriate and nonoffensive manner. Communication skills assisted Mr. Allen to make more "I" statements, pause for responses, maintain appropriate eye contact, and answer with fewer lengthy and detail-ridden sentences. Homework assignments included engaging in conversations with colleagues and practicing not raising his voice, pausing before responding and examining whether what he was about to say could be interpreted as offensive, and pausing for others to respond. As he had identified being a good listener as an attribute of an effective communicator, Mr. Allen tested whether he was truly hearing the others by writing down what they said after the conversation. Possible alternative responses were examined and later role-played in session.

Anger Management

A most fundamental emotional problem of the PAPD patient is maladaptive reactions of anger, hostility, and, in particular, resentment. In treatment of these disordered emotions, therapists need to assist PAPD patients in both managing and examining their ideas of "righteous revenge" and the means planned for getting back at others they perceived to have been rewarded unfair recognition and validation. Associated themes such as "they should be punished" or "no one really understands" should be identified and questioned (Ottaviani, 1990). Core beliefs regarding control should be explored. This may be difficult to do as it requires patients to focus on their own performance and behaviors rather than on their perceived mistreatment from others. In addition, they will be asked to consider the judgments of others in determining realistic expectations. This process will quite likely tap into the narcissistic quality of the core beliefs, compelling schema-related superiority and entitlement of the patient with PAPD. Strategies of treatment with narcissistic personality disorder may prove helpful as well.

Due to core beliefs that others may be attempting to control or devalue their value and worth, the emotional response of anger often drives the behavioral response to a situation of the individual with PAPD. A cognitive interpretation of the situation may not occur; rather, reactions are derived from the immediate visceral response. This process can be labeled for the patient as emotion-based reasoning (Ottaviani, 1990), which often results in mistakes and distortions, despite the popular notion that one should "go with your gut." A cost-benefit analysis can assist in identifying the advantages and disadvantages of impulsive reactions and the benefit of examining the relationship between core beliefs and their associated emotional responses.

MAINTAINING PROGRESS

For the patient with PAPD, core beliefs of control and resistance to plans, following the suggestions of others, or general compliance with structure can be easily reactivated. Situations that place the patient under the direction of an authority can trigger the control/resistance schema and quickly thwart any therapeutic process gained. Creating a list prior to termination that identifies the risks or situations which may predictably activate the old schema helps patients to proactively approach and manage the situation in a healthy way. Returning for follow-up visits to review their behaviors or problem areas can help in retaining alternative productive means of managing difficult situations. Continuing to work on consolidating new skills in other modalities such as group therapy has potential benefits for maintaining progress and supporting the schema modification.

CONCLUSION

PAPD characteristics of negativism, ambivalence, resistance, unwillingness to meet the expectations of others and an overarching goal of retaining autonomy create significant challenges for therapeutic intervention. Therapists must counter unrelenting skepticism and pessimism in their patients with PAPD and yet allow their patients to retain a sufficient degree of control in the therapeutic process. Core beliefs of control and resistance can be elicited and modified through a variety of specific techniques, including assertiveness and communication training, self and other monitoring, and anger management.

CHAPTER 16

Synthesis and Prospects
for the Future

The concept of personality disorders is continuously evolving. Successive editions of the American Psychiatric Association's *Diagnostic and Statistical Manual of Mental Disorders* have marked significant changes in the theoretical view, range of problems, definitions, and terminology used to denote personality disorders. New disorders are identified as others are eliminated. For example, the inadequate personality (301.82) and the asthenic personality (301.7) in DSM-II disappeared in DSM-III. Narcissistic personality disorder (301.81) emerged for the first time in DSM-III. Passive–aggressive personality disorder was declassified from a formal disorder to a provisional diagnosis in DSM-IV-TR, and may be reclassified again in a subsequent revision. Other terms have changed. For example, the emotionally unstable personality (51.0) in DSM-I became the hysterical personality (301.5) in DSM-II, and histrionic personality disorder (301.5) in DSM-III through DSM-IV-TR. Blashfield and Breen (1989) note the low face validity and high levels of overlap in meaning for several of the personality disorders.

Ongoing confusion is compounded when we look at the differences between the DSM-IV-TR criteria and the *International Classification of Diseases* (ICD; World Health Organization, 1998) criteria for personality disorders. It is essential that ongoing research delineate overlapping categories on Axis II and identify factors that will inform a differential diagnosis. Further, it is important that diagnostic categories offer a valid and useful conceptual framework to support effective clinical interventions.

ASSESSMENT

Effective treatment hinges on ongoing assessment and case conceptualization. One overarching objective in this assessment is to ensure that enduring traits are differentiated from more transient states attributable to circumstances or symptomatic disorders, and that maladaptive implications are tested for cultural biases. The cognitive therapist most likely integrates multiple sources of data, including diagnostic interviews, review of collateral data, behavioral observations, and self-report questionnaires. Idiographic details of the patient's operative beliefs can be pinpointed with specifically designed instruments such as the Personality Belief Questionnaire (Beck & Beck, 1991) or the Schema Questionnaire (Young, 2002b), and relative dimensions of personality features can be profiled.

CLINICAL ISSUES

As the preceding chapters show, considerable progress has been made in applying cognitive therapy in the treatment of personality disorders. However, the practitioner faces the challenge of treating a complex disorder without having a reliable, validated treatment protocol. Furthermore, to a large extent the treatment of each of the personality disorders has been considered in isolation. However, individuals seeking treatment rarely fall neatly into a single diagnostic category. When individuals with personality disorders seek treatment, they may present features of several personality disorders without fully meeting diagnostic criteria for any one personality disorder or they may qualify for more than one personality disorder, diagnosis. In addition, they typically have coexisting Axis I disorders as well.

It is not simple to provide effective treatment in the complex situations encountered in clinical practice. Fortunately, therapists do not have to start from scratch in figuring out how to approach treatment planning with patients who have personality disorders. Reviews of the empirical and clinical literature noted in this volume have provided the basis for general guidelines for cognitive therapy with patients who have personality disorders. These applied guidelines are summarized as follows:

1. *Interventions are most effective when based on an individualized conceptualization of the patient's problems.* Patients with personality disorders are complex, and the therapist is often faced with choosing among many possible targets for intervention and a variety of possible intervention techniques. Not only does this present a situation in which treatment can easily become confused and disorganized if the therapist does not have a clear treatment plan, but the interventions that seem appropriate after a superficial examination of the patient can easily prove ineffective or counterproductive. Turkat and his colleagues (especially Turkat & Maisto, 1985) have demonstrated the value of developing an individualized conceptualization based on a detailed evaluation and testing the validity of that conceptualization both through collecting additional data and through observing the effects of clinical interventions.

The conceptualizations presented in this volume can provide a starting point, but it is important to base interventions on an individualized conceptualization rather than presuming that the "standard" conceptualization will fit every patient with a particular diagnosis. Although developing an understanding of a complex patient is not simple, cognitive therapy can be a self-correcting process through which the conceptualization is refined over the course of treatment. When the therapist begins conceptualization on the basis of an initial evaluation and then bases his or her interventions on this conceptualization, the results of these interventions provide valuable feedback. The "litmus test" for any conceptualization is whether it explains past behavior, accounts for present behavior, and predicts future behavior. If the interventions work as expected, this shows that the conceptualization is accurate enough for the time being. If the interventions prove ineffective or produce unexpected results, this shows that the conceptualization is inadequate. Furthermore, examination of the thoughts and feelings evoked by the interventions may provide valuable data for refining the conceptualization and the treatment plan.

2. *It is important for therapist and patient to work collaboratively toward clearly identified, shared goals.* With patients as complex as those with personality disorders, clear, consistent goals for therapy are necessary to avoid skipping from problem to problem without making lasting progress. However, it is important for these goals to be mutually agreed on in order to minimize the noncollaboration and power struggles that often impede treatment of patients with personality disorders. It can sometimes be difficult to develop shared goals for treatment because patients may present numerous vague complaints and, at the same

time, may be unwilling to modify some of the behaviors which the therapist sees as particularly problematic. The time and effort spent developing mutually acceptable goals can be a good investment. It is likely to maximize the patient's motivation for change, minimize resistance, and make it easier to maintain a consistent focus to treatment.

3. *It is important to focus more than the usual amount of attention on the therapist–patient relationship.* A good therapeutic relationship is as necessary for effective intervention in cognitive therapy as in any other approach to therapy. Behavioral and cognitive-behavioral therapists are generally accustomed to being able to establish a straightforward collaborative relationship at the outset of therapy and then to proceed without paying much attention to the interpersonal aspects of therapy. However, when working with patients who have personality disorders, therapy often is not this straightforward. The dysfunctional schemas, beliefs, and assumptions that bias patient's perceptions of others are likely to bias their perception of the therapist, and the dysfunctional interpersonal behaviors manifest in relationships outside therapy are likely to be manifested in the patient–therapist relationship as well. Interpersonal difficulties manifested in the patient–therapist relationship can disrupt therapy if they are not addressed effectively. However, these difficulties also provide the therapist with an opportunity to do *in vivo* observation and intervention rather than having to rely on the patient's report of interpersonal problems occurring between sessions (Freeman, Pretzer, Fleming, & Simon, 1990; Linehan, 1987a; Mays, 1985; Padesky, 1986).

One type of problem in the therapist–patient relationship that is more common among individuals with personality disorders than among other individuals in cognitive therapy is the phenomenon traditionally termed "transference." This term is traditionally used to refer to times when the patient manifests an extreme or persistent misperception of the therapist based on the patient's previous experience in significant relationships, rather than on the therapist's behavior. This phenomenon can be understood in cognitive terms as resulting from the individual overgeneralizing the beliefs and expectancies they acquired in significant relationships. Individuals with personality disorders are typically vigilant for any sign that their fears may be realized and are prone to react quite intensely when the therapist's behavior appears to confirm their anticipations. When these strongly emotional reactions occur, it is important for the therapist to recognize what is happening, to quickly develop an understanding of what the patient is thinking, and to directly but sensitively address these misconceptions within the therapy. Although these reactions can be quite problematic, they also provide opportunities to identify beliefs, expectations, and interpersonal strategies that play an important role in the patient's problems. This also is an opportunity for the therapist to respond to the patient in ways that disconfirm the patient's dysfunctional beliefs and expectancies.

4. *Consider beginning with interventions that do not require extensive self-disclosure.* Many patients with personality disorders are initially uncomfortable with self-disclosure in psychotherapy. They may not trust the therapist, may be uncomfortable with even mild levels of intimacy, may fear rejection, and so on. It is sometimes necessary to begin treatment with interventions that require extensive discussion of the patient's thoughts and feelings, but often treatment can begin with behavioral interventions that gradually introduce self-disclosure. This allows time for the patient to become more comfortable with therapy and for the therapist to gain the patient's trust and explore the reasons for discomfort with self-disclosure.

5. *Interventions that increase the patient's sense of self-efficacy often reduce the intensity of the patient's symptomatology and facilitate other interventions.* The intensity of the emotional and behavioral responses manifested by individuals with personality disorders is often due in part to the individual's doubts regarding his or her ability to cope effectively with particular problem situations. This doubt regarding one's ability to cope effectively not only intensifies emotional responses to the situation but also predisposes the individual to drastic responses. When it is possible to increase the individual's confidence that he or she will be able to handle problem situations as they arise, this often lowers the patient's level of anxiety, moderates his or her symptomatology, enables him or her to react more deliberately, and makes it easier to implement other interventions. The individual's sense of self-efficacy, his or her confidence that he or she can deal effectively with specific situations when they arise, can be increased through interventions that correct any exaggerations of the demands of the situation or minimization of the individual's capabilities, through helping the individual to improve his or her coping skills, or through a combination of the two (Freeman et al., 1990; Pretzer, Beck, & Newman, 1989).

6. *Do not rely primarily on verbal interventions.* The more severe a patient's problems are, the more important it is to use behavioral interventions to accomplish cognitive as well as behavioral change (Freeman et al., 1990). Role playing within the session and a gradual hierarchy of "behavioral experiments" between sessions provides an opportunity for desensitization to occur, helps the patient to master new skills, and can be quite effective in challenging unrealistic beliefs and expectations. When it is necessary to rely on purely verbal interventions, concrete, real-life examples often are more effective than abstract, philosophical discussions.

7. *Try to identify and address the patient's fears before implementing changes.* Patients with personality disorders often have strong, unex-

pressed fears about the changes they seek or that they are asked to make in the course of therapy. Attempts to induce the patient to simply go ahead without addressing these fears are often unsuccessful (Mays, 1985). If the therapist makes a practice of discussing the patient's expectations and concerns before each change is attempted, it is likely to reduce the patient's level of anxiety regarding therapy and to improve compliance.

8. *Help the patient deal adaptively with aversive emotions.* Patients with personality disorders often experience very intense aversive emotional reactions in specific situations. These intense reactions can be a significant problem in their own right, but in addition, the individual's attempts to avoid experiencing these emotions, his or her attempts to escape the emotions, and his or her cognitive and behavioral response to the emotions often play an important role in the patient's problems. Often, the individual's unwillingness to tolerate aversive affect blocks him or her from handling the emotions adaptively and perpetuates fears about the consequences of experiencing the emotions. When this is the case, it can be important to work systematically to increase the patient's ability to tolerate intense affect and cope effectively with it (Farrell & Shaw, 1994).

9. *Help patients cope with aversive emotions that can be elicited by therapeutic interventions.* In addition to the intense emotions patients experience in day-to-day life, therapy itself can elicit strong emotions. When therapy involves facing one's fears, making major life changes, risking self-disclosure, addressing painful memories, and so on, it can provoke a range of emotional responses. It is important for the therapist to recognize painful emotions provoked by therapy and to help the patient understand them and cope with them. Otherwise, there is a risk that these emotions will drive the patient from therapy. If the therapist makes a habit of obtaining feedback from the patient on a regular basis and watches for nonverbal signs of emotional reactions during the therapy session, it usually is not difficult to recognize problematic emotional reactions. When these reactions occur, it is important for the therapist to develop an understanding of the patient's thoughts and feelings and to help the patient understand his or her own reactions. Often the intensity of the patient's reactions can be moderated by collaborating about the pace of therapy and proceeding in smaller steps. It is important to pace therapy so that the benefits of therapy outweigh the drawbacks and to make sure that the patient recognizes this.

10. *Anticipate problems with completion of assignments.* Many factors contribute to a high rate of assignment noncompletion among patients with personality disorders. In addition to the complexities in the therapist–patient relationship and the fears regarding change discussed earlier, the dysfunctional behaviors of individuals with personality disor-

ders are strongly ingrained and often are reinforced by aspects of the patient's environment. However, rather than simply being an impediment to progress, episodes of noncompletion can provide an opportunity for effective intervention. The most important response may be to increase the collaboration and assess for any issues that are interfering with mutual participation in therapy. Through this collaborative process, further issues that block the patient's progress can be addressed. A plan to pinpoint the thoughts that occur at the times when the patient thinks of acting on the therapy assignment but decides not to often reveals the most significant impediments that need to be overcome.

11. *Do not presume that the patient exists in a reasonable environment.* Some behaviors, such as assertion, are so frequently adaptive that it is easy to assume they are always a good idea. However, patients with personality disorders are often the product of seriously atypical families and often live in atypical environments. When implementing changes, it is important to assess the likely responses of significant others in the patient's environment rather than presuming that others will respond in a reasonable way. Often it is useful to have the patient initially experiment with new behaviors in low-risk situations. This arouses less anxiety and provides the patient with a chance to polish his or her skills before facing more challenging situations.

12. *Limit setting is often an essential part of the overall treatment program.* Setting firm, reasonable limits and enforcing them consistently serves several purposes in therapy with Axis II patients. First, it helps patients to organize their lives in more adaptive ways and protects them from behavioral excesses that cause problems for them and others. Second, it provides an opportunity for the therapist to model a structured, reasoned approach to problem solving. Third, it provides a structure for maintaining a long-term and possible stormy therapeutic relationship. Finally, appropriate limits minimize the risk that the therapist will feel taken advantage of and become resentful.

It might seem a good thing for the therapist to be generous and extend him- or herself in attempting to help a patient who is in great distress, but such "generosity" can easily backfire. Special treatment that seems acceptable in the short run can become galling when demands for special treatment persist month after month. If the therapist allows a situation to develop that causes him or her to feel resentful, a major impediment to effective treatment has also developed. It is particularly important not to inadvertently reinforce dysfunctional behavior by responding in ways that reward the patient for being in distress.

13. *Attend to your own emotional reactions during the course of therapy.* Interactions with personality-disordered patients elicit many emotional reactions from the therapist, ranging from empathic feelings

of depression to strong anger, discouragement, fear, or sexual attraction. It is important for the therapist to be aware of these responses so that they can be used as a source of potentially useful data. Therapists may benefit from using cognitive techniques (such as the Dysfunctional Thought Record; Beck, Rush, Shaw, & Emery, 1979), reviewing their case conceptualization, and/or seeking consultation with an objective colleague. Emotions within the therapist should be considered an expected response that can inform the process of therapy, and should not be considered mistakes or errors per se. Attempts to avoid or suppress emotional responses may increase the risk of mismanaging the therapeutic interaction.

Emotional responses do not occur randomly. An unusually strong emotional response on the therapist's part is often a reaction to some aspect of the patient's behavior, although there may well be other more salient determinants, such as the therapist's history or professional issues. Because a therapist may respond emotionally to a pattern in the patient's behavior long before it has been recognized intellectually, accurate interpretation of one's own responses can speed recognition of these patterns.

Careful thought is needed regarding whether or not to disclose these reactions to the patient and how to manage any disclosure therapeutically. On the one hand, patients with personality disorders may react strongly to therapist self-disclosure, easily misinterpreting this information. On the other hand, if the therapist does not disclose an emotional reaction that is apparent to the patient from nonverbal cues or that the patient anticipates on the basis of experiences in other relationships, it can easily lead to misunderstandings or distrust. This decision is best considered within a thoughtful context of the case conceptualization, the patient's current issues, the state of the therapeutic rapport, and the therapist's level of arousal and ability to cope.

14. *Be realistic regarding the length of therapy, goals for therapy, and standards for therapist self-evaluation.* Many therapists using behavioral and cognitive-behavioral approaches are accustomed to accomplishing substantial results relatively quickly. One can easily become frustrated and angry with the "resistant" patient when therapy proceeds slowly, or become self-critical and discouraged when therapy goes badly. When treatment is unsuccessful, it is important to remember that many factors influence outcome, and therapist competence is only one of those factors. When therapy proceeds slowly, it is important neither to give up prematurely nor to perseverate with an unsuccessful approach. Behavioral and cognitive-behavioral interventions can accomplish substantial, lasting changes in some patients with personality disorders, but more modest results are achieved in other cases, and little is accomplished in others, at least in the immediate term.

CONCLUSION

The past decade has marked rapid growth in mapping specific cognitive features of personality disorders. Perhaps the newest frontier for future work, in addition to further establishing clinical efficacy of the cognitive treatment of Axis II disorders, may be in articulating the process of change in disorders of personality. As we move well into the first decade of the 21st century, we have even more hope that personality conditions, once widely considered refractory to therapeutic interventions, will be found to be modifiable in the same way as affective and anxiety disorders.

References

Abraham, K. (1927). The influence of oral eroticism on character formation. In *Selected papers on psychoanalysis*. London: Hogarth Press. (Original work published 1924)

Abraham, K. (1949). Manifestations of the female castration complex. In *Selected papers of Karl Abraham*. London: Hogarth Press. (Original work published 1920)

Abraham, K. (1953). Contributions to the theory of the anal character. In *Selected papers of Karl Abraham* (D. Bryan & A. Strachey, Trans.). New York: Basic Books. (Original work published 1921)

Adams, P. (1973). *Obsessive children: A sociopsychiatric study*. New York: Brunner/Mazel.

Adams, H. E., Bernat, J. A., & Luscher, K. A. (2001). Borderline personality disorder: An overview. In P. B. Sutker & H. E. Adams (Eds.), *Comprehensive handbook of psychopathology* (pp. 491–507). New York: Kluwer Academic/Plenum Press.

Adler, A. (1991). *The practice and theory of individual psychology*. Birmingham, AL: Classics of Psychiatry & Behavioral Sciences Library. (Original work published 1929)

American Psychiatric Association. (1952). *Diagnostic and statistical manual of mental disorders* (1st ed.). Washington, DC: Author.

American Psychiatric Association. (1968). *Diagnostic and statistical manual of mental disorders* (2nd ed.). Washington, DC: Author.

American Psychiatric Association. (1980). *Diagnostic and statistical manual of mental disorders* (3rd ed.). Washington, DC: Author.

American Psychiatric Association. (1987). *Diagnostic and statistical manual of mental disorders* (3rd ed., rev.). Washington, DC: Author.

American Psychiatric Association. (1989). Passive–aggressive personality disorder. In *Treatments of psychiatric disorders: A task force report of the American Psychiatric Association* (pp. 2783–2789). Washington, DC: Author.

American Psychiatric Association. (1994). *Diagnostic and statistical manual of mental disorders* (4th ed.). Washington, DC: Author.

American Psychiatric Association. (2000). *Diagnostic and statistical manual of mental disorders* (4th ed., text rev.). Washington, DC: Author.

American Psychological Association. (2002). *Ethical principles of psychologists and code of conduct*. Washington, DC: Author.

Anderson, R. (1966). *Neuropsychiatry in World War II* (Vol 1). Washington, DC: Office of the Surgeon General, Department of the Army.

Angyal, A. (1965). *Neurosis and treatment: A holistic theory.* New York: Viking Press.

Arntz, A. (1994). Treatment of borderline personality disorder: A challenge for cognitive-behavioural therapy. *Behaviour Research and Therapy, 32,* 419–430.

Arntz, A. (1999a). Do personality disorders exist?: On the validity of the concept and its cognitive-behavioural formulation and treatment. *Behaviour Research and Therapy, 37,* S97–S134.

Arntz, A. (1999b). *Borderline personality disorder.* Invited lecture presented at the 29th annual Congress of the European Association for Behavioural and Cognitive Therapies, Dresden, Germany.

Arntz, A., Appels, C., & Sieswerda, S. (2000). Hypervigilance in borderline personality disorder: A test with the emotional Stroop paradigm. *Journal of Personality Disorders, 14,* 366–373.

Arntz, A., Dietzel, R., & Dreessen, L. (1999). Assumptions in borderline personality disorder: Specificity, stability, and relationship with etiological factors. *Behaviour Research and Therapy, 37,* 545–557.

Arntz, A., Dreessen, L., Schouten, E., & Weertman, A. (in press). Beliefs in personality disorders: A test with the Personality Disorder Belief Questionnaire. *Behavior Research and Therapy.*

Arntz, A., Klokman, J., & Sieswerda, S. (2003). An experimental test of the Schema Mode Model of borderline personality disorder. *Journal of Behavior Therapy and Experimental Psychiatry.* Manuscript accepted pending revision.

Arntz, A., & Veen, G. (2001). Evaluations of others by borderline patients. *Journal of Nervous and Mental Disease, 189,* 513–521.

Arntz, A., & Weertman, A. (1999). Treatment of childhood memories: Theory and practice. *Behaviour Research and Therapy, 37,* 715–740.

Baker, J. D., Capron, E. W., & Azorlosa, J. (1996). Family environment characteristics of persons with histrionic and dependent personality disorders. *Journal of Personality Disorders, 10,* 82–87.

Baker, L., Silk, K. R., Westen, D., Nigg, J. T., & Lohr, N. E. (1992). Malevolence, splitting, and parental ratings by borderlines. *Journal of Nervous and Mental Disease, 180,* 258–264.

Bandura, A. (1977). *Social learning theory.* Englewood Cliffs, NJ: Prentice-Hall.

Barber, J. P., & Muenz, L. R. (1996). The role of avoidance and obsessiveness in matching patients to cognitive and interpersonal psychotherapy: Empirical findings from the Treatment for Depression Collaborative Research Program. *Journal of Consulting and Clinical Psychology, 64*(5), 951–958.

Bartlett, F. C. (1932). *Remembering.* New York: Columbia University Press.

Bartlett, F. C. (1958). *Thinking: An experimental and social study.* New York: Basic Books.

Baumbacher, G., & Amini, F. (1980–1981). The hysterical personality disorder: A proposed clarification of a diagnostic dilemma. *International Journal of Psychoanalytic Psychotherapy, 8,* 501–532.

Baumeister, R. (2001, April). Violent pride. *Scientific American, 284*(4), 96–101.

Baumeister, R., Bushman, B., & Campbell, W. K (2000). Self-esteem, narcissism, and aggression: Does violence result from low self-esteem or from threatened egotism? *Current Directions in Psychological Science, 9,* 26–29.

Baumeister, R., Smart, L., & Boden, J. (1996). Relation of threatened egotism to violence and aggression: The dark side of high self-esteem. *Psychological Review, 103,* 5–33.

Beck, A. T. (1963). Thinking and depression: I. Idiosyncratic content and cognitive distortions. *Archives of General Psychiatry, 9,* 324–344.

Beck, A. T. (1964). Thinking and depression: II. Theory and therapy. *Archives of General Psychiatry, 10,* 561–571.

Beck, A. T. (1967). Depression: Clinical, experimental and theoretical aspects. New York: Harper & Row. (Republished as *Depression: Causes and treatment.* Philadelphia: University of Pennsylvania Press, 1972)

Beck, A. T. (1976). *Cognitive therapy and the emotional disorders.* New York: International Universities Press.

Beck, A. T. (1983). Cognitive therapy of depression: New perspectives. In P. J. Clayton & J. E. Barrett (Eds.), *Treatment of depression: Old controversies and new approaches.* New York: Raven Press.

Beck, A. T. (1988). *Love is never enough.* New York: Harper & Row.

Beck, A. T. (2002, December). *Cognitive therapy of borderline personality disorder and attempted suicide.* Paper presented at the 1st annual conference of the Treatment and Research Advancements Association for Personality Disorders, Bethesda, MD.

Beck, A. T., & Beck, J. S. (1991). *The Personality Belief Questionnaire.* Bala Cynwyd, PA: Beck Institute for Cognitive Therapy and Research.

Beck, A. T., Butler, A. C., Brown, G. K., Dahlsgaard, K. K., Newman, C. F., & Beck, J. S. (2001). Dysfunctional beliefs discriminate personality disorders. *Behaviour Research and Therapy, 39*(10), 1213–1225.

Beck, A. T., & Emery, G., with Greenberg, R. L. (1985). *Anxiety disorders and phobias: A cognitive perspective.* New York: Basic Books.

Beck, A. T., Freeman, A., & Associates. (1990). *Cognitive therapy of personality disorders.* New York: Guilford Press.

Beck, A. T., Rush, A. J., Shaw, B. F., & Emery, G. (1979). *Cognitive therapy of depression.* New York: Guilford Press.

Beck, J. S. (1995). *Cognitive therapy: Basics and beyond.* New York: Guilford Press.

Bentall, R. P., & Kaney, S. (1989). Content-specific information processing and persecutory delusions: An investigation using the emotional Stroop test. *British Journal of Medical Psychology 62,* 355–364.

Bentall, R. P., Kinderman, P., & Kaney, S. (1994). The self, attributional processes and abnormal beliefs: Towards a model of persecutory delusions. *Behaviour Research and Therapy, 32,* 331–341.

Berk, M. S., Forman, E. M., Henriques, G. R., Brown, G. K., & Beck, A. T., (2002, August). *Characteristics of suicide attempters with borderline personality disorder.* Paper presented at the annual conference of the American Psychological Association, Chicago.

Bernstein, D. A., & Borkovec, T. D. (1976). *Progressive relaxation training: A manual for the helping professionals.* Champaign, IL: Research Press.

Bijttebier, P., & Vertommen, H. (1999). Coping strategies in relation to personality disorders. *Personality and Individual Differences, 26,* 847–856.

Bird, J. (1979). The behavioural treatment of hysteria. *British Journal of Psychiatry, 134,* 129–137.

Birtchnell, J. (1984). Dependence and its relationship to depression. *British Journal of Medical Psychology, 57,* 215–225.

Black, D. W., Monahan, P., Wesner, R., Gabel, J., & Bowers, W. (1996). The effect of fluvoxamine, cognitive therapy, and placebo on abnormal personality traits in 44 patients with panic disorder. *Journal of Personality Disorders, 10*(2), 185–194.

Blackburn, R., & Lee-Evans, J. M. (1985). Reactions of primary and secondary psychopaths to anger-evoking situations. *British Journal of Clinical Psychology, 24,* 93—100.

Blashfield, R. K., & Breen, M. J. (1989). Face validity of the DSM-III-R personality disorders. *American Journal of Psychiatry, 146,* 1575–1579.

Bohus, M., Limberger, M., Ebner, U., Glocker, F. X., Schwarz, B., Wernz, M., & Lieb, K. (2000). Pain perception during self-reported distress and calmness in patients with borderline personality disorder and self-mutilating behavior. *Psychiatric Research, 95,* 251–260.

Bornstein, R. F. (1996). Sex differences in dependent personality disorder prevalence rates. *Clinical Psychology: Science and Practice, 3,* 1–12.

Bornstein, R. F. (1999). Histrionic personality disorder, physical attractiveness, and social adjustment. *Journal of Psychopathology and Behavioral Assessment, 21,* 79–94.

Bourne, E. J. (1995). *The anxiety and phobia workbook* (2nd ed.). Oakland, CA: New Harbinger.

Bowlby, J. (1969). *Attachment and loss: Vol. 1. Attachment.* New York: Basic Books.

Bowlby, J. (1977). The making and breaking of affectional bonds. *British Journal of Psychiatry, 130,* 201–210.

Breier, A., & Strauss, J. S. (1983). Self control in psychotic disorders. *Archives of General Psychiatry, 130,* 201–210.

Breuer, J., & Freud, S. (1955). Studies on hysteria. In J. Strachey (Ed. and Trans.), *The standard edition of the complete psychological works of Sigmund Freud* (Vol. 2, pp. 1–311). London: Hogarth Press. (Original work published 1893–1895)

Brown, E. J., Heimberg, R. G., & Juster, H. R. (1995). Social phobia subtype and avoidant personality disorder: Effect on severity of social phobia, impairment, and outcome of cognitive-behavioral treatment. *Behavior Therapy, 26,* 467–486.

Brown, G. K., Newman, C. F., Charlesworth, S., & Crits-Cristoph, P. (in press). An open clinical trial of cognitive therapy for borderline personality disorder. *Journal of Personality Disorders.*

Bushman, B., & Baumeister, R. (1998). Threatened egotism, narcissism, self-esteem, and direct and displaced aggression: Does self-love or self-hate lead to violence? *Journal of Personality and Social Psychology, 75,* 219–229.

Buss, A. H. (1987). Personality: Primitive heritage and human distinctiveness. In J. Aronoff, A. I. Robin, & R. A. Zucker (Eds.), *The emergence of personality* (pp. 13–48). New York: Springer.

Butler, A. C., & Beck, A. T. (2002). *Parallel forms of the Personality Belief Questionnaire.* Manuscript in preparation.

Butler, A. C., Brown, G. K., Beck, A. T., & Grisham, J. R. (2002). Assessment of dysfunctional beliefs in borderline personality disorder. *Behaviour Research and Therapy, 40*(1), 1231–1240.

Cadenhead, K. S., Perry, W., Shafer, K., & Braff, D. L. (1999). Cognitive functions in schizotypal personality disorder. *Schizophrenia Research 37,* 123–132.

Cale, E. M., & Lilienfeld, S. O. (2002). Histrionic Personality Disorder and Antisocial Personality Disorder: Sex-differentiated manifestations of psychopathy? *Journal of Personality Disorders, 16,* 52–72.

Cameron, N. (1963). *Personality development and psychopathology: A dynamic approach.* Boston: Houghton-Mifflin.

Cameron, N. (1974). Paranoid conditions and paranoia. In S. Arieti & E. Brody (Eds.), *American handbook of psychiatry* (Vol. 3, pp. 676–693). New York: Basic Books.

Campbell, R. J. (1981). *Psychiatric dictionary* (5th ed.). New York: Oxford University Press.

Chadwick, P., & Lowe, C. F. (1990). The measurement and modification of delusional beliefs. *Journal of Consulting and Clinical Psychology, 58,* 225–232.

Chambless, D. L., & Hope, D. A. (1996). Cognitive approaches to the psychopathology and treatment of social phobia. In P. M. Salkovskis (Ed.), *Frontiers of cognitive therapy* (pp. 345–382). New York: Guilford Press.

Chambless, D. L., Renneberg, B., Goldstein, A., & Gracely, E. J. (1992). MCMI-diagnosed personality disorders among agoraphobic outpatients: Prevalence and relationship to severity and treatment outcome. *Journal of Anxiety Disorders, 6*(3), 193–211.

Chatham, P. M. (1985). *Treatment of the borderline personality.* New York: Jason Aronson.

Clark, D. A., & Beck, A. T., with Alford, B. A. (1999). *Scientific foundations of cognitive theory and therapy of depression.* New York: Wiley.

Clark, D. M. (1999). Anxiety disorders: Why they persist and how to treat them. *Behaviour Research and Therapy, 37*(Suppl.), 5–27.

Clark, L. A. (1993). *Manual for the Schedule for Nonadaptive and Adaptive Personality.* Minneapolis: University of Minnesota Press.

Clark, L. A. (1999). Dimensional approaches to personality disorder assessment and diagnosis. In C. R. Cloninger (Ed.), *Personality and psychopathology* (pp. 219–244). Washington, DC: American Psychiatric Press.

Clarkin, J. F., Koenigsberg, H., Yeomans, F., Selzer, M., Kernberg, P., & Kernberg, O. F. (1994). Psychodynamische psychotherapie bij de borderline patiënt. (Psychodynamic psychotherapy with borderline patients.) In J. J. L. Derksen & H. Groen (Eds.), *Handboek voor de behandeling van borderline patiënten, (Handbook of treatment of borderline patients)* (pp. 69–82). Utrecht: De Tijdstroom.

Cleckley, H. (1976). *The mask of sanity* (5th ed.). St. Louis: Mosby.

Clifford, C. A., Murray, R. M., & Fulker, D. W. (1984). Genetic and environmental influences on obsessional traits and symptoms. *Psychological Medicine, 14*(4), 791–800.

Colby, K. M. (1981) Modeling a paranoid mind. *Behavioral and Brain Sciences, 4,* 515–560.

Colby, K. M., Faught, W. S., & Parkinson, R. C. (1979). Cognitive therapy of paranoid conditions: Heuristic suggestions based on a computer simulation model. *Cognitive Therapy and Research, 3,* 55–60.

Colvin, C. R., Block, J., & Funder, D. C. (1995). Overly positive self-evaluations and personality: Negative implications for mental health. *Journal of Personality and Social Psychology, 68,* 1152–1162.

Coolidge, F. L., Thede, L. L., & Jang, K. L. (2001). Heritability of personality disorders in childhood: A preliminary investigation. *Journal of Personality Disorders, 15,* 33–40.

Costa, P. T., & McCrae, R. R. (1992). The five-factor model of personality and its relevance to personality disorders. *Journal of Personality Disorders, 6,* 343–359.

Cowdry, R. W., & Gardner, D. (1988). Pharmacotherapy of borderline personality disorder: alprazolam, carmabazepine, trifluoperazine and tranylcypromine. *Archives of General Psychiatry, 45,* 111–119.

Cowdry, R. W., Gardner, D., O'Leary, K., Leibenluft, E., & Rubinow, D. (1991). Mood variability: A study of four groups. *American Journal of Psychiatry, 148,* 1505–1511.

Dattilio, F. M., & Padesky, C. A. (1990). *Cognitive therapy with couples.* Sarasota, FL: Professional Resource Exchange.

Davidson, K. M., & Tyrer, P. (1996). Cognitive therapy for antisocial and borderline personality disorders: Single case study series. *British Journal of Clinical Psychology, 35,* 413–429.

Davis, D., & Hollon, S. (1999). Reframing resistance and noncompliance in cognitive therapy. *Journal of Psychotherapy Integration, 9*(1), 33–55.

Delphin, M. E. (2002, August). Gender and ethnic bias in the diagnosis of antisocial and borderline personality disorders. *Dissertation Abstracts International, Humanities and Social Sciences, 63,* 767A.

Diaferia, G., Sciuto, G., Perna, G., Bernardeschi, L., Battaglia, M., Rusmini, S., & Bellodi, L. (1993). DSM-III-R personality disorders in panic disorder. *Journal of Anxiety Disorders, 7,* 153–161.

DiGiuseppe, R. (1986). The implication of the philosophy of science for rational-emotive theory and therapy. *Psychotherapy, 23*(4), 634–639.

DiGiuseppe, R. (1989). Cognitive therapy with children. In A. Freeman, K. M. Simon, L. Beutler, & H. Arkowitz (Eds.), *Comprehensive handbook of cognitive therapy* (pp. 515–533). New York: Plenum Press.

DiGiuseppe, R. (2001). *Redirecting anger toward self change.* World Rounds Video. New York: AABT.

Dimeff, L. A., McDavid, J., & Linehan, M. M. (1999). Pharmacotherapy for borderline personality disorder: A review of the literature and recommendations for treatment. *Journal of Clinical Psychology in Medical Settings, 6,* 113–138.

Dlugos, R. F., & Friedlander, M. L. (2001). Passionately committed psychotherapists: A qualitative study of their experience. *Professional Psychology: Research and Practice, 32*(3), 298–304.

Dobson, K. S., & Pusch, D. (1993). Towards a definition of the conceptual and empirical boundaries of cognitive therapy. *Australian Psychologist, 28,* 137–144.

Dowd, E. T. (2000). *Cognitive hypnotherapy.* Northvale, NJ: Jason Aronson.

Dowrick, P. W. (Ed.). (1991) *Practical guide to using video in the behavioural sciences.* New York: Wiley.

Dreessen, L., & Arntz, A. (1998). The impact of personality disorders on treatment outcome of anxiety disorders: Best-evidence synthesis. *Behaviour Research and Therapy, 36,* 483–504.

Dreessen, L., Arntz, A., Luttels, C., & Sallaerts, S. (1994). Personality disorders do not influence the results of cognitive behavior therapies for anxiety disorders. *Comprehensive Psychiatry, 35,* 265–274.

Dumas, P., Souad, M., Bouafia, S., Gutknecht, C., Ecochard, R., Dalery, J., Rochet, T., & d'Amato, T. (2002). Cannabis use correlates with schizotypal personality traits in healthy students. *Psychiatry Research, 109,* 27–35.

Dutton, D. G., & Hart, S. D. (1992). Risk markers for family violence in a federally incarcerated population. *International Journal of Law and Psychiatry, 15,* 101–112.

D'Zurilla, T. J., & Goldfried, M. R. (1971). Problem solving and behavior modification. *Journal of Abnormal Psychology, 78,* 107–126.

Easser, B. R., & Lesser, S. R. (1965). Hysterical personality: A reevaluation. *Psychoanalytic Quarterly, 34,* 390–415.

Eisely, L. (1961). *Darwin's century.* Garden City, NY: Doubleday/Anchor.

Ellis, A. (1962). *Reason and emotion in psychotherapy.* New York: Lyle Stuart.

Ellis, A. (1985). *Overcoming resistance: Rational-emotive therapy with difficult clients.* New York: Springer.

Ellis, H. (1898). Auto-eroticism: A psychological study. *Alienist and Neurologist, 19,* 260–299.

Erikson, E. (1950). *Childhood and society.* New York: Norton.

Esman, A. H. (1986). Dependent and passive–aggressive personality disorders. In A. M. Cooper, A. J. Frances, & M. H. Sacks (Eds.), *The personality disorders and neuroses* (pp. 283–289). New York: Basic Books.

Fagan, T. J., & Lira, F. T. (1980). The primary and secondary sociopathic personality: Differences in frequency and severity of antisocial behavior. *Journal of Abnormal Psychology, 89*(3), 493–496.

Fahy, T. A., Eisler, I., & Russell, G. F. (1993). Personality disorder and treatment response in bulimia nervosa. *British Journal of Psychiatry, 162,* 765–770.

Farrell, J. M., & Shaw, I. A. (1994). Emotion awareness training: A prerequisite to effective cognitive-behavioral treatment of borderline personality disorder. *Cognitive and Behavioral Practice, 1,* 71–91.

Felske, U., Perry, K. J., Chambless, D. L., Renneberg, B., & Goldstein, A. J. (1996). Avoidant personality disorder as a predictor for treatment outcome among generalized social phobics. *Journal of Personality Disorders, 10,* 174–184.

Fenichel, O. (1945). *The psychoanalytic theory of neuroses.* New York: Norton.

First, M. B., Spitzer, R. L., Gibbon, M., & Williams, J. B. W. (1995). The Structured Clinical Interview for DSM-III-R Personality Disorders (SCID-II): Part I. Description. *Journal of Personality Disorders, 9,* 83–91.

Fleming, B., & Pretzer, J. (1990). Cognitive-behavioral approaches to personality disorders. In M. Hersen, R. M. Eisler, & P. M. Miller (Eds.), *Progress in behavior modification* (Vol. 25, pp. 119–151). Newbury Park, CA: Sage.

Fonagy, P., Leigh, T., Steele, M., Steele, H., Kennedy, R., Mattoon, G., et al. (1996). The relation of attachment status, psychiatric classification, and response to psychotherapy. *Journal of Consulting and Clinical Psychology, 64*, 22–31.

Fossati, A., Madeddu, F., & Maffei, C. (1999). Borderline personality disorder and childhood sexual abuse: A meta-analytic study. *Journal of Personality Disorders, 13*, 268–280.

Fossati, A., Maffei, C., Bagnato, M., Donati, D., Donini, M., Fiorelli, M., & Norella, L. (2000). A psychometric study of DSM-IV passive–aggressive (negativistic) personality disorder criteria. *Journal of Personality Disorders, 14*(1), 72–83.

Frances, A. (1980). The DSM-III personality disorders section: A commentary. *American Journal of Psychiatry, 137*(9), 1050–1054.

Frances, A. (1988). Dependency and attachment. *Journal of Personality Disorders, 2*, 125.

Freeman, A. (1987). Understanding personal, cultural, and religious schema in psychotherapy. In A. Freeman, N. Epstein, & K. Simon (Eds.), *Depression in the family* (pp. 79–99). New York: Haworth Press.

Freeman, A. (1988) Cognitive therapy of personality disorders. In C. Perris & M. Eismann (Eds.), *Cognitive psychotherapy: An update* (pp. 49–52). Umea: DOPW Press.

Freeman, A. (1990). *Clinical applications of cognitive therapy.* New York: Plenum Press.

Freeman, A. (2002). *Cognitive-behavioral therapy for severe personality disorders.* In S. G. Hofmann & M. C. Thompson (Eds.), *Treating chronic and severe mental disorders* (pp. 382–402). New York: Guilford Press.

Freeman, A., & Datillio, F. M. (Eds.). (1992). *Comprehensive casebook of clinical psychology.* New York: Plenum Press.

Freeman, A., & Dolan, M. (2001). Revisiting Prochaska and DiClemente's stages of change theory: An expansion and specification to aid in treatment planning and outcome evaluation. *Cognitive and Behavioral Practice, 8*(3), 224–234.

Freeman, A., & Leaf, R. (1989). Cognitive therapy applied to personality disorders. In A. Freeman, K. Simon, L. Beutler, & H. Arkowitz (Eds.), *Comprehensive handbook of cognitive therapy* (pp. 403–433). New York: Plenum Press.

Freeman, A., Pretzer, J., Fleming, B., & Simon, K. M. (1990). *Clinical applications of cognitive therapy.* New York: Plenum Press.

Freeston, M. H., Rheaume, J., & Ladoucer, R. (1996). Correcting faulty appraisals of obsessional thoughts. *Behaviour Research and Therapy, 34*, 433–446.

Freud, S. (1953). Three essays on the theory of sexuality. In J. Strachey (Ed. and Trans.), *The standard edition of the complete psychological works of Sigmund Freud* (Vol. 7, pp, 255–268). London: Hogarth Press. (Original work published 1905)

Freud, S. (1955). Notes upon a case of obsessional neurosis. In J. Strachey (Ed. and Trans.), *The standard edition of the complete psychological works of Sigmund Freud* (Vol. 10, pp. 151–320). London: Hogarth Press. (Original work published 1909)

Freud, S. (1957). On narcissism: An introduction. In J. Strachey (Ed. and Trans.), *The standard edition of the complete psychological works of Sigmund Freud* (Vol. 14, pp. 67–102). London: Hogarth Press. (Original work published 1914)

Freud, S. (1989). Character and anal eroticism. In P. Gay (Ed.), *The Freud Reader* (pp. 293–297). New York: Norton. (Original work published 1908)

Gardner, D. L., & Cowdry, R. W. (1985). Alprazolam-induced dyscontrol in borderline personality disorder. *American Journal of Psychiatry, 142*, 98–100.

Gasperini, M., Provenza, M., Ronchi, P., Scherillo, P., Bellodi, L., & Smeraldi, E. (1989). Cognitive processes and personality disorders in affective patients. *Journal of Personality Disorders, 3*, 63–71.

Giesen-Bloo, J., & Arntz, A. (2003). World assumptions and the role of trauma in borderline personality disorder. *Journal of Behavior Therapy and Experimental Psychiatry.* Manuscript accepted pending revision.

Giesen-Bloo, J., Arntz, A., van Dyck, R., Spinhoven, P., & van Tilburg, W. (2001, July). *Outpatient treatment of borderline personality disorder: Analytical psychotherapy versus cognitive behavior therapy.* Paper presented at the World Congress of Behavioral and Cognitive Therapies, Vancouver.

Giesen-Bloo, J., Arntz, A., van Dyck, R., Spinhoven, P., & van Tilburg, W. (2002, November). *Outpatient treatment of borderline personality disorder: Schema focused therapy vs. transference focused psychotherapy, preliminary results of an ongoing multicenter trial.* Paper presented at the symposium on "Transference Focused Psychotherapy for Borderline Personality," New York.

Gilbert, P. (1989). *Human nature and suffering.* Hillsdale, NJ: Erlbaum.

Gilligan, C. (1982). *In a different voice.* Cambridge, MA: Harvard University Press.

Gilson, M. L. (1983). Depression as measured by perceptual bias in binocular rivalry. *Dissertation Abstracts International, 44*(8B), 2555 (University Microfilms No. AAD83–27351)

Goldstein, A. P., Martens, J., Hubben, J., Van Belle, H. A., Schaaf, W., Wirsma, H., & Goedhart, A. (1973). The use of modeling to increase independent behavior. *Behaviour Research and Therapy, 11,* 31–42.

Goldstein, W. (1985). *An introduction to the borderline conditions.* Northvale, NJ: Jason Aronson.

Gradman, T. J., Thompson, L. W., & Gallagher-Thompson, D. (1999). Personality disorders and treatment outcome. In E. Rosowsky, R. C. Abrams, & R. A. Zweig (Eds.), *Personality disorders in older adults: Emerging issues in diagnosis and treatment* (pp. 69–94). Mahwah, NJ: Erlbaum.

Greenberg, D., & Stravynski, A. (1985). Patients who complain of social dysfunction: I. Clinical and demographic features. *Canadian Journal of Psychiatry, 30,* 206–211.

Greenberg, R. P., & Bornstein, R. F. (1988). The dependent personality: I. Risk for physical disorders. *Journal of Personality Disorders, 2,* 126–135.

Greenberg, R. P., & Dattore, P. J. (1981). The relationship between dependency and the development of cancer. *Psychosomatic Medicine, 43,* 35–43.

Greenberger, D., & Padesky, C. A. (1995). *Mind over mood: Change how you feel by changing the way you think.* New York: Guilford Press.

Gresham, F. M., MacMillan, D. L., Bocian, K. M., Ward, S. L., & Forness, S. R. (1998). Comorbidity of hyperactivity–impulsivity–inattention and conduct problems: Risk factors in social, affective, and academic domains. *Journal of Abnormal Child Psychology, 26,* 393–406.

Guidano, V. F., & Liotti, G. (1983). *Cognitive processes and emotional disorders.* New York: Guilford Press.

Gunderson, J. G. (1996). The borderline patient's intolerance of aloneness: Insecure attachments and therapist availability. *American Journal of Psychiatry, 153,* 752–758.

Gunderson, J. G., Frank, A. F., Ronningstam, E. F., Wachter, S., Lynch, V. J., & Wolf, P. J. (1989). Early discontinuance of borderline patients from psychotherapy. *Journal of Nervous and Mental Disease, 177,* 38–42.

Gunderson, J. G., & Singer, M. (1975). Defining borderline patients: An overview. *American Journal of Psychiatry, 132,* 1–9.

Gunderson, J. G., Triebwasser, J., Phillips, K. A., & Sullivan, C. N. (1999). Personality and vulnerability to affective disorders. In C. Robert Cloninger (Ed.), *Personality and psychopathology* (pp. 3–32). Washington, DC: American Psychiatric Press.

Habel, U., Kuehn, E., Salloum, J. B., Devos, H., & Schneider, F. (2002). Emotional processing in the psychopathic personality. *Aggressive Behavior, 28*(5), 394–400.

Hardy, G. E., Barkham, M., Shapiro, D. A., Stiles, W. B., Rees, A., & Reynolds, S. (1995). Impact of Cluster C personality disorders on outcomes of contrasting brief psychotherapies for depression. *Journal of Consulting and Clinical Psychology, 63*(6), 997–1004.

Hare, R. (1985). A checklist for the assessment of psychopathy. In M. H. Ben-Aron, S. J. Hucker, & C. Webster (Eds.), *Clinical criminology* (pp. 157–167). Toronto: M. & M. Graphics.

Hare, R. (1986). Twenty years of experience with the Cleckley psychopath. In W. Reid, D. Dorr, J. Walker, & J. Bonner (Eds.), *Unmasking the psychopath* (pp. 3–27). New York: Norton.

Hawton, K., & Kirk, J. (1989). Problem-solving. In K. Hawton, P. Salkovskis, J. Kirk, & D. Clark (Eds.), *Cognitive behavior therapy for psychiatric problems* (pp. 406–449). Oxford, UK: Oxford University Press.

Head, S. B., Baker, J. D., & Williamson, D. A. (1991). *Journal of Personality Disorders, 5,* 256–263.

Heimberg, R. G. (1996). Social phobia, avoidant personality disorder and the multiaxial conceptualization of interpersonal anxiety. In P. M. Salkovskis (Ed.), *Trends in cognitive and behavioural therapies* (pp. 43–61). London: Wiley.

Herbert, J. D., Hope, D. A., & Bellack, A. S. (1992). Validity of the distinction between generalized social phobia and avoidant personality disorder. *Journal of Abnormal Psychology, 101,* 332–339.

Herman, J. L., Perry, J. C., & van der Kolk, B. A. (1989). Childhood trauma in borderline personality disorder. *American Journal of Psychiatry, 146,* 490–495.

Herman, J. L., & van der Kolk, B. A. (1987). Traumatic origins of borderline personality disorder. In B. A. van der Kolk (Ed.), *Psychological trauma*. Washington, DC: American Psychiatric Press.

Herpertz, S. C., Dietrich, T. M., Wenning, B., Krings, T., Erberich, S. G., Willmes, K., et al. (2001). Evidence of abnormal amygdala functioning in borderline personality disorder: A functional MRI study. *Biological Psychiatry, 50,* 292–298.

Herpertz, S. C., Schwenger, U. B., Kunert, H. J.. Lukas, G., Gretzer, U., Nutzmann, J., et al. (2000). Emotional responses in patients with borderline as compared with avoidant personality disorder. *Journal of Personality Disorders, 14,* 328–337.

Herpertz, S. C., Werth, U., Lukas, G., Qunaibi, M., Schuerkens, A., Kunert, H.-J., et al. (2001). Emotion in criminal offenders with psychopathy and borderline personality disorder. *Archives of General Psychiatry, 58,* 737–745.

Heumann, K. A., & Morey, L. C. (1990). Reliability of categorical and dimensional judgments of personality disorder. *American Journal of Psychiatry, 147,* 498–500.

Hill, A. B. (1976). Methodological problems in the use of factor analysis: A critical review of the experimental evidence for the anal character. *British Journal of Medical Psychology, 49,* 145–159.

Hill, D. C. (1970). Outpatient management of passive-dependent women. *Hospital and Community Psychiatry, 21,* 38–41.

Hinkle, L. E. (1961). Ecological observations on the relation of physical illness, mental illness and the social environment. *Psychosomatic Medicine, 23,* 289–296.

Hogan, R. (1987). Personality psychology: Back to basics. In J. Aronoff, A. I Robin, & R. A. Zucker, (Eds.), *The emergence of personality* (pp. 141–188). New York: Springer.

Hollandsworth, J., & Cooley, M. (1978). Provoking anger and gaining compliance with assertive versus aggressive responses. *Behavior Therapy, 9,* 640–646.

Hollon, S. D., Kendall, P. C., & Lumry, A. (1986). Specificity of depressogenic cognitions in clinical depression. *Journal of Abnormal Psychology, 95*(1), 52–59.

Horney, K. (1945). *Our inner conflicts.* New York: Norton.

Horney, K. (1950). *Neurosis and human growth.* New York: Norton.

Horowitz, M. (Ed.). (1977). *Hysterical personality.* New York: Jason Aronson.

Hyler, S. E., & Rieder, R. O. (1987). *PDQ-R: Personality Diagnostic Questionnaire—Revised.* New York: New York State Psychiatric Institute.

Ingram, R. E., & Hollon, S. D. (1986). Cognitive therapy for depression from an information processing perspective. In R. E. Ingram (Ed.), *Information processing approaches to clinical psychology* (pp. 261–284). New York: Academic Press.

Janssen, S. A., & Arntz, A. (2001). Real-life stress and opioid-mediated analgesia in novice parachute jumpers. *Journal of Psychophysiology, 15,* 106–113.

Johnson, J. J., Cohen, P., Smailes, E. M., Skodol, A. E., Brown, J., & Oldham, J. M. (2001). Childhood verbal abuse and risk for personality disorders during adolescence and early adulthood. *Comprehensive Psychiatry, 42,* 16–23.

Johnson, J. J., Smailes, E. M., Cohen, P., Brown, J., & Bernstein, D. P. (2000). Associations between four types of childhood neglect and personality disorder symptoms during adolescence and early adulthood: Findings of a community-based longitudinal study. *Journal of Personality Disorders, 14,* 171–187.

Johnson, S. (1987). *Humanizing the narcissistic style.* New York: Norton.

Jones, E. (1961). Anal erotic character traits. In *Papers on psychoanalysis.* Boston: Beacon Press. (Original work published 1918)

Juni, S., & Semel, S. R. (1982). Person perception as a function or orality and anality. *Journal of Social Psychology, 118,* 99–103.

Kagan, J. (1989). Tempermental contributions to social behavior. *American Psychologist, 44*(4), 668–674.

Kass, D. J., Silvers, F. M., & Abrams, G. M. (1972). Behavioral group treatment of hysteria. *Archives of General Psychiatry, 26,* 42–50.

Kegan, R. (1986). The child behind the mask: Sociopathy as a developmental delay. In W. Reid, D. Dorr, J. Walker, & J. Bonner (Eds.), *Unmasking the psychopath* (pp. 45–77). New York: Norton.

Kelly, G. (1955). *The psychology of personal constructs.* New York: Norton.

Kemperman, I., Russ, M. J., Clark, W. C., Kakuma, T., Zanine, E., & Harrison, K. (1997). Pain assessment in self-injurious patients with borderline personality disorder using signal detection theory. *Psychiatry Research, 70,* 175–183.

Kendler, K. S., & Gruenberg, A. M. (1982). Genetic relationship between Paranoid Personality Disorder and the "schizophrenic spectrum" disorders. *American Journal of Psychiatry, 139,* 1185–1186.

Kernberg, O. F. (1975). *Borderline conditions and pathological narcissism.* New York: Jason Aronson.

Kernberg, O. F. (1976). *Object relations theory and clinical psycho-analysis.* New York: Jason Aronson.

Kernberg, O. F. (1984). *Severe personality disorders: Psychotherapeutic strategies.* New Haven: Yale University Press.

Kernberg, O. F. (1996). A psychoanalytic theory of personality disorders. In J. F. Clarkin & M. F. Lenzeweger (Eds.), *Major theories of personality disorder* (pp. 106–137). New York: Guilford Press.

Kernberg, O. F., Selzer, M. A., Koenigsberg, H. W., Carr, A. C., & Appelbaum, A. H. (1989). *Psychodynamic psychotherapy of borderline patients.* New York: Basic Books.

Kernis, M. H., Grannemann, B. D., & Barclay, L. C. (1989). Stability and level of self-esteem as predictors of anger arousal and hostility. *Journal of Personality and Social Psychology, 56,* 1013–1022.

Kimmerling, R., Zeiss, A., & Zeiss, R. (2000). Therapist emotional responses to patients: Building a learning-based language. *Cognitive and Behavioral Practice, 7,* 312–321.

Kingdon, D. G., & Turkington, D. (1994). *Cognitive-behavioral therapy of schizophrenia.* New York: Guilford Press.

Klein, M. H., Benjamin, L. S., Rosenfeld, R., Treece, C., Husted, J., & Greist, J. H. (1993). The Wisconsin Personality Disorders Inventory: Development, reliability, and validity. *Journal of Personality Disorders, 7,* 285–303.

Klonsky, E. D., Oltmanns, T. F., Turkheimer, E., & Fiedler, E. R. (2000). Recollections of conflict with parents and family support in the personality disorders. *Journal of Personality Disorders, 14,* 327–338.

Kochen, M. (1981). On the generality of PARRY, Colby's paranoia model. *The Behavioral and Brain Sciences, 4,* 540–541.

Koenigsberg, H., Kaplan, R., Gilmore, M., & Cooper, A. (1985). The relationship between syndrome and personality disorder in DSM-III: Experience with 2,462 patients. *American Journal of Psychiatry, 142,* 207–212.

Kohlberg, L. (1984). *The psychology of moral development.* New York: Harper & Row.

Kohut, H. (1971). *The analysis of the self.* New York: International Universities Press.

Kolb, L. C. (1968). *Noyes' clinical psychiatry* (7th ed.). Philadelphia: Saunders.

Koocher, G., & Keith-Spiegel, P. (1998). *Ethics in psychology: Professional standards and cases* (2nd ed.). New York: Oxford University Press.

Koons, C. R., Robbins, C. J., Tweed, J. L., Lynch, T. R., Gonzalez, A. M., Morse, J. Q., et al. (2001). Efficacy of dialectical behavior therapy in women with borderline personality disorder. *Behavior Therapy, 32,* 371–390.

Kraeplin, E. (1913). *Psychiatrie: Ein lehrbuch* (8th ed., Vol. 3). Leipzig: Barth.

Kretschmer, E. (1936). *Physique and character.* London: Routledge & Kegan Paul.

Kuyken, W., Kurzer, N., DeRubeis, R. J., Beck, A. T., & Brown, G. K. (2001). Response to cognitive therapy in depression: The role of maladaptive beliefs and personality disorders. *Journal of Consulting and Clinical Psychology, 69*(3), 560–566

Layden, M. A., Newman, C. F., Freeman, A., & Morse, S. B. (1993). *Cognitive therapy of borderline personality disorder.* Boston: Allyn & Bacon.

Lazare, A., Klerman, G. L., & Armor, D. (1966). Oral, obsessive and hysterical personality patterns. *Archives of General Psychiatry, 14,* 624–630.

Lazare, A., Klerman, G. L., & Armor, D. (1970). Oral, obsessive and hysterical personality patterns: Replication of factor analysis in an independent sample. *Journal of Psychiatric Research, 7,* 275–290.

Lee, C. W., Taylor, G., & Dunn, J. (1999). Factor structure of the Schema Questionnaire in a large clinical sample. *Cognitive Therapy and Research, 23,* 441–451.

Levy, D. (1966). *Maternal overprotection.* New York: Norton.

Liberman, R., De Risis, W., & Mueser, K. (1989). *Social skills training for psychiatric patients.* New York: Pergamon Press.

Like, R., & Zyzanski, S. J. (1987). Patient satisfaction with the clinical encounter: Social psychological determinants. *Social Science in Medicine, 24*(4), 351–357.

Lilienfeld, S. O., VanValkenburg, C., Larntz, K., & Akiskal, H. S. (1986). The relationship of histrionic personality disorder to antisocial personality and somatization disorders. *American Journal of Psychiatry, 143,* 718–722.

Linehan, M. M. (1987a). Dialectical behavior therapy in groups: Treating borderline personality disorders and suicidal behavior. In C. M. Brody (Ed.), *Women in groups.* New York: Springer.

Linehan, M. M. (1987b). Dialectical behavioral therapy: A cognitive behavioral approach to parasuicide. *Journal of Personality Disorders, 1,* 328–333.

Linehan, M. M. (1993). *Cognitive-behavioral treatment of borderline personality disorder.* New York: Guilford Press.

Linehan, M. M., Armstrong, H. E., Suarez, A., Allmon, D., & Heard, H. L. (1991). Cognitive-behavioral treatment of chronically parasuicidal borderline patients. *Archives of General Psychiatry, 48,* 1060–1064.

Linehan, M. M., & Heard, H. L. (1999). Borderline personality disorder: Costs, course, and treatment outcomes. In N. E. Miller & K. M. Magruder (Eds.), *Cost-effectiveness of psychotherapy: A guide for practitioners, researchers, and policymakers* (pp. 291–305). New York: Oxford University Press.

Linehan, M. M., Heard, H. L., & Armstrong, H. E. (1993). Naturalistic follow-up of a behavioral treatment for chronically parasuicidal borderline patients. *Archives of General Psychiatry, 50,* 971–974.

Linehan, M. M., Schmidt, H., Dimeff, L. A., Craft, J. C., Kanter, J., & Comtois, K. (1999). Dialectical behavior therapy for patients with borderline personality disorder and drug-dependence. *American Journal on Addictions, 8,* 279–292.

Linehan, M. M., Tutek, D. A., & Heard, H. L. (1992, November). *Interpersonal and social treatment outcomes in borderline personality disorder.* Paper presented at the 26th annual conference of the Association for Advancement of Behavior Therapy, Boston.

Lion, J. R. (Ed.). (1981). *Personality disorders: Diagnosis and management.* Baltimore: Williams & Wilkens.

Livesley, W. J. (1990). *Dimensional Assessment of Personality Pathology—Basic Questionnaire.* Unpublished manuscript, University of British Columbia.

Livesley, W. J., Jang, K., Schroeder, M. L., & Jackson, D. N. (1993). Genetic and environmental factors in personality dimensions. *American Journal of Psychiatry, 150,* 1826–1831.

Loranger, A. W. (1991). Diagnosis of personality disorders: General considerations. In R. Michels (Ed.), *Psychiatry* (Vol. 1, pp. 1–14). Philadelphia: Lippincott.

Loranger, A. W. (1999). Categorical approaches to assessment and diagnosis of personality disorders. In C. Robert Cloninger (Ed.), *Personality and psychopathology* (pp. 201–217). Washington, DC: American Psychiatric Press.

Loranger, A. W., Lenzenweger, M. F., Gartner, A. F., Lehman, S. V., Herzig, J., Zammit, G. K., et al. (1991). Trait–state artifacts and the diagnosis of personality disorders. *Archives of General Psychiatry, 48,* 720–728.

Loranger, A. W., Susman, V. L., Oldham, J. M., & Russakoff, L. M. (1987). The Personality Disorder Examination: A preliminary report. *Journal of Personality Disorders, 1,* 1–13.

Luborsky, L., McLellan, A. T., Woody, G. E., O'Brien, C. P., & Auerbach, A. (1985). Therapist success and its determinants. *Archives of General Psychiatry, 42,* 602–611.

MacKinnon, R. A., & Michaels, R. (1971). *The psychiatric interview in clinical practice* (pp. 110–146). Philadelphia: Saunders.

Maffei, C., Fossati, A., Agnostoni, I., Barraco, A., Bagnato, M., Deborah, D., et al. (1997). Interrater reliability and internal consistency of the Structured Clinical Interview for DSM-IV Axis II Personality Disorders (SCID-II), version 2.0. *Journal of Personality Disorders, 11*(3), 279–284.

Mahoney, M. (1984). Behaviorism, cognitivism, and human change processes. In M. A. Reda & M. Mahoney (Eds.), *Cognitive psychotherapies: Recent developments in theory, research, and practice* (pp. 3–30). Cambridge, MA: Ballinger.

Malinow, K. (1981). Passive–aggressive personality. In J. Lion (Ed.), *Personality disorders diagnosis and management (revised for DSM III)* (2nd ed., pp. 121–132). Baltimore: Williams & Wilkins.

Malmquist, C. P. (1971). Hysteria in childhood. *Postgraduate Medicine, 50,* 112–117.

Marchand, A., Goyer, L. R., Dupuis, G., & Mainguy, N. (1998). Personality disorders and the outcome of cognitive behavioural treatment of panic disorder with agoraphobia. *Canadian Journal of Behavioural Science, 30,* 14–23.

Marmor, J. (1953). Orality in the hysterical personality. *Journal of the American Psychoanalytic Association, 1,* 656–671.

Martin, J., Martin, W., & Slemon, A. G. (1987). Cognitive mediation in person-centered and rational-emotive therapy. *Journal of Counseling Psychology, 34*(3), 251–260.

Masterson, J. F. (1985). *Treatment of the borderline adolescent: A developmental approach.* New York: Brunner/Mazel.

Mavissakalian, M., & Hamman, M. S. (1987). DSM-III personality disorder in agoraphobia: II. Changes with treatment. *Comprehensive Psychiatry, 28,* 356–361.

Mays, D. T. (1985) Behavior therapy with borderline personality disorders: One clinician's perspective. In D. T. Mays & C. M. Franks (Eds.), *Negative outcome in psychotherapy and what to do about it* (pp. 301–311). New York: Springer.

McCann, J. (1988). Passive–aggressive personality disorder: A review. *Journal of Personality Disorders, 2*(2), 170–179.

McCown, W., Galina, H., Johnson, J., DeSimone, P., & Posa, J., (1993). Borderline personality disorder and laboratory induced cold pressor pain: Evidence of stress-induced analgesia. *Journal of Psychopathology and Behavioral Assessment, 15,* 87–95.

McCreery, C., & Claridge, G. (2002). Healthy schizotypy: The case of out-of-the-body experiences. *Personality and Individual Differences, 32,* 141–154.

McDougall, W. (1921). *An introduction to social psychology* (14th ed.). Boston: John W. Luce.

McGinn, L. K., & Young, J. E. (1996). Schema-focused therapy. In P. M. Salkovskis (Ed.), *Frontiers of cognitive therapy* (pp. 182–207). New York: Guilford Press.

McKay, D., Neziroglu, F., Todaro, J., & Yaryura-Tobias, J. A. (1996). Changes in personality disorders following behavior therapy for obsessive-compulsive disorder. *Journal of Anxiety Disorders, 10*(1), 47–57.

Merbaum, M., & Butcher, J. N. (1982). Therapists' liking of their psychotherapy patients: Some issues related to severity of disorder and treatability. *Psychotherapy: Theory, Research and Practice, 19*(1), 69–76.

Mersch, P. P. A., Jansen, M. A., & Arntz, A. (1995). Social phobia and personality disorder: Severity of complaint and treatment effectiveness. *Journal of Personality Disorders, 9,* 143–159.

Millon, T. (1969). *Modern psychopathology: A biosocial approach to maladaptive learning and functioning.* Philadelphia: Saunders.

Millon, T. (1981). *Disorders of personality: DSM-III, Axis II.* New York: Wiley.

Millon, T. (1983). *Manual for the Millon Clinical Multiaxial Inventory–I (MCMI-I).* Minneapolis: National Computer Systems.

Millon, T. (1985). *Personality and its disorders.* New York: Wiley.

Millon, T. (1993). Negativistic (passive–aggressive) personality disorder. *Journal of Personality Disorders, 7*(1), 78–85.

Millon, T. (1996). *Disorders of personality: DSM-IV and beyond* (2nd ed.). New York: Wiley.

Millon, T., & Davis, R. (1996). Negativistic personality disorders: The vacillating pattern. In T. Millon, *Disorders of personality: DSM-IV and Beyond* (2nd ed., pp. 541–574). New York: Wiley.

Millon, T., Davis, R. D., & Millon, C. (1996). *The Millon Clinical Multiaxial Inventory–III manual.* Minnetonka, MN: National Computer System.

Millon, T., Davis, R., Millon, C., Escovar, L., & Meagher, S. (2000). *Personality disorders in modern life.* New York: Wiley.

Millon, T., Millon, C., & Davis, R. D. (1994). *Millon Clinical Multiaxial Inventory–III.* Minneapolis: National Computer Systems.

Mooney, K. A., & Padesky, C. A. (2000). Applying client creativity to recurrent problems: Constructing possibilities and tolerating doubt. *Journal of Cognitive Psychotherapy: An International Quarterly, 14*(2), 149–161.

Morey, L. C., Waugh, M. H., & Blashfield, R. K. (1985). MMPI scores for the DSM-III personality disorders: Their derivation and correlates. *Journal of Personality Assessment, 49,* 245–251.

Morrison, A. P. (1998). A cognitive analysis of the maintenance of auditory hallucinations: Are voices to schizophrenia what bodily sensations are to panic? *Behavioural and Cognitive Psychotherapy, 26,* 289–302.

Morrison, A. P., & Renton, J. C. (2001). Cognitive therapy for auditory hallucinations: A theory-based approach. *Cognitive and Behavioral Practice, 8,* 147–169.

Najavits, L. (2000). Researching therapist emotions and countertransference. *Cognitive and Behavioral Practice, 7,* 322–328.

Nakao, K., Gunderson, J. G., Phillips, K. A., Tanaka, N., Yorifuji, K., Takaishi, J., & Nishimura, T. (1992). Functional impairment in personality disorders. *Journal of Personality Disorders, 6,* 24–33.

Nelson-Gray, R. O., Johnson, D. Foyle, L. W., Daniel, S. S., & Harmon, R. (1996). The effectiveness of cognitive therapy tailored to depressives with personality disorders. *Journal of Personality Disorders, 10,* 132–152.

Nestadt, G., Romanoski, A. J., Chahal, R., Merchant, A., Folstein, M. F., Gruenberg, E. M., & McHugh, P. R. (1990). An epidemiological study of histrionic personality disorder. *Psychological Medicine, 20,* 413–422.

Newman, C. (1997). Maintaining professionalism in the face of emotional abuse from clients. *Cognitive and Behavioral Practice, 4,* 1–29.

Newman, C. F. (1999). Showing up for your own life: Cognitive therapy of avoidant personality disorder. *In Session: Psychotherapy in Practice, 4*(4), 55–71.

Neziroglu, F., McKay, D., Todaro, J., & Yaryura-Tobias, J. A. (1996). Effect of cognitive behavior therapy on persons with body dysmorphic disorder and comorbid axis II diagnosis. *Behavior Therapy, 27,* 67–77.

Norcross, J. C., Prochaska, J. O., & Gallagher, K. M. (1989). Clinical psychologists in the 1980's: II. Theory, research, and practice. *The Clinical Psychologist, 42*(3), 45–53.

Ogata, S. N., Silk, K. R., Goodrich, S., Lohr, N. E., Westen, D., & Hill, E. M. (1990). Childhood sexual and physical abuse in adult patients with borderline personality disorder. *American Journal of Psychiatry, 147,* 1008–1013.

O'Leary, K. M., Cowdry, R. W., Gardner, D. L., Leibenluft, E., Lucas, P. B., & deJong-Meyer, R. (1991). Dysfunctional attitudes in borderline personality disorder. *Journal of Personality Disorders, 5,* 233–242.

Olin, S. S., Raine, A., Cannon, T. D., & Parnas, J. (1997). Childhood behavior precursors of schizotypal personality disorder. *Schizophrenia Bulletin, 23,* 93–103.

O'Reilly, T., Dunbar, R., & Bentall, R. P. (2001). Schizotypy and creativity: An evolutionary connection? *Personality and Individual Differences, 31,* 1067–1078.

Ottaviani, R. (1990). Passive–aggressive personality disorder. In A. T. Beck, A. Freeman, & Associates, *Cognitive therapy of personality disorders* (pp. 333–349). New York: Guilford Press.

Overholser, J. C. (1987). Facilitating autonomy in passive-dependent persons: An integrative model. *Journal of Contemporary Psychotherapy, 17,* 250–269.

Overholser, J. C. (1991). Categorical assessment of the dependent personality disorder in depressed inpatients. *Journal of Personality Disorders, 5,* 243–255.

Overholser, J. C. (1992). Interpersonal dependency and social loss. *Personality and Individual Differences, 13,* 17–23.

Overholser, J. C., Kabakoff, R., & Norman, W. H. (1989). Personality characteristics in depressed and dependent psychiatric inpatients. *Journal of Personality Assessment, 53,* 40–50.

Padesky, C. A. (1986, September 18–20). *Personality disorders: Cognitive therapy into the 90's.* Paper presented at the Second International Conference on Cognitive Psychotherapy, Umeå, Sweden.

Padesky, C. A. (1993). Schema as self prejudice. *International Cognitive Therapy Newsletter, 5/6,* 16–17.

Padesky, C. A. (1994). Schema change processes in cognitive therapy. *Clinical Psychology and Psychotherapy, 1,* 267–278.

Padesky, C. A., with Greenberger, D. (1995). *Clinician's Guide to Mind Over Mood.* New York: Guilford Press.

Paris, J. (1993). The treatment of borderline personality disorder in light of the research on its long term outcome. *Canadian Journal of Psychiatry, 38*(Suppl. 1), S28–S34.

Patrick, M., Hobson, R. P., Castle, D., Howard, R., & Maughan, B. (1994). Personality disorder and the mental representation of early social experience. *Developmental Psychopathology, 6,* 375–388.

Perez, M., Pettit, J., David, C., Kistner, J., & Joiner, T. (2001). The interpersonal consequences of inflated self-esteem in an inpatient psychiatric youth sample. *Journal of Consulting and Clinical Psychology, 69*(4), 712–716.

Perris, C., & McGorry, P. D. (1998). *Cognitive psychotherapy of psychotic and personality disorders: Handbook of theory and practice.* New York: Wiley.

Perry, J., & Flannery, R. (1982). Passive–aggressive personality disorder treatment implications of a clinical typology. *Journal of Nervous and Mental Disease, 170*(3), 164–173.

Person, E. S. (1986). Manipulativeness in entrepreneurs and psychopaths. In W. Reid, D. Dorr, J. Walker, & J. Bonner (Eds.), *Unmasking the psychopath* (pp. 256–273). New York: Norton.

Persons, J. (1986). The advantages of studying psychological phenomena rather than psychiatric diagnoses. *American Psychologist, 41,* 1252–1260.

Persons, J. B., Burns, B. D., & Perloff, J. M. (1988). Predictors of drop-out and outcome in cognitive therapy for depression in a private practice setting. *Cognitive Therapy and Research, 12,* 557–575.

Peselow, E. D., Sanfilipo, M. P., & Fieve, R. R. (1994). Patients' and informants' reports of personality traits during and after major depression. *Journal of Abnormal Psychology, 103*(4), 819–824.

Peters, E. R., Joseph, S. A., & Garety, P. A. (1999). Measurement of delusional ideation in the normal population: Introducing the PDI (Peters et al. Delusions Inventory). *Schizophrenia Bulletin, 25,* 553–576.

Pfohl, B. (1991). Histrionic personality disorder: A review of available data and recommendations for DSM-IV. *Journal of Personality Disorders, 5*(2), 150–166.

Pfohl, B. (1999). Axis I and Axis II: Comorbidity or confusion? In C. Robert Cloninger (Ed.), *Personality and psychopathology* (pp. 83–98). Washington, DC: American Psychiatric Press.

Pfohl, B., Blum, N., Zimmerman, M., & Stangl, D. (1989). *Structured Interview for DSM-III-R Personality (SIDP-R).* Iowa City: University of Iowa, Department of Psychiatry.

Piaget, J. (1926). *The language and thought of the child.* New York: Harcourt, Brace.

Piaget, J. (1952). *The origin of intelligence in children.* New York: International Universities Press. (Original work published 1936)

Pilkonis, P. (1988). Personality prototypes among depressives: Themes of dependency and autonomy. *Journal of Personality Disorders, 2,* 144–152.

Pilkonis, P. A., Heape, C. L., Proietti, J. M., Clark, S. W., McDavid, J. D., & Pitts, T. E. (1995). The reliability and validity of two structured diagnostic interviews for personality disorders. *Archives of General Psychiatry, 52*(12), 1025–1033.

Pilkonis, P. A., Heape, C. L., Ruddy, J., & Serrao, P. (1991). Validity in the diagnosis of personality disorders: The use of the LEAD standard. *Psychological Assessment, 3*(1), 46–54.

Pitman, R. K., van der Kolk, B. A., Orr, S. P., & Greenberg, M. S. (1990). Naloxone-reversible analgesic response to combat-related stimuli in posttraumatic stress disorder. *Archives of General Psychiatry, 47,* 541–544.

Pollack, J. M. (1979). Obsessive–compulsive personality: A review. *Psychological Bulletin, 86,* 225–241.

Pretzer, J. L. (1985, November). *Paranoid personality disorder: A cognitive view.* Paper presented at the meeting of the Association for the Advancement of Behavior Therapy, Houston, TX.

Pretzer, J. L. (1988). Paranoid personality disorder: A cognitive view. *International Cognitive Therapy Newsletter,* 4(4), 10–12.

Pretzer, J. (1990). Borderline personality disorder. In A. T. Beck, A. Freeman, & Associates, *Cognitive therapy of personality disorders* (pp. 176–207). New York: Guilford Press.

Pretzer, J. L., & Beck, A. T. (1996). A cognitive theory of personality disorders. In J. F. Clarkin & M. F. Lenzenweger (Eds.), *Major theories of personality disorder* (pp. 36–105). New York: Guilford Press.

Pretzer, J., Beck, A. T., & Newman, C. F. (1989). Stress and stress management: A cognitive view. *Journal of Cognitive Psychotherapy: An International Quarterly, 3,* 163–179.

Pretzer, J., & Hampl, S. (1994). Cognitive behavioural treatment of obsessive compulsive personality disorder. *Clinical Psychology and Psychotherapy,* 1(5), 298–307.

Prochaska, J. O., & DiClemente, C. C. (1982). Transtheoretical therapy: Toward a more integrative model of change. *Psychotherapy: Theory, Research and Practice,* 19(3), 276–288.

Prochaska, J. O., & Norcross, J. C. (2003). *Systems of psychotherapy: A transtheoretical analysis* (5th ed.). Pacific Grove, CA: Brooks/Cole.

Prout, M., & Platt, J. (1983). The development and maintenance of passive-aggressiveness: The behavioral approach. In R. Parsons & R. Wicks (Eds.), *Passive aggressiveness theory and practice* (pp. 25–43). New York: Brunner/Mazel.

Quay, H. C., Routh, D. K., & Shapiro, S. K. (1987). Psychopathology of childhood: From description to validation. *Annual Review of Psychology, 38,* 491–532.

Rabins, P. V., & Slavney, P. R. (1979). Hysterical traits and variability of mood in normal men. *Psychological Medicine, 9,* 301–304.

Rakos, R. F. (1991). *Assertive behavior: Theory, research, and training.* New York: Routledge.

Raskin, R., Novacek, J., & Hogan, R. (1991). Narcissistic self-esteem management. *Journal of Personality and Social Psychology, 60,* 911–918.

Rasmussen, S., & Tsuang, M. (1986). Clinical characteristics and family history in DSM-III obsessive–compulsive disorder. *American Journal of Psychiatry, 143,* 317–322.

Rehm, L. (1977). A self-control model of depression. *Behavior Therapy, 8,* 787–804.

Reich, J. H. (1987). Instruments measuring DSM-III and DSM-III-R personality disorders. *Journal of Personality Disorders, 1,* 220–240.

Reich, W. (1972). *Character analysis.* New York: Farrar, Straus, & Giroux.

Reich, J., & Noyes, R. (1987). A comparison of DSM-III personality disorders in acutely ill panic and depressed patients. *Journal of Anxiety Disorders, 1,* 123–131.

Reich, J., Noyes, R., & Troughton, E. (1987). Dependent personality disorder associated with phobic avoidance in patients with panic disorder. *American Journal of Psychiatry, 144,* 323–326.

Reid, W. H. (Ed.). (1981). *The treatment of the antisocial syndromes.* New York: Van Nostrand.

Reid, W. H. (1988). *The treatment of psychiatric disorders: Revised for the DSM-III-R.* New York: Brunner/Mazel.

Renneberg, B., Heyn, K., Gebhard, R., & Bachmann, S. (in press). Facial expression of emotions in borderline personality disorder and depression. *Journal of Behavior Therapy and Experimental Psychiatry.*

Rhodewalt, F., & Morf, C. (1995). Self and interpersonal correlates of the Narcissistic Personality Inventory: A review and new findings. *Journal of Research in Personality, 29,* 1–23.

Robins, L. N. (1966). *Deviant children grow up: A sociological and psychiatric study of sociopathic personality.* Oxford: Williams & Wilkens.

Rossi, A., & Daneluzzo, E. (2002). Schizotypal dimensions in normals and schizophrenic patients: A comparison with other clinical samples. *Schizophrenia Research, 54,* 67–75.

Russ, M. J., Roth, S. D., Lerman, A., Kakuma, T., Harrison, K., Shindledecker, R. D., Hull, J., & Mattis, S. (1992). Pain perception in self-injurious patients with borderline personality disorder. *Biological Psychiatry, 32,* 501–511.

Russ, M. J., Roth, S. D., Kakuma, T., Harrison, K., Shindledecker, R. D., & Hull, J. W. (1994). Pain perception in self-injurious borderline patients: nalaxone effects. *Biological Psychiatry, 35,* 207–209.

Salkovskis, P. (Ed.). (1996). *Frontiers of cognitive therapy.* New York: Guilford Press.

Sanderson, W. C., Beck, A. T., & McGinn, L. K. (1994). Cognitive therapy for generalized anxiety disorder: Significance of co-morbid personality disorders. *Journal of Cognitive Psychotherapy: An International Quarterly, 8,* 13–18.

Saul, L. J., & Warner, S. L. (1982). *The psychotic personality.* New York: Van Nostrand.

Scarr, S. (1987). Personality and experience: Individual encounters with the world. In J. Aronoff, A. I. Robin, & R. A. Zucker (Eds.), *The emergence of personality* (pp. 66–70). New York: Springer.

Schmidt, N. B., Joiner, T. E., Young, J. E., & Telch, M. J. (1995). The Schema Questionnaire: Investigation of psychometric properties and the hierarchical structure of a measure of maladaptive schemas. *Cognitive Therapy and Research, 19,* 295–321.

Schneider, K. (1958). *Psychopathic personalities* (M. Hamilton, Trans.). Springfield, IL: Charles C. Thomas. (Original work published 1923)

Sciuto, G., Diaferia, G., Battaglia, M., Perna, G. P., Gabriele, A., & Bellodi, L. (1991). DSM-III-R personality disorders in panic and obsessive compulsive disorder: A comparison study. *Comprehensive Psychiatry, 32*(5), 450–457.

Scrimali, T., & Grimaldi, L. (1996). Schizophrenia and Cluster A personality disorders. *Journal of Cognitive Psychotherapy: An International Quarterly, 10*(4), 291–304.

Shapiro, D. (1965). *Neurotic styles.* New York: Basic Books.

Shea, M. T., Pilkonis, P. A., Beckham, E., Collins, J. F., Elkins, I., Sotsky, S. M., & Docherty, J. P. (1990). Personality disorders and treatment outcome in the NIMH Treatment of Depression Collaborative Research Program. *American Journal of Psychiatry, 147,* 711–718.

Shelton, J. L., & Levy, R. L. (1981). *Behavioral assignments and treatment compliance: A handbook of clinical strategies.* Champaign, IL: Research Press.

Sieswerda, S., & Arntz. A. (2001, July 17–21). *Schema-specific emotional STROOP effects in BPD patients.* Paper presented at the World Congress of Behavioral and Cognitive Therapies, Vancouver.

Skodol, A., Buckley, P., & Charles, E. (1983). Is there a characteristic pattern to the treatment history of clinical outpatients with borderline personality disorder? *Journal of Mental and Nervous Disease, 171,* 405–410.

Slavney, P. R. (1978). The diagnosis of hysterical personality disorder: A study of attitudes. *Comprehensive Psychiatry, 19,* 501–507.

Slavney, P. R. (1984). Histrionic personality and antisocial personality: Caricatures of stereotypes? *Comprehensive Psychiatry, 25,* 129–141.

Slavney, P. R., Breitner, J. C. S., & Rabins, P. V. (1977). Variability of mood and hysterical traits in normal women. *Journal of Psychiatric Research, 13,* 155–160.

Slavney, P. R., & McHugh, P. R. (1974). The hysterical personality. *Archives of General Psychiatry, 30,* 325–332.

Slavney, P., & Rich, G. (1980). Variability of mood and the diagnosis of hysterical personality disorder. *British Journal of Psychiatry, 136,* 402–404.

Small, I., Small, J., Alig, V., & Moore, D. (1970). Passive–aggressive personality disorder: A search for a syndrome. *American Journal of Psychiatry, 126*(7), 973–983.

Smokler, I. A., & Shevrin, H. (1979). Cerebral lateralization and personality style. *Archives of General Psychiatry, 36,* 949–954.

Smucker, M. R., Dancu, C., Foa, E. B., & Niederee, J. L. (1995). Imagery rescripting: A new treatment for survivors of childhood sexual abuse suffering from posttraumatic stress. *Journal of Cognitive Psychotherapy, 9,* 3–17.

Soloff, P. H. (1994). Is there any drug treatment of choice for the borderline patient? *Acta Psychiatrica Scandinavica, 379,* 50–55.

Spitzer, R. L. (1983). Psychiatric diagnosis: Are clinicians still necessary? *Comprehensive Psychiatry, 24,* 399–411.

Spivack, G., & Shure, M. B. (1974). *Social adjustment of young children: A cognitive approach to solving real-life problems.* San Francisco: Jossey-Bass.

Springer, T., Lohr, N. E., Buchtel, H. A., & Silk, K. R. (1995). A preliminary report of short-term cognitive-behavioral group therapy for inpatients with personality disorders. *Journal of Psychotherapy Practice and Research, 5,* 57–71.

Standage, K., Bilsbury, C., Jain, S., & Smith, D. (1984). An investigation of role-taking in histrionic personalities. *Canadian Journal of Psychiatry, 29,* 407–411.

Stanley, B., Bundy, E., & Beberman, R. (2001). Skills training as an adjunctive treatment for personality disorders. *Journal of Psychiatric Practice, 7*(5), 324–335. Stein, K. F. (1996). Affect instability in adults with a borderline personality disorder. *Archives of Psychiatric Nursing, 10,* 32–40.

Steiner, J. L., Tebes, J. K., Sledge, W. H., & Walker, M. L. (1995). A comparison of structured clinical interview for DSM-III-R and clinical diagnoses. *Journal of Nervous and Mental Disease, 183*(6), 365–369.

Steiner, J. L., Tebes, J. K., Sledge, W. H., Walker, W. H., & Loukides, M. (1995). A comparison of the Structured Clinical Interview for DSM-III-R and clinical diagnoses. *Journal of Nervous and Mental Disease, 183*(6), 365–369.

Stern, A. (1938). Psychoanalytic investigations and therapy in the borderline group of neuroses. *Psychoanalytic Quarterly, 7,* 467–489.

Stone, M. (1993a). *Abnormalities of personality: Within and beyond the realm of treatment.* New York: Norton.

Stone, M. (1993b). Long-term outcome in personality disorders. *British Journal of Psychiatry, 162,* 299–313.

Stone, M. H. (2000). Gradations of antisociality and rersponsiveness to psychosocial therapies. In J. G. Gunderson & G. O. Gabbard (Eds.), *Psychotherapy for personality disorders* (pp. 95–130). Washington, DC: American Psychiatric Press.

Stravynski, A., Marks, I., & Yule, W. (1982). Social skills problems in neurotic outpatients: Social skills training with and without cognitive modification. *Archives of General Psychiatry, 39,* 1378–1385.

Sullivan, H. S. (1956). *Clinical studies in psychiatry.* New York: Norton.

Swann, W. B., Jr. (1990). To be known or to be adored: The interplay of self-enhancement and self-verification. In E. T. Higgins & R. M. Sorrentino (Eds.), *Handbook of motivation and cognition* (Vol. 2, pp. 408–448). New York: Guilford Press.

Tellegen, A. (1993). *Multidimensional Personality Questionnaire.* Minneapolis: University of Minnesota Press.

Temoshok, L., & Heller, B. (1983). Hysteria. In R. J. Daitzman (Ed.), *Diagnosis and intervention in behavior therapy and behavioral medicine* (pp. 204–294). New York: Springer.

Torgerson, S. (1980). The oral, obsessive and hysterical personality syndromes. *Archives of General Psychiatry, 37,* 1272–1277.

Trull, T. J. (2001). Structural relations between borderline personality disorder features and putative etiological correlates. *Journal of Abnormal Psychology, 110*, 471–481.

Trull, T. J., Goodwin, A. H., Schopp, L. H., Hillenbrand, T. L., & Schuster, T. (1993). Psychometric properties of a cognitive measure of personality disorders. *Journal of Personality Assessment, 61*(3), 536–546.

Trull, T. J., Widiger, T. A., & Guthrie, P. (1990). Categorical versus dimensional status of borderline personality disorders. *Clinical Psychology Review, 7*, 49–75.

Turkat, I. D. (1985). Formulation of paranoid personality disorder. In I. D. Turkat (Ed.), *Behavioral case formulation* (pp. 157–198). New York: Plenum Press.

Turkat, I. D. (1986). The behavioral interview. In A. R. Ciminero, K. S. Calhoun, & H. E. Adams (Eds.), *Handbook of behavioral assessment* (2nd ed., pp. 109–149). New York: Wiley.

Turkat, I. D. (1987). The initial clinical hypothesis. *Journal of Behavior Therapy and Experimental Psychiatry, 18*, 349–356.

Turkat, I. D. (1990). *The personality disorders: A psychological approach to clinical management.* New York: Pergamon Press.

Turkat, I. D., & Banks, D. S. (1987). Paranoid personality and its disorder. *Journal of Psychopathology and Behavioral Assessment, 9*, 295–304.

Turkat, I. D., & Carlson, C. R. (1984). Data-based versus symptomatic formulation of treatment: The case of a dependent personality. *Journal of Behavioral Therapy and Experimental Psychiatry, 15*, 153–160.

Turkat, I. D., & Maisto, S. A. (1985). Personality disorders: Application of the experimental method to the formulation and modification of personality disorders. In D. H. Barlow (Ed.), *Clinical handbook of psychological disorders: A step-by-step treatment manual* (pp. 503–570). New York: Guilford Press.

Turner, R. M. (1987). The effects of personality disorder diagnosis on the outcome of social anxiety symptom reduction. *Journal of Personality Disorders, 1*, 136–143.

Turner, R. M. (1989). Case study evaluations of a bio-cognitive-behavioral approach for the treatment of borderline personality disorder. *Behavior Therapy, 20*, 477–489.

Vaillant, G. E. (1978). Natural history of male psychological health: IV. What kinds of men do not get psychosomatic illness? *Psychosomatic Medicine, 40*, 420–431.

Van Asselt, A. D. I., Dirksen, C. D., Severens, J. L., & Arntz, A. (2002). *Societal costs of illness in BPD patients: results from bottom-up and top-down estimations.* Manuscript submitted for publication.

van den Bosch, L. M. C., Verheul, R., Schippers, G. M., & van den Brink, W. (2002). Dialectical behavior therapy of borderline patients with and without substance use problems: Implementation and long term effects. *Addictive Behaviors, 900*, 1–13.

Van IJzendoorn, M. H., Schuengel, C., & Bakermans-Kranenburg, M. J. (1999). Disorganized attachment in early childhood: Meta-analysis of precursors, concomitants, and sequelae. *Development and Psychopathology, 11*, 225–249.

van Os, J., Hanssen, M., Bijl, R. V., & Ravelli, A. (2000). Strauss (1969) revisited: A psychosis continuum in the normal population? *Schizophrenia Research, 45*, 11–20.

van Velzen, C. J. M., & Emmelkamp, P. M. G. (1996). The assessment of personality disorders: Implications for cognitive and behavior therapy. *Behaviour Research and Therapy, 34*(8), 655–668.

Veen, G., & Arntz, A. (2000). Multidimensional dichotomous thinking characterizes borderline personality disorder. *Cognitive Therapy and Research, 24*, 23–45.

Ventura, J., Liberman, R. P., Green, M. F., Shaner, A., & Mintz, J. (1998). Training and quality assurance with Structured Clinical Interview for DSM-IV (SCID-I/P). *Psychiatry Research, 79*(2), 163–173.

Vereycken, J., Vertommen, H., & Corveleyn, J. (2002). Authority conflicts and personality disorders. *Journal of Personality Disorders, 16*(1), 41–51.

Veterans Administration. (1951). *Standard classification of diseases*. Washington, DC: Author.

Vieth, I. (1963). *Hysteria: History of a disease*. Chicago: University of Chicago Press.

Wachtel, P. L. (Ed.). (1982). *Resistance: Psychodynamic and behavioral approaches*. New York: Plenum Press.

Waldinger, R. J., & Gunderson, J. C. (1984). Completed psychotherapies with borderline patients. *American Journal of Psychiatry, 38*, 190–202.

Waldinger, R. J., & Gunderson, J. G. (1987). *Effective psychotherapy with borderline patients: Case studies*. New York: Macmillan.

Waller, G., & Button, J. (in press). Processing of threat cues in borderline personality disorder. *Behavioural and Cognitive Psychotherapy*.

Ward, L. G., Freidlander, M. L., & Silverman, W. K. (1987). Children's depressive symptoms, negative self-statements, and causal attributions for success and failure. *Cognitive Therapy and Research, 11*(2), 215–227.

Weaver, T. L., & Clum, G. A. (1993). Early family environment and traumatic experiences associated with borderline personality disorder. *Journal of Consulting and Clinical Psychology, 61*, 1068–1075.

Weertman, A., & Arntz, A. (2001, July 17–21). *Treatment of childhood memories in personality disorders: A controlled study contrasting methods focusing on the present and methods focusing on childhood memories*. Paper presented at the World Congress of Behavioral and Cognitive Therapies, Vancouver.

Weiss, M., Zelkowitz, P., Feldman, R. B., Vogel, J., Heyman, M., & Paris, J. (1996). Psychopathology in offspring of mothers with borderline personality disorder: A pilot study. *Canadian Journal of Psychiatry, 41*, 285–290.

Wellburn, K., Coristine, M., Dagg, P., Pontefract, A., & Jordan, S. (2002). The Schema Questionnaire—Short Form: Factor analysis and relationship between schemas and symptoms. *Cognitive Therapy and Research, 26*(4), 519–530.

Wellburn, K., Dagg, P., Coristine, M., Dagg, P., & Pontefract, A. (2000). Schematic change as a result of an intensive group-therapy day-treatment program. *Psychotherapy, 37*(2), 189–195.

Wells, A. (1997). *Cognitive therapy for anxiety disorders*. London, Wiley.

West, M., & Sheldon, A. E. R. (1988). Classification of pathological attachment patterns in adults. *Journal of Personality Disorders, 2*, 153–159.

Westen, D. (1991). Social cognition and object relations. *Psychological Bulletin, 109*, 429–455.

Wetzler, S., & Morey, L. (1999). Passive–aggressive personality disorder: The demise of a syndrome. *Psychiatry, 62*(1), 49–59.

Whitman, R., Trosman, H., & Koenig, R. (1954). Clinical assessment of passive–aggressive personality. *Archives of Neurology and Psychiatry, 72*, 540–549.

Widiger, T. A. (1992). Categorical versus dimensional classification: Implications from and for research. *Journal of Personality Disorders, 6*, 287–300.

Widiger, T. A., & Frances, A. (1987). Interviews and inventories for the measurement of personality disorders. *Clinical Psychology Review, 7*, 49–75.

Wilkins, S., & Venables, P. H. (1992). Disorder of attention in individuals with schizotypal personality. *Schizophrenia Bulletin, 18*, 717–723.

Wink, P. (1991). Two faces of narcissism. *Journal of Personality and Social Psychology, 61* 590–597.

Woody, G. E., McLellan, A. T., Luborsky, L., & O'Brien, C. P. (1985) Sociopathy and psychotherapy outcome. *Archives of General Psychiatry, 42*, 1081–1086.

Woolson, A. M., & Swanson, M. G. (1972). The second time around: Psychotherapy with the "hysterical woman." *Psychotherapy: Theory, Research and Practice, 9*, 168–175.

World Health Organization. (1998). *International classification of diseases* (9th rev., 5th ed.). Geneva: Author.

Wright, J., & Davis, D. (1994). The therapeutic relationship in cognitive behavioral therapy: Patient perceptions and therapist responses. *Cognitive and Behavioral Practice, 1*, 25–45.

Yalom, I. (1985). *The theory and practice of group psychotherapy* (3rd ed.). New York: Basic Books.

Yeomans, F. E., Selzer, M. A., & Clarkin, J. F. (1993). Studying the treatment contract in intensive psychotherapy with borderline patients. *Psychiatry, 56*, 254–263.

Young, J. E. (1984, November). *Cognitive therapy with difficult patients.* Workshop presented at the meeting of the Association for Advancement of Behavior Therapy, Philadelphia.

Young, J. E. (1990). *Cognitive therapy for personality disorders: A schema-focused approach.* Sarasota, FL: Professional Resource Exchange.

Young, J. E. (1994). *Cognitive therapy for personality disorders: A schema-focused approach* (rev. ed.). Sarasota, FL: Professional Resource Exchange.

Young, J. E. (2002a). *Schema theory.* http://www.schematherapy.com/id30.htm.

Young, J. E. (2002b). *Overview of schema inventories.* http://www.schematherapy.com/id49.htm.

Young, J. E., & Brown, G. (1994). Schema Questionnaire. In J. E. Young (Ed.), *Cognitive therapy for personality disorders: A schema-focused approach* (rev. ed., pp. 63–76). Sarasota, FL: Professional Resource Exchange.

Young, J. E., Klosko, J., & Weishaar, M. E. (2003). *Schema therapy: A practitioner's guide.* New York: Guilford Press.

Zanarini, M.C. (1997). *Role of sexual abuse in the etiology of borderline personality disorder.* Washington, DC: American Psychiatric Press.

Zanarini, M. C. (2000). Childhood experiences associated with the development of borderline personality disorder. *Psychiatric Clinics of North America, 23*, 89–101.

Zetzel, E. (1968). The so-called good hysteric. *International Journal of Psycho-Analysis, 49*, 256–260.

Zimmerman, M. (1994). Diagnosing personality disorders: A review. *Archives of General Psychiatry, 51*, 225–245.

Zimmerman, M., Pfohl, B., Coryell, W., Stangl, D., & Corenthal, C. (1988). Diagnosing personality disorder in depressed patients. *Archives of General Psychiatry, 45*, 733–737.

Zimmerman, M., Pfohl, B., Stangl, D., & Corenthal, C. (1986). Assessment of DSM-III personality disorders: The importance of interviewing an informant. *Journal of Clinical Psychiatry, 47*, 261–263.

Zimmerman, M., Pfohl, B., Stangl, D., & Coryell, W. (1985). The validity of DSM-III Axis IV. *American Journal of Psychiatry, 142*(12), 1437–1441.

Zlotnick, C., Rothschild, L., & Zimmerman, M. (2002). The role of gender in the clinical presentation of patients with borderline personality disorder. *Journal of Personality Disorders, 16*(3), 277–282.

Zuroff, D., & Mongrain, M. (1987). Dependency and self-criticism: Vulnerability factors for depressive affective states. *Journal of Abnormal Psychology, 96*, 14–22.

Zwemer, W. A., & Deffenbacher, J. L. (1984). Irrational beliefs, anger, and anxiety. *Journal of Counseling Psychology, 31*(3), 391–393.

Index